D1706926

THE FRONTAL LOBES

The Frontal Lobes

Donald T. Stuss, Ph.D.
Associate Professor
Schools of Medicine (Neurology)
and Psychology
University of Ottawa
Clinical Neuropsychologist
Ottawa General Hospital
Ottawa, Ontario, Canada

D. Frank Benson, M.D.
The Augustus S. Rose Professor
of Neurology
Department of Neurology
Reed Neurological Institute
UCLA School of Medicine
Los Angeles, California

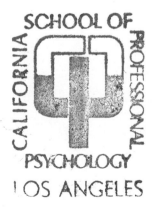

CALIFORNIA SCHOOL OF PROFESSIONAL PSYCHOLOGY
LOS ANGELES

Raven Press New York

Raven Press, 1185 Avenue of the Americas, New York, New York 10036

Made in the United States of America

Library of Congress Cataloging-in-Publication Data

Stuss, Donald T.
  The frontal lobes.

  Includes bibliographies.
  1. Frontal lobes.   I. Benson, D. Frank (David Frank), 1928–   II. Title.
QP382.F7S78   1986   612'.825   85-24474
ISBN 0-88167-153-3

The material contained in this volume was submitted as previously unpublished material, except in the instances in which credit has been given to the source from which some of the illustrative material was derived.
  Great care has been taken to maintain the accuracy of the information contained in the volume. However, Raven Press cannot be held responsible for errors or for any consequences arising from the use of the information contained herein.

9 8 7 6 5 4 3 2

Encouragement and assistance were provided by the ladies in our lives, our wives and mothers. In gratitude, this book is dedicated to Kaaren Stuss, Donna Benson, and Anne Stuss.

Preface

This book was first conceived as a study of frontal lobe anatomy and connections and the relationship of these facts to the exploration of complex human behavior. The material in the book has been developed through the authors' collaboration on clinical investigations of patients with frontal lobe damage, most particularly through the fortunate opportunity to be investigators in the Northampton Veterans Administration Medical Center Leukotomy Study. An early conceptualization of this material and frontal lobe functioning was published in the January 1984 issue of *Psychological Bulletin*; the outline and background data developed for that presentation acted as the direct impetus for the present volume.

The Frontal Lobes is written primarily for neurologists and neuropsychologists, but the material described is fully pertinent for other professionals interested in the complex functioning of the as yet poorly understood anterior cortical regions. The purpose of the book is to fill a perceived void of any recent collection of basic clinical neurological and neuropsychological information on human frontal lobe functioning. References to the animal literature, excellently summarized in other recent publications, are held to a minimum in order to emphasize the clinical features. At the same time, we have attempted to provide a scientific and theoretical basis for our clinical presentation.

Donald T. Stuss
D. Frank Benson

Acknowledgment

The concepts presented in this book reflect not only our own ideas but, to a great degree, the research and concepts of our colleagues and other investigators with an interest in the same phenomena. We have attempted to represent the ideas of others faithfully and apologize if we have not succeeded. Our gratitude is extended to our friends and colleagues from the Boston Veterans Administration Medical Center, the Boston University Department of Neurology, the UCLA Department of Neurology, and the University of Ottawa Division of Neurology for their input during discussions and rounds. In particular, the exceptional cooperation of the Northampton Veterans Administration Medical Center must be acknowledged for its role in the investigation of the leukotomy subjects. Primary associates in that study were Drs. W. Weir, E. Kaplan, M. Naeser, and H. Levine (see Appendix). Joaquin Fuster, M.D., graciously assisted with Chapter 2.

This book would not have been possible without the assistance of many others. Library assistance, typing, and other help were shared by (in alphabetical order): A. Cerri, C. Della Malva, S. LaRochelle, V. McFarlane, J. O'Farrell, C. Poirier, B. Porch, A. Proulx, and F. Sarazin. Those to whom we are most indebted, and who are well aware of this status, are particularly thanked. Art and photographic work were completed by the University of Ottawa Medical Communications Department and the Medical Center of the UCLA School of Medicine.

Financial assistance during the preparation of this book was received from the Medical Research Council of Canada, the Ontario Mental Health Foundation, and the Augustus S. Rose Endowment Fund. Funding of various sections of research on frontal lobe completed by the authors and included in this book was provided by the National Research Council of Canada, the UCLA Augustus S. Rose Endowment Fund, the University of Ottawa Faculty of Social Sciences, and the Research Services of the Veterans Administration. This assistance is gratefully acknowledged.

Contents

THE FRONTAL LOBES

1

Introduction

In a number of ways, study of the frontal lobes might be described as the study of the qualities that differentiate a human being from other animals. As far back as 1928 the American neurologist Tilney suggested that the entire period of human evolutionary existence could be viewed as the "age of the frontal lobe."

Most early discussions, often leading to stormy debates, centered on whether the frontal association cortex did or did not subserve the highest intellectual and moral functions that characterized the human (Feuchtwanger, 1923; Goldstein, 1944; Halstead, 1947a; Hebb, 1945; Mettler, 1949; Rylander, 1939; Teuber, 1959; Weinstein and Teuber, 1957). Recent research has prudently abstained from this degree of theoretical polemics but continues to describe the functions of the frontal lobes in terms suggesting superordinate control. Most agree that study of the frontal lobes represents an important aspect of the investigation of higher mental function in man.

Clinically, frontal lobe damage has been recognized as a source of significant and unique behavioral alterations for well over a century. Patients with frontal lobe trauma or tumor have been studied extensively and many abnormalities described. The pathology has varied in both variety and extent, and the observed behavioral alterations have included a sizable proportion of all recognized human brain activities. Although certain features are seen more often than others, no single, consistent behavior pattern can be called a frontal syndrome. Nonetheless, frontal lobe impairment, at least when moderately severe, is readily recognized by clinicians. Correlation of the clinical features with damage to specific frontal areas has demanded a careful research approach.

The importance of the frontal lobes for human brain activity is reflected in their neuroanatomy. The human frontal lobe is considerably different from that of other animals. First, the size of the frontal lobes in humans, usually estimated at between 24 and 33% of the total cortical surface (Batuyev, 1969; Goldman-Rakic, 1984b), is far larger than that of any of the higher apes; they, in turn, have more prefrontal cortex than dogs, which have more than cats, which have more than rats, and so on. Phylogenetically, the human frontal lobe is the latest area to develop, reflecting its unique status in the evolutionary ladder. That portion of the frontal lobe called prefrontal cortex has undergone far greater development in the human than in any other species. These differences present a problem for research, as the more available animals for research have relatively minute amounts of the pertinent type of cortex. Finally, the complexity of the reciprocal connections with cortical, limbic, and subcortical areas (the blueprints on which brain functions can be mapped) also suggests a key role for the frontal lobes in higher human functioning.

Despite the accepted importance and the obvious challenge to investigators of human mental activities, firm data concerning frontal lobe function are minimal when compared to the accumulated knowledge of other brain areas. Teuber (1964) voiced concern and suggested study of the human brain from the front rather than the prevalent study of posterior (sensory-motor) functions with attempt to move forward. It is easy to suggest that the frontal lobe is involved in memory, intelligence, attention, visual-spatial functions, language, and in fact virtually every human function. Yet most formal research demonstrates that the frontal lobes have little relevance to these recognized functions; large portions of the frontal lobe may be damaged or removed without producing striking changes. Even with the broader theoretical concepts positing "executive" or "supervisory" roles for the frontal lobes, it has been difficult to define and develop a task that adequately reflects these activities. The practical difficulties of research design have made frontal lobe investigation a quagmire for many researchers.

Many practical difficulties plague human frontal lobe research. Frontal lobe pathology rarely respects anatomical boundaries; pathoanatomical conclusions about specific areas within the frontal lobes, or even about the frontal lobes themselves, must be made with caution. Even when patients have clearly delineated frontal lobe pathology secondary to surgery (e.g., frontal leukotomy), postoperative behavior is difficult to isolate from premorbid psychiatric or epileptogenic problems. Laboratory techniques such as computed tomography (CT) scans and electroencephalography (EEG) remain inadequately sensitive to the location and extent of pathology; most commonly used neuropsychological tests are insensitive to frontal lobe deficits.

With improvements in clinical investigations, laboratory procedures, psychological assessments, and theoretical concepts, the study of frontal lobe function has advanced. There is a need to correlate and review current knowledge with particular stress on human frontal lobe functions. The decision to focus on human research was based on the presence of a number of previous publications with a primary if not exclusive focus on animal frontal lobe functions (Fuster, 1980; Konorski, Teuber, and Zernicki, 1972; Pribram and Luria, 1973), the demonstration of significant anatomical discrepancies of human frontal lobe, and finally the perceived absence of a summary work on human frontal lobe functions with a focus on clinical and research information. The more immediate impetus derived from the authors' investigations of the neuropsychological residuals of prefrontal leukotomy.

HISTORICAL BACKGROUND

As a backdrop for exploring the functions of the human frontal lobes in subsequent chapters, the data and the theoretical approaches produced by early investigators are reviewed. This information is categorized in several arbitrarily devised sections.

Holistic Versus Localization Approach

In 1922 Bianchi wrote: "What is the function of that large and excitable mass of brain situated in front of the motor zone?" This is a question that has intrigued and challenged thinkers for centuries. One troublesome problem in investigating frontal lobe function has been the tendency to utilize only a single approach to brain activity. Some investigators consider sensory-motor and mental activity as a unitary function; others parcel these activities, with certain areas of the brain (centers) considered dominant for specific activities. Disagreement between the holistic and localization approaches has more often obscured than aided investigation of brain function.

Those who look at brain function as a single, whole activity represent a larger group and provide a far richer background. The mind–body dichotomy formalized by Descartes had actually been present for several millenia, always with mental activity discussed as a single, independent activity. Although theologians and philosophers routinely discussed mental activity as an abstract, most came to recognize the brain as the seat of these activities. Mental activity was invariably treated as a single function, however, with the brain acting as a whole, much like the kidney or liver. This attitude prevails in many current approaches to brain function. The brain is viewed as a passive organ, responsive to external stimuli but with the response dependent to a considerable degree on the background (training) of prior response to stimuli. Through most of the history of mankind, there has been little evidence to suggest that differences in mental function depended on involvement of focal brain areas. Without such information, the holistic approach to mental activity represented the most advanced thinking and became deeply entrenched.

The first broad objection to the widely accepted holistic approach came from Francis Joseph Gall, the first true neuroscientist, whose ideas, though naive, were at least a century ahead of those of his contemporaries. Gall and Spurzheim (1809) posited that discrete mental activities were performed in separate areas of the brain. Based on correlations of primitive neuroanatomy and gross behavioral characteristics, they developed the pseudoscience of phrenology. Although based on inadequate knowledge of anatomy and psychology, their efforts introduced several important theoretical propositions for discussion and investigation: (1) the cerebral convolutions are the organs of the intellectual faculty, the parts of the human brain that subserve instincts, sentiments, tendencies, talents, affective qualities, and, in general, the moral and intellectual forces; (2) particular forms of intelligence such as memory, imagination, and behavioral tendencies exist, and each cerebral organ has its own particular variation of these; (3) "the qualities common to man and to animals have their seats in the lateral posterior parts of the head (brain). In proportion and as animals have been endowed with a share of certain anterior and superior encephalic parts so they enjoy certain intellectual faculties . . . man is the more intelligent, the more the anterior superior brain is developed" (Soury, 1899, p. 68). In addition to what were radical and heretical theories, Gall had produced an exciting new avenue through which to approach the problems of brain function, the correlation of behavioral observations with brain anatomy. The neuroanatomy available to Gall was limited almost entirely to the shape of the skull, but the proposition that behavior could be correlated with anatomy represented a major advance.

Gall's statements were radical, and the leading minds of the day refused to accept them. Fleurens (1842) considered Gall's notions fantastic and maintained that "there is no such thing as a different site for the different faculties and the different perceptions" (p. 68). Hitzig (1874), one of the earliest experimentalists to face the questions of cerebral localization, also disagreed. He emphatically demanded that the cortical centers are merely collecting centers and later stated that "intelligence, or more correctly, the treasury of ideas, is to be sought for in all parts of the cortex, or rather, in all parts of the brain" (p. 70).

The localization of mental functions within selective portions of the brain remains a subject for debate. Many investigators continue to demand that the brain acts as an integrated whole, as demonstrated by the fact that damage to almost any portion of the brain alters mental function. Also, there is a general rule, basically supported by observation, that the greater the area of damage, the greater the degree of mental decline. The latter point has been championed by numerous twentieth century investigators, most adequately by Lashley (1929) and Chapman and Wolff (1959). Nonetheless, almost all investigators now agree with Gall that different areas of the brain do subserve different functions, albeit the areas are closely interrelated and their functions integrated. The precise anatomical delineation of the motor and sensory cortices and the focal nature of certain language functions offer strong examples. Even more convincing, the features of mental decline that follow brain damage appear to depend on the anatomical sites of damage; major damage in one portion of the brain may produce a considerably different symptom picture than a quantitatively similar amount of damage in another site. When reviewing the background of the investigation of frontal lobe activity, the ongoing holistic versus localization controversy deserves consideration. Neither view is entirely correct, and neither is entirely wrong; information of value is available from both approaches. In a degree that varies with current modes and fashions, belief in one approach is in ascendancy at a given time. This variability has been clearly reflected in the investigations of frontal lobe functions.

Physiological Approach

Many of the earliest attempts to study frontal lobe functions were carried out by nineteenth century physiologists. The work was crude, the animals examined had only limited amounts of frontal lobe, and, without antiseptic techniques, the complication rate was enormous. Nevertheless, some important investigations were performed and key observations made.

Ferrier (1886), by means of animal experimentation, suggested that a center for movements of the head and eyes was located in the frontal lobes, and he postulated that the frontal lobes were the organ of attention. Ferrier's experimental observations were confirmed by demonstrations using either stimulation or ablation (Crosby, Humphrey, and Lauer, 1962; Grünbaum and Sherrington, 1903). His attention theory was challenged, however, when it was demonstrated that animals deprived of both frontal lobes can move both the head and eyes (Crosby et al., 1962). Although these animals lack normal curiosity, there is no paralysis of head or eye movement.

Following experiments on a variety of animal species, Bianchi (1895) added a series of observations on frontal lobe function:

1. Restlessness—Animals with bilateral mutilating frontal lobe injuries move about consistently and aimlessly.
2. Indifference—Such animals show suppression of curiosity and interest.
3. Decreased affect—Bilateral frontal animals show little interest or concern toward other animals.
4. Emotionality—These animals suffer a strong fear of noise, other animals, and so on, stimuli which did not disturb them prior to surgery. In addition, they are very slow in returning to a state of calm.
5. Abnormal mental state—Such animals show defective reflection, judgment, and memory and have an incapacity for new adaptation.
6. Instincts—Certain instincts have been weakened.
7. Activity—There is a tendency toward stereotypic and automatic activities.

Based on these observations, Bianchi concluded that the frontal lobe is *an* organ of intellect but was careful to avoid stating that it is *the* organ of intellect.

A number of early investigators opposed suggestions that the frontal lobe was of particular importance in higher functions. Munk (1890) maintained that there was no relationship between intelligence and the frontal lobes and, to support his contention, demonstrated that damage to either the occipital or the parietal-temporal areas produced far greater intellectual disturbance than quantitatively comparable frontal lobe damage. Goltz (1884) also denied that intelligence had a specific relationship with the anterior lobes of the brain and stated that: (1) lesions confined to the frontal lobes are followed by consequences that are less significant than those due to lesions of other parts of the brain; and (2) lesions limited to one frontal lobe produce no appreciable defect.

Loeb (1886) denied psychic functions for the frontal lobes; Luciani (1912) and Horsley and Schafer (1888) did not believe that, after destruction of the prefrontal lobes, dogs or apes differed in any appreciable way from intact animals, at least so far as intelligence was concerned. These investigators produced alterations of basic motor and sensory functions by affecting the more posterior portions of animal brains, whereas anterior (frontal) manipulation produced no dramatic behavioral changes.

By this time, new approaches and a new lexicon were added to the investigations. One important step was the introduction of the term *apperception* (Wundt, 1873–1874). Wundt distinguished sensory perception, the noting of a simple perception of an object, from an attentive perception, the recognition and association of that perception. There was an implication that apperception was a function of the frontal lobe. This idea was advanced by Flechsig (1896), who suggested that the frontal lobes play a predominant part in the formation of the ego insofar as that activity composed feelings, voluntary acts, and mnemonic traces. He posited that the centers of association dominate the intellectual life, are the true organs of thought, and are primarily frontal in location. Flechsig carefully separated aphasia and agnosia, considering them intellectual disturbances of a lesser degree that indicated a more posterior cerebral disturbance. In 1905 Flechsig proposed "the frontal lobe as a center of apperception," that a relationship existed between the frontal lobes and the attributes of sociability and social sentiments, and finally that "the most important factors of will are connected with the frontal associative centers" (p. 83).

Italian physiologists Fano (1895) and Polimanti (1906) considered the frontal lobes to be inhibitory organs and proposed that frontal lobe symptomatology was based on the absence, to a greater or lesser extent, of a restraining influence on motor activity.

Another major step came from the work of Franz (1907), who adopted the psychological testing techniques originated by Thorndike (1911). The animals used by Franz for experimentation were trained to acquire new associations and then were reexamined following mutilation of the frontal lobes. His findings can be summarized as three major points:

1. When the frontal lobes are destroyed, recent acquisitions are lost.
2. The loss of associations does not result from lesions of other parts of the brain.
3. The loss of associations is not due to shock.

Flechsig's notions and Franz's ideas were carried further by Lugaro (1908), who stated, "The frontal lobes are the organ which registers the story of the acts of all one's life (experience), the organ which feels the most intimate impulses of the organism, and elaborates the particular individual mode of reaction to external stimuli" (p. 91). Thus lesions of the frontal lobe would damage the personality and alter the individual's character.

A respected contemporary, Monakow (1905), disagreed and stated that observations on neither humans nor animals could furnish data sufficiently strong to prove the functional role of the frontal lobes. He believed that inflammatory processes secondary to surgical damage explained many of the experimental observations and suggested that secondary degeneration occurred in the more posterior areas (particularly the optic thalamus) following mutilation of frontal lobes in animals. Frontal lobe damage was thought to alter subcortical and posterior cortical centers by means of diaschisis, and the observed behavioral alterations apparently reflected the entire array of damaged areas. The holistic/localization disagreement continued, albeit with a more scientific basis.

Anatomical Approach

During the time of the early physiological observations and continuing to the present, ongoing improvement in the techniques used to study the anatomical connections of frontal lobe structures has been important. Utilizing a variety of techniques (Marchi stain, Nauta stain, horseradish peroxidase), anatomists have continued to discover important anatomical relationships of frontal lobe structures (Goldman and Nauta, 1976; Krieg, 1949; Nauta, 1971, 1972; Pandya, Dye, and Butters, 1971; Van Hoesen, Pandya, and Butters, 1975). In general, most studies have demonstrated the remarkable richness and diversity of both the frontal lobe structures and their connections. Understanding this complex matrix is crucial for attempts to delineate the role of the frontal lobes in mental life.

Unfortunately, most nonanatomists, even investigators trained in the neurosciences, tend to accept the frontal lobe as a single functional center, a holistic entity. Anatomical studies have shown numerous strikingly specific connections that imply important functional correlations, but this material is not widely appreciated. Chapter 2 reviews some of the important anatomical demonstrations of the frontal lobes and their connections.

Although the anatomical work has consistently increased in sophistication, most inferences concerning frontal lobe function based on these anatomical findings remain just that—inferences. The ability to correlate the anatomical composition with the function of the human frontal lobe remains limited, demanding sophisticated clinical/pathological correlation studies.

Clinical Observation Approach

Because of the lack of appropriate animal models and the difficulty performing either physiological or anatomical studies on humans, most observations of frontal function have been made on individuals suffering brain damage. Many such reports have been presented, but the results are far from clear. Important among the clinical observations are the case reports on severe frontal injury, the classic cases such as Phineas Gage (Harlow, 1868) and those of Welt (1888) and Brickner (1936). Following the demonstration by Jacobsen (1935) of considerable alteration in the anxiety levels of several chimpanzees whose frontal lobes were partially removed, Moniz (1937) and many others (Freeman, 1949; Scoville, 1949) used similar techniques to treat human psychiatric disorders, thereby providing additional observations on the psychic functions of the frontal lobes. Luria, Pribram, and Homskaya (1964), Hécaen (1964), and many others have studied frontal and prefrontal tumors and correlated the observed behavioral abnormalities with anatomical localization. Finally, many investigators (Feuchtwanger, 1923; Kleist, 1934a; Lishman, 1968; Weinstein and Teuber, 1957) have correlated the behavioral activities and sites of damage of individuals who sustained brain injuries in the two world wars.

Limitations of the clinical observation approach are obvious. Variations in site and type of pathology, premorbid education and behavior of the subject, and testing techniques used for investigation yield disparate observations. Clear proof has remained evasive. Nonetheless, some consistency has been noted, and these observations represent a sizable portion of current knowledge of the functions of the human frontal lobe.

Neuropsychological Approach

Neuropsychology is a relatively recent subdivision of psychological investigation, and the neuropsychological approach represents the newest approach to the study of human frontal function. In large degree the neuropsychological approach has evolved from clinical observations. Investigators such as Goldstein (1944), Luria (1965, 1969, 1973a), Milner (1963, 1964, 1982), and Teuber (1964) observed many patients with frontal pathology and against this background developed increasingly more specific procedures to investigate human frontal lobe functioning. In many respects, this book is an organized review of the clinical observations and neuropsychological approaches that have been used to study the behavioral functions subserved by the frontal lobes.

Despite the large quantity of collected information and the continuous advance of knowledge, the debate concerning holistic versus localization approaches continues. In fact, it is only in relatively recent times that any evidence supporting true localization within the human frontal lobe has been offered. From any approach, the question raised by Bianchi concerning the functions of the frontal lobes still beckons.

PERSONAL BACKGROUND

The information presented in this book reflects the particular backgrounds of the two authors. The focus is on human frontal lobe functions, with particular emphasis on the activities of the prefrontal granular cortex. References to the animal and physiological literature are not emphasized but are presented in the context of corroborating evidence where considered appropriate.

Northampton Veterans Administration Leukotomy Study

In addition to clinical observations, the authors' experience with frontal lobe damage derives from a follow-up study of schizophrenics who had undergone prefrontal leukotomy as a treatment for psychiatric disorder. The Northampton Veterans Administration (VA) leukotomy series was made possible through the active cooperation of the administration and staff (Chief of Neurology, Dr. William Weir) of the Northampton Veterans Administration Medical Center. The study itself was undertaken at the Boston Veterans Administration Medical Center with the encouragement and cooperation of the administration, the Department of Neurology (Dr. Robert Feldman), Department of Radiology (Dr. Harvey Levine), and Research Psychology section (Dr. Harold Goodglass). Many of the colleagues who were involved in the study are coauthors on various publications. The Appendix presents a listing of published articles and chapters that describe the Northampton VA Leukotomy Study, along with the names of coauthors who worked on portions of the study. In addition, the research would have been impossible without the assistance of residents, fellows, neuropsychologists, research assistants, and the dedicated and accomplished nursing staff of Ward 7D of the Boston Veterans Administration Medical Center.

Although the results of the Northampton study can never conclusively deny the influence of ongoing schizophrenia, the advent of the CT scan allowed demarcation of localized orbital frontal pathology, an opportunity rarely available in previous frontal lobe research. By use of selected control groups and the division by varying degrees of psychiatric recovery among the leukotomized patients, a number of hypotheses concerning frontal lobe functions could be raised. An outline of the methodology and general results of the Northampton study are presented here as an introduction to results chronicled in subsequent chapters. These are further delineated in a number of publications (see Appendix).

Sixteen schizophrenics who had undergone prefrontal leukotomy more than 25 years earlier (between 1948 and 1952) were available for study. They were selected from 56 patients still followed out of the approximately 180 patients originally treated at the Northampton VA hospital by leukotomy. Prior to surgery each patient had been assigned a diagnosis of schizophrenia and institutionalized a minimum of 1 year. After unsuccessful treatment for the psychosis (medications, electroconvulsive therapy, insulin shock, hydrotherapy, and others), all underwent prefrontal leukotomy. To study the long-term effects, the leukotomized schizophrenics were divided into three groups that reflected the degree of recovery as defined by: (1) postsurgery duration of hospitalization; (2) number of years since discharge; (3) amount of hospital contact after discharge.

Group I was the good recovery group. These five patients had a mean duration of 14 years since last discharge from hospital. Each had been successful in returning to some kind of work and to living independently.

Group II consisted of five patients with a more limited recovery; they had been free of hospital care for at least 6 years prior to study, but none had successfully returned to work and all continued to have a more notable degree of psychotic symptomatology than those in group I.

Group III, six patients considered to show "no improvement," had been hospitalized continually from time of leukotomy to the time of assessment; leaves from the hospital were either infrequent and unsuccessful or never permitted.

Two control groups were selected in an attempt to isolate the effects of prefrontal pathology.

Group IV was a psychiatric control group comparable to group III, the poor recovery leukotomized patients, in virtually every consideration except that they had not undergone psychosurgery. They also had been institutionalized continuously for about 25 years.

Group V, a normal control group, matched to the other four groups in age, education, socioeconomic status, and military history, but with no evident central nervous system dysfunction and no psychiatric history.

Two additional control groups were sought: (1) psychiatric patients diagnosed as schizophrenic at the same time as the patients in the study but who had spontaneously recovered; (2), leukotomized schizophrenics who had recovered to the extent that they had remained totally free of hospital care. Although it was believed that patients in both of these categories did exist, they were long lost to hospital follow-up procedures and could not be found.

When the findings from the x-ray CT scans were correlated with the status of recovery, a totally unexpected result was evident. The good recovery group had the largest prefrontal lesions, whereas the poor recovery group had the smallest lesions (Benson, Stuss, Naeser, et al., 1981). These results indicated that the greater the size of frontal lobe destruction, particularly if slightly asymmetrical, the better the psychiatric outcome (Naeser, Levine, Benson, et al., 1981). Not so unexpectedly, the neuropsychological results also correlated with the degree of recovery, the good recovery group performing best (frequently at a level equivalent to that of the normal control group). The isolation of specific deficits that could be hypothesized to reflect frontal lobe functioning occurred when all three leukotomized groups were significantly inferior to the normal control group on tests thought to tap frontal lobe function. The overall conclusion, tempered by awareness of the small sample size and the continuing presence of ongoing psychiatric disease, is that some specific deficits secondary to orbital frontal lesions can be demonstrated. These findings are reported throughout the book, always in context with clinical observations and the neuropsychological investigations reported by others.

SUMMARY

The book is organized as follows. Chapters 2 through 4 present basic knowledge of the frontal lobes, their neuroanatomy, the mechanisms by which they may be damaged, and the various tools used to measure the extent, location, and effect of the damage. Chapters 5 through 8 report the more obvious, most sensational, and/or most frequently described findings following frontal lobe damage. This discussion covers frontal motor disorders, apparent problems with attention, and disturbances of awareness, personality, and emotion. Chapters 9 and 10 examine how supposedly nonfrontal activities—sensory-perceptual and visual-spatial functions—can be affected by damage to the frontal lobes or its direct connections.

The remainder of the book deals with more complex mental activities that are often considered vulnerable to frontal, particularly prefrontal, lobe damage, Chapters 11 and 12 deal with the influence of frontal damage on language and memory.

Chapters 13 and 14 address the role of frontal lobes in "intelligence" and "cognitive" functions by reviewing and discussing effects of frontal malfunction on what are loosely termed cognitive and executive abilities. Chapter 15 presents the localization of frontal lobe functions suggested by the findings reviewed in this volume. Although this material is closely related to the context of the introductory chapters on neuroanatomy, pathology, and assessment, it is logically reviewed after all specific functions have been presented. Moreover, the presentation of our concept of brain organization in relationship to higher mental functions prefaces the final two chapters, which discuss theories of frontal lobe function. In Chapter 16 a selected number of contemporary theories concerning the functions and mode of operations of the frontal lobes in relationship to other brain activities are presented. Finally, in Chapter 17 the authors present their own postulations. This represents our attempt to understand the concepts emerging from the previous chapters and our proposal of a model for future research.

2

Neuroanatomical Considerations

Advances in knowledge of the functions of the frontal lobes depend, to a great extent, on knowledge of the neuroanatomy of this cortical area. For review, the subject of the neuroanatomy of the frontal lobes is divided into four sections. The first section defines the frontal lobes morphologically including external description; division of cortical areas; cytoarchitectural divisions; frontal-thalamic definitions; vascular distribution; and some gross subdivisions based on apparent functions. The second major section summarizes the known connections of the frontal lobe with sensory and association cortices, olfactory and limbic systems, thalamus, motor cortex, basal ganglia, cerebellum, tectum, brainstem and reticular systems, and commissural connections. The final two sections present the biochemical systems serving the frontal lobes and give an introduction to the changes with development. The morphological descriptions, including blood supply and separation into cytoarchitectonic and functional subdivisions, are based primarily on human anatomy whereas much of the remainder is derived from animal (especially primate) research.

ANATOMICAL CLASSIFICATIONS

External Description

In the most elementary approach, the frontal lobes may be divided into three surface areas: lateral, medial, and inferior. On the lateral surface (Fig. 2-1), the frontal lobe is defined as the entire brain area lying in front of the central sulcus and above the lateral fissure. Medially (Fig. 2-2), it surrounds the anterior section of the corpus callosum and is defined posteriorly by an imaginary line dropped from the medial portion of the central sulcus down to the corpus callosum. The anterior part of the cingulate gyrus may or may not be considered part of the medial frontal lobe (Pandya, Van Hoesen, and Mesulam, 1981). From the inferior viewpoint (Fig. 2-3), the lateral-posterior borders are the temporal poles, whereas more medially the frontal lobe is arbitrarily defined by a line drawn from side to side at the level of the optic chiasm.

Each surface area has its own sulcal demarcations. On the lateral external surface (Fig. 2-1), the precentral sulcus runs parallel to the central sulcus. The precentral sulcus can usually be divided into two parts, a superior part which rarely intersects

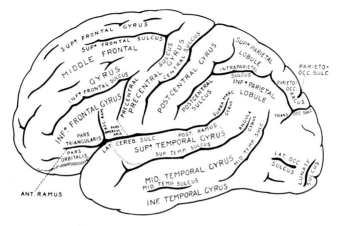

FIG. 2-1. Lateral surface of the left cerebral hemisphere. (From Williams and Warwick: *Functional Neuroanatomy of Man.* Churchill Livingstone, Edinburgh, 1975, with permission.)

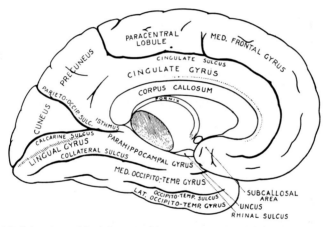

FIG. 2-2. Medial surface of the left cerebral hemisphere, with removal of the brainstem. (From Williams and Warwick: *Functional Neuroanatomy of Man.* Churchill Livingstone, Edinburgh, 1975, with permission.)

the superior border of the lobe and an inferior section which may run inferiorly to the lateral sulcus. Extending forward horizontally from the superior and inferior sections of the precentral sulcus run the superior and inferior frontal sulci. These divide the lateral convexity of the frontal lobes into three sections of approximately equal width. These two sulci do not reach the anterior border of the frontal lobe and are frequently interrupted by small bridging gyri. Between them an intermediate sulcus is present in some specimens. The lateral fissure, which forms the inferior border of the lateral aspect of the frontal lobe, is most frequently divided into three rami. The main section of the fissure, which runs laterally and divides the frontal lobe from the temporal lobe, is called the posterior ramus. Two smaller

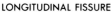
LONGITUDINAL FISSURE

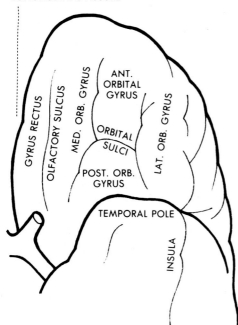

FIG. 2-3. Inferior (basal) aspect of the left hemisphere of the brain. Note that the pictured orbital gyral pattern is not consistently seen. (From Williams and Warwick: *Functional Neuroanatomy of Man.* Churchill Livingstone, Edinburgh, 1975, with permission.)

rami, extending horizontally and superiorly from the lateral fissure, project upward for a short distance into the frontal lobe and are called the anterior horizontal ramus and the anterior ascending ramus. Some anatomists consider the sulci that cut into the frontal lobe from the lateral sulcus as being too variable to be useful (Gardner, 1975).

The sulci divide the lateral surface area into distinct divisions or gyri. The precentral gyrus is the strip of cortex that runs vertically between the central and precentral sulci. Anterior to the precentral sulcus are three horizontal gyri (superior, middle, and inferior frontal gyri) defined by the superior and inferior frontal sulci. Finally, the rami of the lateral fissure intrude into the inferior frontal gyrus, dividing it into three parts: the pars opercularis is posterior, the pars triangularis is in the middle, and the pars orbitalis is anterior. All three divisions of the inferior frontal gyrus lie in front of the precentral gyrus, extending anteriorly and inferiorly.

On the medial surface of the frontal lobe (Fig. 2-2), the central fissure may be seen as a posterior boundary, but it extends only a small distance. Most of the posterior boundary of the frontal lobe on the medial surface is an imaginary line dropped from the end of the central fissure. The precentral sulcus, as noted, does not normally extend to the medial surface. Frequently, however, there is a small, vertical paracentral sulcus lying on the superior border of the medial frontal lobe, anterior to the central fissure. The major defining sulcus on the medial surface is the cingulate sulcus which begins beneath the rostrum of the corpus callosum and arches up and around the genu of the corpus callosum, extends backward, and finally terminates close to the anterior edge of the parietal lobe. These sulci divide the medial surface of the frontal cortex as follows: the superior frontal gyrus, which overlaps from the lateral surface, lies between the anterior part of the cingulate gyrus and the superior edge of the hemisphere. It extends posteriorly to the arbitrary line dropped from the central fissure. This part of the superior frontal gyrus is occasionally labeled the medial frontal gyrus. Beneath the cingulate sulcus is the cingulate gyrus, separated from the corpus callosum by the callosal sulcus. This gyrus extends posteriorly and is considered part of the limbic system. Finally, the medial portion of the frontal lobe, which is an extension of the precentral and postcentral gyri and is bordered anteriorly by the paracentral sulcus, is called the paracentral lobule.

The inferior surface (Fig. 2-3) faces both inferiorly and laterally as it meets the lateral frontal cortex. The most prominent feature of the inferior frontal cortex is the attachment of the olfactory bulb and its tract, lying in the olfactory sulcus and leading posteriorly. These pathways, labeled the olfactory tract, are situated medially, lying near and running parallel to the longitudinal cerebral fissure that divides the two frontal lobes. The olfactory tract courses to the posterior end of the inferior surface, dividing at the olfactory trigone, which lies approximately 1 cm in front of the notch for the diencephalon. The olfactory pathways then travel either medially (to the medial olfactory stria and septal area) or laterally (to the lateral olfactory stria and to the piriform cortex) (Gardner, 1975). The olfactory sulcus is the dividing point for the two major sections of the inferior surface. Medial to the olfactory sulcus and adjacent to the longitudinal cerebral fissure lies the gyrus rectus. Lateral to the olfactory sulcus are a series of irregular orbital gyri subdivided by an inconsistent number of orbital sulci. The orbital gyri are not normally specifically defined.

Division of Cortical Areas

Over the years a number of schemes have been developed to differentiate various segments of cortex, including frontal and prefrontal areas (Brodmann, 1909, 1914; von Bonin and Bailey, 1947). The Brodmann system, depicted in Fig. 2-4, is the most widely used for identifying specific cortical areas. Although not exact, this division has proved a useful guide to a global differentiation of both anatomical

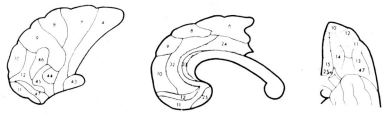

FIG. 2-4. Brodmann areas of the lateral *(left)*, medial *(central)*, and orbital *(right)* aspects of the frontal lobe. (From Robin and Macdonald: *Lessons of Leucotomy*. Henry Kimpton, London, 1975, with permission.)

and functional subdivisions. The Brodmann areas for the three frontal surfaces are as follows: The lateral surface contains Brodmann areas 4, 6, 8–12, and 43–47; the medial surface consists of areas 6, 8–12, 24, 25, 32, and 33; and the inferior surface includes areas 10–15, 25, and 47 (Robin and Macdonald, 1975). Even more useful is a functional subdivision based on the Brodmann numbers. Area 4 denotes the primary motor area; the premotor area is designated by areas 6, 8, 43, 44, and 45; and the prefrontal cortex is denoted by areas 9–15, 46, and 47 (with the possible addition of areas 13–15) (Jouandet and Gazzaniga, 1979). Riegele (1931), however, suggested that areas 43 to 45 are cytoarchitectonically more similar to prefrontal cortex. Walsh (1978) presented four major divisions of frontal cortex: motor (area 4); premotor (6 and part of 8); prefrontal (9, 10, 45, and 46); and basomedial (9–13, 24, and 32), the latter two frequently grouped into one prefrontal division.

A second, less commonly used means of subdividing the frontal cortex is von Bonin and Bailey's (1947) cytoarchitectural map. There is an approximate comparison to the Brodmann areas. Frontal agranular cortex (Brodmann areas 4 and 6) (see below) corresponds to FA, FB, and FC of von Bonin and Bailey (Akert, 1964), whereas frontal granular cortex, labeled FD by von Bonin and Bailey, corresponds to Brodmann areas 8–12. The transitional zone, area 8, is similar to the von Bonin and Bailey areas FDr and FD△. The von Bonin and Bailey labeling is most frequently used in primate research, whereas the Brodmann numbers are used more often in reference to human functions.

Cytoarchitectural Divisions

Although the cerebral hemispheres are frequently defined by the underlying cytoarchitectural cortical structure (Brodmann, 1914; von Bonin and Bailey, 1947), the various cell layers also have significant functional attributes. Neocortex consists of six cell layers; the names of these six layers give the defining characteristics: I, molecular layer; II, external granular layer; III, external pyramidal layer; IV, internal granular layer; V, internal pyramidal layer; VI, polymorphic layer.

The relative proportion of each cell layer in a specific part of neocortex is used to define that cortex into one of five distinct compositions (von Economo, 1929). Frontal neocortex has three such subdivisions based on cell layer percentages (Fig. 2-5). The motor and premotor cortex (primarily Brodmann areas 4 and 6) is known as heterotypical frontal agranular cortex. The presence of cells with long nerve fibers to carry impulses to the brainstem produce a significantly increased layer of pyramidal cells, i.e., enlarged external pyramidal layer III and internal layer V, whereas layers II and IV are virtually absent. Layers III and V become fused into one deep layer with a high concentration of large pyramidal cells. Although Brodmann areas 4 and 6 are both considered agranular cortex, they are differentiated from each other by the presence of the giant pyramidal cells of Betz, which appear to be limited to the motor cortex (area 4) of the precentral gyrus. Areas 44 and 45, lying in the inferior frontal convolution, have been considered cytoar-

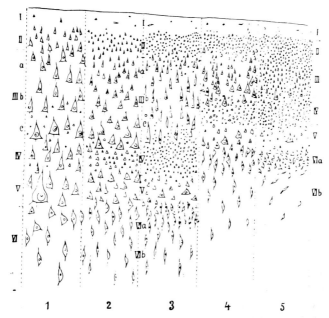

FIG. 2-5. The five basic types of cortical structure. **1:** Agranular motor. **2:** Frontal granular or frontal homotypical (prefrontal). **3:** Parietal homotypical. **4:** Polar. **5:** Granular koniocortex. Frontal cortex essentially consists of types 1 and 2 and transitional cortex (primarily frontal eye fields) between them. (From Von Economo: *The Cytoarchitectonics of the Human Cerebral Cortex.* Oxford University Press, Oxford, 1929, with permission.)

chitecturally continuous with area 6 (Jouandet and Gazzaniga, 1979) or as part of prefrontal cortex (Riegele, 1931). These two areas lie immediately anterior to primary motor regions for the face, lips, tongue, and pharynx.

The second major cytoarchitectonic division of the frontal cortex is the granular homotypical cortex, an area that is virtually identical to the prefrontal cortex. Here, layers II and IV, i.e., the granular cell layers, increase in size whereas the layers of medium and large pyramidal cells (III and V) are decreased. Granular cortex is normally found in sensory cortical areas. However, the frontal granular cortex appears somewhat different than the granular koniocortex of the posterior sensory areas—hence the term granular homotypical cortex. In general, the prefrontal granular cortex is a phylogenetically recent structure, prominent only in primates and reaching its largest size in man (Nauta, 1971). The lateral frontal granular cortex is one of the last cortical areas to become myelinated (Jouandet and Gazzaniga, 1979).

Lying between the granular and agranular frontal cortical areas is a band of transitional cortex with a gradient of granularization of layer IV and pyramidalization of layers III and V. It is roughly equivalent to Brodmann area 8. In the rhesus monkey it lies in the cradle of the arcuate sulcus, whereas in man it represents the posterior end of the middle frontal gyrus. Area 8 coincides in general with the frontal eye fields, although the physiological boundaries of the latter appear to exceed area 8 (Smith, 1944). Low threshold frontal eye field definition, however, appears to be smaller than area 8 (Bruce and Goldberg, 1984).

The prefrontal cortex has also been architectonically divided based on a concept of "dual origin" of cerebral cortex phylogenetic development (Barbas and Pandya, 1982). One section is a bilaminar proisocortical region, consisting of areas 25 and 32 (around the rostral tip of the cingulate sulcus). From here, there is a progressive laminar differentiation on a dorsal course through areas 9, 10, 46, and 8. A second similar rudimentary proisocortical region begins in the caudal orbital surface near the olfactory tubercle, with progressive differentiation through areas 13, 12, 10, 46, and 8. Commissural fibers originating from regions with similar architectonic features have a common place in the corpus callosum (Barbas and Pandya, 1984).

Frontal-Thalamic Definition

The frontal cortex can also be divided according to its thalamic connections (Akert, 1964; Goldman, 1979; Nauta, 1971), and this division appears to have important phylogenetic and functional correlates. The two major thalamic afferents to the frontal cortex derive from the dorsal-medial (MD) nucleus and the ventroanterior (VA) and ventrolateral (VL) nuclei (Fig. 2-6). Areas 4 and 6 of Brodmann (agranular cortex) are recipients from the lateral and anterior ventral nuclei, respectively. The prefrontal granular cortex is defined by projections from the MD nucleus and appears to be divisible into several distinct regions. The lateral parvocellular section of the MD nucleus projects to Brodmann areas 9 and 10 but not to orbital cortex. The medial magnocellular portion of the MD nucleus sends afferents to orbital cortex. Projections to the rostral bank of the arcuate sulcus (frontal eye field, area 8) derive from the paralamellar section of the MD nucleus. If connections with the MD nucleus are considered the defining characteristic of the prefrontal cortex, the frontal eye fields would be labeled prefrontal, even though they do not entirely fill the anatomical or cytoarchitectonic definition (Nauta, 1971). Nauta (1971) stated that the entire prefrontal cortex should be considered association cortex as no prefrontal area can be identified with a particular sensory modality.

There are also a number of connections between frontal areas and nonspecific thalamic structures, particularly the nucleus reticularis and the midline region of the intralaminar thalamic complex (Nauta, 1964). Although the primary connections of this nonspecific thalamic projection system appear to go to the orbital frontal cortex, the projection is not sufficiently definitive to define this area (Scheibel and Scheibel, 1967).

Vascular Distribution

Another anatomical division of the frontal lobes is through their blood supply. Differentiation is less sharp and less consistent, but alterations, both developmental

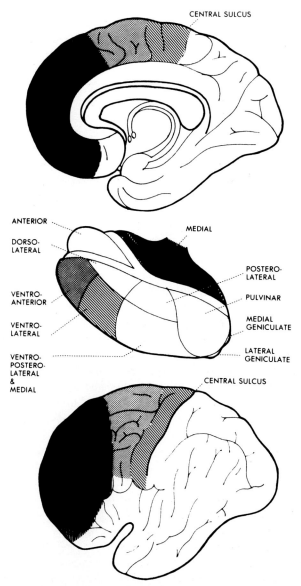

FIG. 2-6. Thalamic-frontal connections, as indicated by matched shading. The thalamus, subdivided into regions, is presented in the center, with the medial view of the cortex represented at the top and the left lateral cortex represented on the bottom. (From Curtis, Jacobson, and Marcus: *An Introduction to the Neurosciences.* Saunders, Philadelphia, 1972, with permission.)

and acquired, may prove significant. Most attention is given to the patterns of cortical branches, but distribution to subcortical structures active in so-called frontal system activities is also of significance.

The frontal lobes receive vascular supply exclusively from the bilateral anterior cerebral and the anterior branches of the middle cerebral arteries, all originating from the internal carotid artery (Carpenter and Sutin, 1983; Chusid, 1970).

The anterior cerebral artery is said to have two major divisions: central and cerebral (Perlmutter and Rhoton, 1978). The central (basal perforating) branches travel somewhat posteriorly to supply the anterior hypothalamus, septum pellucidum, anterior commissure, fornix, anterior-inferior striatum, and anterior diencephalon. The cerebral division may be subdivided into cortical, subcortical, and callosal arteries, the cortical branches having most relevance to the prefrontal cortex. The cortical branch of the anterior cerebral artery primarily traverses the medial surface of the frontal lobe, skirting up and around the genu of the corpus callosum and coursing caudally along the superior surface of the corpus callosum. Along this path, it sends out branches that feed the rectus and internal orbital gyri, the cingulate gyrus, and the mesial section of the superior frontal and precentral gyri. These branches extend over the edge of the medial surface of the hemisphere to feed the superior frontal gyrus, the frontal pole, and the most superior sections of the middle frontal gyrus. This cortical anterior cerebral artery may be subdivided into orbital frontal, frontal polar, and internal frontal arteries, each of which supplies specific frontal areas. The anterior cerebral arteries of each hemisphere are joined mesially by the short anterior communicating artery which lies just anterior to the optic chiasm. The anterior communicating artery, uniting the two anterior cerebral arteries, forms the anterior arc of the circle of Willis, the ring of blood vessels around the optic chiasm and pituitary stock that allows collateral flow.

Distal to the anterior communicating artery, the anterior cerebrals send out a number of penetrating branches. Most are short terminals feeding medial structures including the anterior corpus callosum. The most significant penetrating branch, the recurrent artery of Heubner, may arise either just proximal or just distal to the anterior communicating branch. It courses into the anterior penetrating substance and courses to the anterior caudate and putamen and the anterior limb of the internal capsule, fulfilling a function analogous to that of the lenticular and lateral striate branches of the middle cerebral arteries.

The middle cerebral artery is the larger of the two branches of the internal carotid artery (Gibo, Carver, Rhoton, et al., 1981). Once it divides from the internal carotid artery, it travels to the lateral portion of the cerebral hemispheres, giving rise en route to the lateral (lenticular) and medial striate arteries (Stephens and Stillwell, 1969). The main artery continues laterally and posteriorly within the sylvian fissure, breaking over the cortical surface in all directions. Doing so, it provides the vascular supply for most of the lateral portion of each cerebral hemisphere. Within the frontal lobes, it supplies the lateral orbital gyrus, the inferior and middle frontal gyrus, and anterior central gyrus of the dorsal-lateral convexity but stops short of the frontal tip anteriorly.

In summary, the vascular territories provide one relatively simple means of dividing the frontal lobes. The dorsal-lateral convexity is served by the middle cerebral artery, whereas the medial frontal area and the frontal tips are supplied by the anterior cerebral artery. Both feed the orbital surface, the division occurring between the lateral (middle cerebral) and medial (anterior cerebral) sections. Utilization of vascular territories in conjunction with the particular Brodmann areas irrigated may be an even more useful localization procedure (Marino, 1977).

Gross Functional Subdivisions

Yet another way to subdivide the frontal lobe is by the major functions generated. Most differentiation of function for the frontal lobes has been proposed for the lateral surface. The precentral gyrus (Brodmann area 4), the agranular motor cortex, is a major source of cortical-spinal and cortical-bulbar pyramidal fibers (Carpenter and Sutin, 1983; Gardner, 1975). It has reciprocal connections with the postcentral gyrus and receives a major input from the cerebellum and basal ganglia by way of the lateral ventral thalamic nucleus. Area 6, the premotor area, receives input from the cerebellum and basal ganglia by means of the anterior ventral thalamic nucleus and also gets significant input from association cortex. Area 6 projects primarily to subcortical structures such as the basal ganglia and is important for major extrapyramidal functions. Continuing on the lateral surface, areas 44 and 45, the opercular and triangular portions of the inferior frontal gyrus, are considered to represent the motor memories for speech patterns. Some authors (Jouandet and Gazzaniga, 1979) consider this section, known as Broca's area, and also area 43, as continuations of premotor area 6, primarily because they are cytoarchitectonically similar. Others do not (Walsh, 1978). One section of area 8, the posterior end of the middle frontal gyrus, contains the motor area for eye movements, allowing deviation of the eyes to the contralateral side. That is, the left frontal eye field is important for visual examination in the right visual field. The cortical mass anterior to areas described above, the prefrontal granular cortex, is in general considered association cortex. Functions associated with this region are the major topic of this book.

Functions associated with the inferior and medial surface of the frontal lobes are described in a more general fashion. The inferior surface is referred to as the orbital cortex and is considered to be an integral part of the limbic system.

On the medial surface, the paracentral lobule is an extension of the motor and sensory cortices onto the medial aspect of the hemisphere. Specific localizable functions according to the homunculus have been described. The supplementary motor area (SMA) is situated anterior to the paracentral lobule and contains the medial extension of the homunculus where perineal and leg movements are mediated. Corresponding Brodmann areas are 6 and (at least partially) 8. The SMA has bilateral reciprocal connections with areas 4, 6, and 8 and the anterior cingulate regions. It projects bilaterally to the striatum and receives input from areas 7, 5, 3, 1, 2, and SII (Damasio and Van Hoesen, 1980; Williams and Warwick, 1975). The SMA is considered by some to be a second speech area and also appears to be important in voluntary movements (Damasio and Van Hoesen, 1980; Penfield and Welch, 1951). Specific functional differentiation of the superior frontal gyrus on the medial surface is yet to be made.

A general overview of the functional differentiation of the frontal cortex has been proposed by Akert (1964) based on granular and agranular subdivisions. The agranular cortex has, by way of long axons to the brainstem and spinal cord, control over the pyramidal motor system. The granular cortex is "nonmotor," with only indirect influence on motor function.

CONNECTIONS OF THE FRONTAL LOBES

Although this section emphasizes connections between the prefrontal cortex and other cerebral areas, it must be noted that separation of gross cortical anatomy and its connections is artificial. Each is totally dependent on and influenced by the other.

Frontal-Cortical Sensory Connections

Much of the suggested importance of the prefrontal cortex in relationship to the external milieu derives from its reciprocal connections and central position to input from all three major sensory modalities (Chavis and Pandya, 1976; Jones and Powell, 1970; Kuypers, Szwarcbart, Mishkin, et al., 1965; Nauta, 1971, 1972; Pandya and Kuypers, 1969) (Fig. 2-7). Direct primary sensory field to prefrontal cortex pathways are virtually nonexistent, however. Rather, the visual, auditory, and somatic sensory areas connect with immediately adjoining association zones (e.g., primary visual cortex 17 to visual association cortex 18 or 19). From these areas of sensory association cortex, pathways project to many distant areas including motor association cortex. Most significant for the prefrontal cortex are pathways coursing to either or both the inferior parietal lobule and the rostral (anterior) half of the temporal cortex. The connecting pathways are primarily long neuronal chains, formed either in linear sequence or in parallel lines. The number of connections initiating from a particular cortical area increases the more distal the association area is from the primary sensory cortical area. There is at least partial overlap of information from the three main sensory modalities in the inferior parietal lobule (cross-modal associations) (Butters, Barton, and Brody, 1970; Geschwind, 1965), particularly in the human. Both the parietal area and the rostral temporal cortex are important origins of direct cortical-frontal connections, both projecting in relatively specific pathways to a large area of the frontal convexity, as well as the lateral orbital sulcus (Nauta, 1971, 1972; Petrides and Pandya, 1984; Schwartz and Goldman-Rakic, 1984). The pathway from the anterior temporal cortex traverses the uncinate bundle, and that from the inferior parietal area joins the superior longitudinal fasciculus.

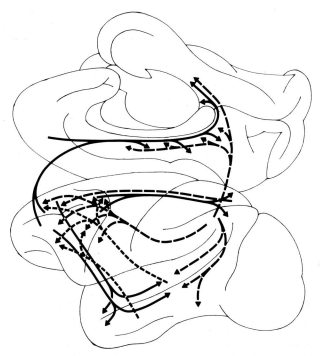

FIG. 2-7. Afferent and efferent frontal cortical and limbic connections. Multimodal association zones in both the parietal and temporal areas have direct cortical/dorsal-lateral frontal connections. Inferior parietal connections to cingulate and hippocampal zones are also present. In turn, various areas of the frontal lobe project to both parietal and temporal lobules, cingulate and hippocampal gyri, and upper and middle temporal gyri. (From Nauta: *J. Psychiatr. Res.*, 8:167–187, 1971, with permission.)

The middle temporal area, in the posterior bank of the superior temporal sulcus, receives visual input from both striate and superior colliculus via the inferior pulvinar (Maioli, Squatrito, Galletti, et al., 1983). This in turn has direct connections to the frontal eye field, which, as suggested by the authors, may consist of several functional units based on specific connections between these two areas.

Information from the inferior parietal lobule also projects to the cingulate, hippocampal, and temporal gyri, and via callosal connections to a homologous area in the contralateral hemisphere (Nauta, 1971, 1972, 1973; Schwartz and Goldman-Rakic, 1984). The connection with the temporal region creates another trimodality sensory information overlap.

To some extent at least, these afferent pathways are reciprocal (Nauta, 1971, 1972). Fibers originating in the caudal frontal convexity, i.e., frontal eye fields, project back to the inferior parietal zone. Although there is no anatomical evidence for direct connections between area 8 and oculomotor nuclei (Astruc, 1971), there is some evidence of connections between the frontal eye fields and occipital cortex (Chusid, Sugar, and French, 1948). Frontal-temporal connections consist of two pathways deriving from the temporal convexity: (1) pathways from areas dorsal to the principal sulcus course to rostral superior temporal areas; and (2) the ventral half of the dorsal bank of the principal sulcus projects to the ventral (middle and inferior gyri) temporal area via the uncinate fasciculus. Much of the information from these frontal-temporal connections may be further transferred medially to the MD nucleus (see below).

Knowledge of the afferent pathways has been refined by animal research (Goldman and Nauta, 1977b). In the monkey the midregion of the dorsal bank of the dorsal-lateral convexity (sulcus principalis) has four main ipsilateral projections. One runs in a ventral bank of the principal sulcus inferiorly to the convexity ventral to this sulcus, reaching the medial orbital gyrus and the superior temporal cortex. A second pathway crosses dorsally to the frontal eye fields and to the dorsal half of the frontal convexity. A third rostral connection goes to the entire medial surface. Finally, connections join the medial wall to the cingulate and gyrus fornicatus. Contralateral projections from the sulcus principalis cross the genu of the corpus callosum to join the homotypical area of the other frontal lobe. In addition, many contralateral projections course to the same areas as the ipsilateral projections, apparently allowing the two hemispheres to respond simultaneously.

The posterior-medial orbital frontal area has ipsilateral connections that course laterally to the lateral orbital frontal cortex and medially to the gyrus rectus. A contralateral projection crosses the rostrum of the corpus callosum to the homotypical area and also goes to the sites served by the ipsilateral projections.

Frontal-Olfactory Connections

Although other association areas receive information from the three major sensory modalities, only the prefrontal cortex also receives projections from olfactory areas and is the only cortical area receiving information from all sensory modalities (Nauta, 1971, 1972, 1973; Potter and Nauta, 1979; Powell, Cowan, and Raisman, 1965) (Fig. 2-8). The olfactory tract projects to the piriform cortex and then to the medial, magnocellular portion of the MD nucleus, which (see below) sends information to more anterior sections of the orbital frontal cortex as well as to the lateral posterior orbital frontal (LPOF) quadrant of the same area. The olfactory cortex also projects to the amygdala, which may have connections with the MD nucleus (Nauta, 1971). A second olfactory frontal pathway has been described that bypasses the thalamus and travels by the lateral entorhinal (prorhinal) area directly to the LPOF quadrant (Potter and Nauta, 1979). This area appears to be important for the processing of olfactory information as bilateral ablation results in decreased ability to distinguish odors.

Frontal-Limbic Connections

In the broadest concept limbic mechanisms consist of activities carried out through three independent but functionally linked systems (Nauta, 1971, 1973). The first, the primarily cortical limbic lobe, consists of the gyrus fornicatus (gyrus

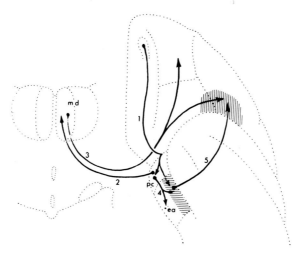

FIG. 2-8. Olfactory-orbital frontal associations in the monkey. PC, piriform cortex; md, medial-dorsal thalamic nucleus; ea, entorhinal area; *horizontal lines*, prorhinal cortex; *vertical lines*, lateral posterior orbital frontal cortex (LPOF). Five connections are demonstrated: 1, olfactory tract; 2, pc to medial md; 3, medial md to orbital frontal surface; 4, pc to ea; 5, prorhinal cortex (lateral ea) to LPOF. (From Potter and Nauta: *Neuroscience*, 4:361–367, 1979, with permission.)

cinguli and parahippocampal gyrus, including the uncal olfactory cortex), hippocampus proper (Ammon's horn, dentate gyrus, and fimbria fornicis), and the only subcortical component, the amygdala. This cortical limbic lobe is linked to a second, a subcortical system, that includes a limbic midbrain area called the septohypothalamo-mesencephalic (SHM) continuum. This continuum has a relatively distinct circuitry connecting the hypothalamus, a section rostral to the hypothalamus (preoptic and septal region), and a caudal section, the limbic midbrain area composed of the ventral tegmental area of Tsai, Bechterow's composite nucleus centralis superior tegmenti, Gudden's nucleus tegmenti profundus, and the ventral part of the central gray substance. The SHM continuum receives afferents from the amygdala, hippocampus, spinal cord, and lower brainstem and sends efferents to the thalamus, visceral motor system, and hypophyseal complex. Finally, the third system linked with limbic function is the visceroendocrine periphery, consisting of ill-defined visceral-sensory pathways ascending from the spinal cord and medulla oblongata. The functions of this third system appear to be reflected in mood and motivational changes (Nauta, 1971, 1973).

The frontal lobe is unique among cortical areas in having the greatest variety of connections to these three limbic areas, and the fact that the frontal lobe can influence and be influenced by these limbic zones is of considerable importance (Nauta, 1971, 1973). The dorsal part of the frontal convexity and possibly the medial surface send a pathway dorsally along the cortex of the cingulate gyrus, giving off collaterals along the way to the retrosplenial cortex and the presubiculum with the longest fibers apparently entering the subiculum next to Ammon's horn (Fig. 2-7). A second pathway starts in the posterior orbital area and moves caudally over a ventral route into the entorhinal area (Fig. 2-8). Orbital frontal cortex may exert hippocampal control via entorhinal-hippocampal projections. Although no direct frontal-amygdala projection exists, there are known connections to the amygdala from the frontal convexity via a cortical intermediary station in the middle and inferior temporal gyri.

Of the entire isocortex, only the prefrontal lobe has direct connections with the SHM continuum. Nauta (1973) postulated two direct frontal-SHM pathways. One pathway, with origins in the caudal orbital frontal area, passes caudally via the internal capsule or through the substantia innominata to the lateral hypothalamus and septal areas. A second pathway starts in the dorsal convexity, apparently areas 9 and 46 (dorsal to the monkey's principal sulcus), and travels via the medial internal capsule to rostral lateral hypothalamus, dorsal hypothalamus, and paramedian zone of the mesencephalic continuum.

Afferent limbic-frontal connections are a means by which the frontal cortex monitors and is affected by the internal milieu, especially the visceroendocrine periphery. The caudal pole of the SHM continuum and the mammillary bodies project to the cingulate via the anterior thalamic nuclei and are thus connected to the frontal convexity dorsal to the principal sulcus (Nauta, 1973). It is recalled that this area in turn projects to the gyrus fornicatus and hypothalamus.

A second view of frontal-limbic organization was proposed by Livingston and Escobar (1973; Livingston, 1977). They posited two limbic circuits, medial and basolateral, with separate anatomical relationships and functions. The medial limbic circuit (Papez, 1937), composed of the hippocampal gyrus, fornix, cingulate gyrus, anterior thalamic nuclei, septal nuclei, and mammillary bodies, is connected with the reticular core of the diencephalic-hypothalamic-tegmental regions, and is primarily concerned with activity in the brainstem reticular core and hypothalamus. The basolateral limbic circuit, composed of the orbital frontal cortex, dorsal medial thalamic nucleus, amygdala, and anterior temporal cortex, participate in general sensory activities mediated by the dorsal medial thalamus. The frontal lobe plays a dominant role in modulating the two circuits, and normal behavior is hypothesized as a relative balance between the activities of both circuits.

More recent research has further defined the cingulate connection, especially to the frontal cortex (Pandya et al., 1981) (Fig. 2-9). The cingulate cortex may be divided into three sections. The rostral cingulate, i.e., Brodmann areas 25 and 32, in front of the genu of the corpus callosum, has connections with the frontal convexity dorsal to the principal sulcus (area 9, middle orbital frontal areas 11, 12, and 13) and the rostral superior temporal gyrus (area 2). Pandya and colleagues suggested that this cingulate area may be more correctly considered part of the prefrontal cortex. Cingulate areas 24 and 23 have more widespread cortical connections. Cingulate area 24 receives input from midline and intralaminar thalamic nuclei and projects to frontal premotor cortex (area 6), periarcuate "eye field" cortex (area 8), and orbital frontal cortex (area 12). In addition, the caudal part of area 24 is connected to area 7, a rostral section of the inferior parietal cortex,

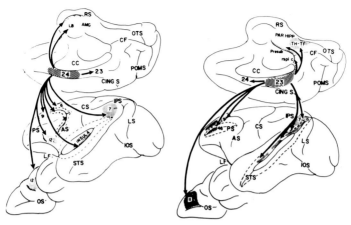

FIG. 2-9. Summary of the numerous projections from areas 23 and 24 of the cingulate gyrus to the medial-lateral and basal surfaces of the cerebral hemispheres. AMG, amygdala; AS, arcuate sulcus; CC, corpus callosum; CF, calcarine fissure; CINGS, cingulate sulcus; CA, central sulcus; IOS, inferior occipital sulcus; IPS, intraparietal sulcus; LB, latero-basal nucleus; LF, lateral (sylvian) fissure; LS, lunate sulcus; OS, orbital sulcus; OTS, occipital-temporal sulcus; POMS, parietal-occipital medialis sulcus; Presub, presubiculum; PS, principal sulcus; RS, rhinal sulcus; rspl c, retrosplenial cortex; STS, superior temporal sulcus; TH-TF, parahippocampal gyrus. (From Pandya, Van Hoesen, and Mesulam: *Exp. Brain Res.*, 42:319–330, 1981, with permission.)

whereas the rostral part of area 24 has connections with insular cortex, perirhinal cortex, and the laterobasal amygdaloid complex. Area 23, which receives projections from the anterior thalamic nuclei, is joined with prefrontal area 9 as well as the rostral orbital frontal cortex (area 11). Other connections from cingulate area 23 include the caudal section of the inferior parietal lobule (area 7, superior temporal sulcus, parahippocampal gyrus, retrosplenial cortex, and presubiculum).

Reciprocal prefrontal-hippocampal connections are now known to occur indirectly and directly through two pathways starting in the dorsal-lateral prefrontal cortex (Goldman-Rakic, Selemon, and Schwartz, 1984). A lateral pathway courses in the frontal-occipital fasciculus ventral-lateral to the striatum, ventrally into the temporal lobe along the border of the amygdala, into the posterior parahippocampal gyrus, with some fibers extending to the presubiculum. A larger medial pathway traverses within the cingulate to the caudal presubiculum and adjacent transitional cortices, forming heavy connections between the frontal and caudal-medial temporal lobe. Both pathways converge in the occipital lobe. These two pathways may provide the basis for understanding functional connections of frontal and hippocampal zones, perhaps as related to memory.

A large portion of limbic afferent connections to the frontal cortex are transferred via the MD nucleus (see below) (Fig. 2-10). The olfactory sensorium and the SHM continuum, represented by the olfactory cortex of the uncus, septum, amygdala, and ventromedial midbrain tegmentum, are all associated with the medial magnocellular division of the MD nucleus.

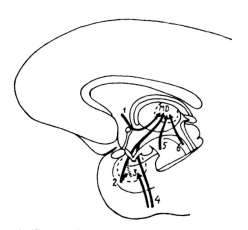

FIG. 2-10. Six of the subcortical afferents to the medial-dorsal thalamic nucleus (MD): 1, septum; 2, olfactory cortex; 3, amygdala (shaded due to uncertainty); 4, inferior temporal region (2, 3, and 4 are components of the inferior thalamic peduncle); 5, ventral-medial area of midbrain tegmentum; 6, dorsal region of tegmentum. (From Nauta: *J. Psychiatric Res.*, 8:167–187, 1971, with permission.)

Frontal-Thalamic Connections

Ipsilateral frontal-thalamic connections have been reported primarily for the reticular, ventral-anterior, and MD thalamic nuclei (Fig. 2-6). The largest number of projections arise from the MD nucleus (Akert, 1964; Goldman, 1979; Nauta, 1971). Three separate MD nucleus-frontal connections have been described in the rhesus monkey. The middle third of the principal sulcus on the dorsal-lateral prefrontal convexity is connected with the lateral parvocellular portion of the MD nucleus and is the primary source of important thalamic-dorsal-lateral prefrontal connections. It has been suggested that this is an extension of the tract of the nucleus solitarius (Nauta, 1964). The more medially placed magnocellular portion of the MD nucleus primarily connects to the orbital frontal cortex and provides information from many sources (Fig. 2-10) (Nauta, 1971). The temporal-frontal convexity cortical–cortical connections via the uncinate bundle are paralleled by a medial projection from the lower temporal regions via the inferior thalamic peduncle to the medial magnocellular MD nucleus. Pathways to the medial part of the MD nucleus also come from the olfactory cortex via the amygdala or directly from septal regions, the ventromedial midbrain tegmenta, and from fibers passing through the dorsal tegmentum. This information passes through the magnocellular portion of the MD nucleus as it is projected to orbital frontal cortex, which itself has connections with the hippocampus, septum, and hypothalamus. A third major frontal-MD nucleus connection is to the frontal eye field (area 8), a projection from the pars multiformis paralamellaris. Goldman (1979) also reported connections of the inferior frontal convexity with the MD nucleus cells that lie next to and overlap the medial magnocellular and the lateral parvocellular portions of the MD nucleus.

Important connections exist between frontal and nonspecific thalamic system nuclei (Goldman, 1979; Scheibel and Scheibel, 1967). In general, the axons of the nonspecific thalamic system nuclei are similar to those of the brainstem reticular formation: literally no short axon cells but extensive branching and collaterals. The nuclei may be divided into two types. First, those with paired nuclear areas include center median, parafascicular, centrolateral, paracentral, anterior-medial, ventral-medial, reticular (nucleus reticularis thalami), and possibly parataenial flank midline. The second type includes smaller, unpaired, midline-bridging nuclei such as the periventricular complex, rhomboidal reuniens, submedial, central-medial, and a complex of more anterior nuclei: interanteromedial, dorsal, and ventral.

Afferents to the nonspecific thalamic system derive from several sources (Scheibel and Scheibel, 1967): the dorsal branch of the ascending brainstem reticular neurons, the spinothalamic system, the mesencephalic tectal and pretectal regions, the basal forebrain area, and the neocortex, particularly the orbital frontal cortex. The efferent projections of the nonspecific thalamic system have been described as follows: the intralaminar portion projects to the medial, ventral anterior area and the nucleus reticularis, where it has intensive collateralization. This pathway then courses along the medial part of the caudate through the inferior thalamic peduncle to the base of the ventral, medial, and orbital cortex, apparently continuing as far as the anterior frontal pole. Other connections travel to the anterior section of the nucleus accumbens septi. These massive reciprocal orbital frontal connections have been suggested as the most important pathway for cortical synchronous wave activity (Skinner and Lindsley, 1967). The thalamic intralaminar nuclei must travel through the sheet-like field of the nucleus reticularis thalami, which surround the rostrolateral surface of the thalamus (Scheibel, 1980; Scheibel and Scheibel, 1967) (Fig. 2-11).

An opposing but complementary interaction between the brainstem reticular core and the frontal granular cortex is postulated to occur by means of this grid, which modulates thalamic cortical interaction, apparently by a feedback control mechanism (Scheibel, 1980). The nucleus reticularis is suggested as being a mosaic of balanced gatelets, each with its own specific input from three sources: (1) sensory input and feedback from the sensory motor cortex; (2) general information concerning stimulus novelty or danger arising via the mesencephalic reticular core; and (3) frontal-thalamic projections providing the possibility of imposition of higher-level monitoring, planning, and decision-making.

Not all information from the brainstem reticular core must undergo the frontal-thalamic modulation suggested above (Scheibel and Scheibel, 1967). The ventral branch of the brainstem ascending system bypasses the controlled route by traversing ventrally through the zona incerta and hypothalamus with projections to many cortical areas. The paths for cortical desynchronization and for cortical recruitment are distinct; the former has a ventral brainstem route, and the latter passes via the dorsal thalamic system.

In addition to ipsilateral frontal thalamic connections, evidence has been presented for direct monosynaptic contralateral routes (Goldmann, 1979). In general, the contralateral routes parallel the ipsilateral connections, providing the possibility of both ipsi- and contralateral mediation of incoming information. Ipsilateral projections are always dominant. In addition, dorsal convexity, inferior convexity, and orbital frontal zones project contralaterally to the dorsal section of the nucleus centralis densocellularis, a midline thalamic nucleus surrounding the nucleus an-

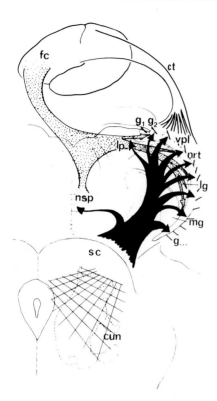

FIG. 2-11. Some of the systems influencing the gating operations of the nucleus reticularis thalami (nrt). sc, superior colliculus; cun, nucleus cuneiformis of the mesencephalic tegmentum underlying sc; fc, frontal granular cortex; nsp, medial nonspecific thalamus; g, gatelets of the nrt; ct, cortical thalamic projections. Three systems are shown in the opposed but complementary role of the nrt. The blackened arrow is the ascending projection from sc and cun; the dotted arrows are projections from fc and nsp; the clear pathway represents the descending cortical-thalamic projections. (From Scheibel: In: *The Reticular Formation Revisited*, edited by Hobson and Brazier. Raven Press, New York, 1980, with permission.)

terior medialis. No contralateral projections are reported to pulvinar, ventroanterior nucleus, or nucleus reticularis.

Frontal-Motor Connections

Frontal-motor connections may be grouped into three divisions. Primary motor cortex (area 4), involved with direct pyramidal output, is not of direct concern to this book and is not reviewed. The second division concerns prefrontal-motor connections. Early results suggested that cortical-caudate projections were topographically specific, frontal cortex projecting to the head of the caudate with parietal, occipital, and temporal projections occurring progressively more caudally over the body and tail of the caudate (Kemp and Powell, 1970, 1971). More recent evidence suggests that Brodmann area 9, the middle one-third of the dorsal bank of the principal sulcus, projects ipsilaterally to the entire caudate (Goldman and Nauta, 1977a). This frontal-caudate projection is indeed maximum to the head of the caudate, with the distribution throughout the remainder of the nucleus being uneven with clusters. The projection appears to enter the caudate by the head and then extend within the nuclear body. This connection appears to be part of a "complex" loop involving as well the rostrodorsal globus pallidus internal segment and the rostromedial substantia nigra pars reticulata, with output to the ventroanterior thalamic nucleus (DeLong, Georgopoulos, and Crutcher, 1983; Evarts, Kimura, Wurtz, et al., 1984). In animal studies this complex loop appears to be involved in more complex motor behaviors such as delayed alternation tasks (DeLong et al., 1983).

Yeterian and Van Hoesen (1978) found that cortical-caudate connections are predictable from the reciprocal cortical-cortical connections, such that interrelated cortical areas project, at least in part, to similar caudate areas. For example, frontal area 46 and temporal area 21 both project to the similar caudate area; rostral cingulate area 24 and inferior parietal area 7 are similarly connected through a specific caudate region.

Between the primary motor and prefrontal cortex is situated the nonprimary motor cortex, important in the control of skilled movements. At least two separate nonprimary motor regions may be described [Muakassa and Strick (1979) described four] with distinct subcortical-thalamic inputs (Wise and Strick, 1984). The striatum and globus pallidus project to the supplementary motor cortex via the oral (rostral) nucleus of the ventrolateral complex of the thalamus. A second nonprimary motor field is the premotor cortex, which receives inputs from caudal portions of deep cerebellar nuclei through thalamic nucleus X, another section of the ventrolateral complex. The nonprimary motor cortex appears to be important in the preparation and sensory guidance of movement (Wise and Strick, 1984). The premotor and the sensory-motor cortices appear to be involved in a more strictly "motor" loop for finer movement of individual body parts (e.g., leg, face) (DeLong et al., 1983; Evarts et al., 1984). The motor loop involves the putamen, projecting to caudal-ventral portions of the globus pallidus internal segment and the caudal-lateral region of the substantia nigra pars reticulata with distinctive outputs to the ventral-lateral thalamic nucleus.

Frontal-Cerebellar Connections

Connections from the frontal lobe to the cerebellum appear to be indirect, the vast majority being related via the brainstem (Wiesendanger, 1983). Projections from the forelimb area of motor, premotor, and frontal association cortex travel to the cerebellum via pontine nuclei, pontine tegmental reticular nuclei, the lateral reticular nucleus, and the inferior olive (Ito, 1984). In contrast to these extensive projections, perhaps reflecting the greater control required for hand movements, pathways from the trunk and hindlimb areas of the motor cortex and from parietal association cortex primarily go to the anterior cerebellar lobe. A number of cortical-cerebellar loops have been described (Wiesendanger, 1983).

Reciprocal connections from cerebellum to cerebral cortex traverse the thalamus (Ito, 1984). Fastigial cerebellar nuclei project bilaterally to the hindlimb area of the motor cortex and to the parietal cortex. Contralateral pathways move from the interpositus nuclei to premotor and trunk motor areas. Forelimb motor, premotor, and prefrontal cortex receive contralateral afferents from the dentate nuclei.

The cerebellum is also involved in visually triggered saccades and head movements. The mechanism appears to be cerebellar side paths associated with connections from prefrontal eye fields to pontine reticular formation and/or posterior medial thalamus (Ito, 1984).

Frontal-Tectal Connections

Fiber degeneration subsequent to lesions of the frontal eye fields of the arcuate fasciculus (monkey) revealed a frontal-tectal connection that was once considered to be unique (Astruc, 1971; Kuypers and Lawrence, 1967). The latter study also suggested the possibility of a frontal-polar-tectal relationship. Investigation of frontal-tectal connections other than from area 8 have confirmed that the middle third of the dorsal bank of the principal sulcus also projects to the superior colliculus, but only to the more caudal regions with density of connections increasing caudally (Goldman and Nauta, 1976). This frontal area also is related to the dorsal-lateral region of the central gray substance and the dorsal region of the pontine nuclei. In addition, connecting pathways from the principal sulcus to the nearby frontal eye fields are present. Contralateral projections to the tectum were reported from prefrontal eye fields, principal sulcus, rostral-dorsal convexity, and medial prefrontal areas (Leichnetz, Spencer, Hardy, et al. 1981). Injection in the posterior part of the medial orbital gyrus in the hand-arm area of the primary motor cortex did not reveal tectal connections (Goldman and Nauta, 1976), but area 6 has bilateral connections to the superior colliculi (Distel and Fries, 1982).

Reciprocal connections also exist between the pretectal region (in particular the nucleus limitans) and the frontal eye fields, suggesting that visual input could also reach frontal eye fields through the pretectum, bypassing the visual cortex (Barbas and Mesulam, 1981; Leichnetz, 1982).

Frontal-Brainstem Connections

The connections between the brainstem and the frontal lobe have been discussed to some extent in the preceding sections; these include the frontal-limbic and frontal-thalamic connections. As a general concept, Luria (1973a) noted that an activating input to the brainstem reticular formation arises from the orbital and medial frontal cortex. Thus the frontal cortex is involved in regulating the general state of arousal and tone. Connections from the dorsal-lateral prefrontal (and cingulate) cortex to three main brainstem locations are listed (Porrino and Goldman-Rakic, 1982). The first is to the ventral midbrain including the following areas: anterior-ventral tegmental area, retrorubral nucleus, and the medial one-third portion of the substantia nigra pars compacta. The second is a dorsal-lateral prefrontal-brainstem connection to the central superior nucleus and the caudal subdivision of the dorsal raphe nucleus (bilateral distribution); the third is to the locus ceruleus (bilateral) and nearby medial parabrachial nucleus. Connections from the orbital prefrontal cortex to the brainstem were similar, with the absence of connections to the substantia nigra. The demonstrated relationship of many of these brainstem areas to sleep and arousal (Luria, 1973a; Moruzzi and Magoun, 1949) suggests a close relationship of the prefrontal cortex to these states. In addition, these pathways correspond to known monoamine pathways.

Descending cortical afferents to the noradrenergic locus ceruleus and serotonergic dorsal and central superior raphe nuclei of the brainstem may be specific to dorsal-medial and in particular dorsal-lateral prefrontal cortex (Arnsten and Goldman-Rakic, 1984). Less dense descending ipsilateral and contralateral projections were found from these two cortical areas but not from orbital prefrontal, parietal association, somatosensory, or inferior temporal zones. The possible specificity is all the more striking upon noting the lack of projections from parietal association cortex, which shares so many other efferent projections with the prefrontal cortex. The absence of orbital frontal afferents may reflect the functional heterogeneity of the frontal lobes (Goldman, 1971; Rosenkilde, 1979; Rosvold, 1972).

A number of functional implications of these connections can be suggested. The locus ceruleus has been noted to fire in response to relevant stimuli and to quickly habituate to irrelevant stimuli. The prefrontal cortex may be important among cortical areas for indicating relevance to the locus ceruleus; lesions of dorsal prefrontal cortex and/or ascending locus ceruleus axons result in increased distractibility with response to irrelevant stimuli (Grueninger and Pribram, 1969; Roberts, Price, and Fibiger, 1975). The correlation of the raphe nuclei to general modulation of behavior (sleep–waking, eating, aggression, depression) (Heninger, Charney, and Sternberg, 1984; McGinty and Siegel, 1983; Wurtman and Growdon, 1980; Yamamoto and Ueki, 1977) may explain the role of dorsal-lateral prefrontal cortex in these functions.

Commissural Connections

In general, ablation-degeneration experiments indicated that frontal commissural fibers run in the rostral corpus callosum in a topographically organized fashion: precentral in the posterior portion of rostral half; premotor in the dorsal and ventral; prefrontal in the central (Pandya, Karol, and Heilbronn, 1971). Autoradiographic techniques have further specified the topographical organization (Barbas and Pandya, 1984) (Fig. 2-12). The rostral-caudal position of frontal commissural fibers apparently depends on the relative architectonic differentiation (Barbas and Pandya, 1982) of the origin. Connections originating in caudal-orbital and medial-frontal areas traverse the anterior genu and rostrum of the corpus callosum. Commissural fibers springing from the arcuate sulcus were identified in the rostral corpus callosum. Injections in the lateral principal sulcus region course through an intermediate position.

FRONTAL NEUROTRANSMITTER SYSTEMS

Knowledge concerning frontal neurotransmitter systems is relatively limited. First, as the field is relatively new, only limited research has involved human prefrontal neurotransmitter activity (Ross and Stewart, 1981). Second, there are many neurotransmitters, and those with which we are most familar may make only

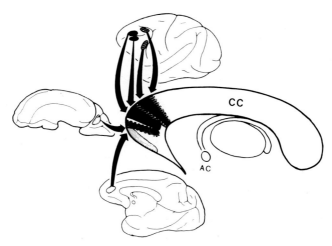

FIG. 2-12. Frontal origin and corpus callosum localization and general overlap of frontal commissural fibers. *Solid area*, principal sulcus region; *horizontal area*, medial prefrontal and caudal orbital regions; *hatched area*, arcuate sulcus concavity; CC, corpus callosum; AC, anterior commissure. (From Barbas and Pandya: *Exp. Brain Res.*, 55:187–191, 1984, with permission.)

a " modest contribution to the total synaptic complement of the neocortex" (Coyle, 1982). The relationship of neurotransmitter characteristics and subsequent symptomatology to brain functioning is just beginning.

The best established relationship of a neurotransmitter to frontal lobe functioning at the present time appears to be with dopamine. Among the various dopamine systems, dopamine-containing axons from the ventral tegmental area and substantia nigra appear to have a focal and predominant distribution to prefrontal and cingulate cortex, particularly to the mesial frontal area (Bannon and Roth, 1983; Bjorklund, Divac, and Lindvall, 1978; Coyle, 1982; Moore, 1982; Simon, 1981). Based on the relative concentration of their terminations in different layers, it appears that there may be two or three separate mesocortical dopamine systems (Emson and Koob, 1978; Lindvall, Bjorklund, and Divac, 1978; Lindvall, Bjorklund, Moore, et al., 1974). A medial prefrontal or anteromedial dopamine system runs from the ventral tegmental area to deep frontal layers, having a projection zone corresponding roughly to the projection zone of the dorsal-medial nucleus, i.e., to the prefrontal cortex. An anterior cingulate system travels from the tegmentum and substantia nigra to the outer layers of the cingulate gyrus. A third perirhinal system derives from other cells in the ventral tegmental area and terminates in the suprarhinal cortex. This third system appears to be a direct but lateral continuation of the anteromedial system. In general, the first two dopamine systems appear to correspond to dorsal-lateral and orbital cortices, suggesting two dopamine systems to the frontal cortex.

Within the frontal lobes, the medial cortex has the highest dopamine concentration, the perirhinal area somewhat lower, with dorsal and lateral cortices containing the least (Lindvall et al., 1978). There is also an anterior-caudal difference, motor and premotor areas having lower dopamine levels than the prefrontal cortex but higher than the posterior cortical areas (Bjorklund et al., 1978).

Dopamine appears to be essential for normal frontal lobe function [see Glowinski, Tassin, and Thierry (1984) for a concise review]. If dopamine innervation is disrupted, a deficit similar to that seen after focal frontal damage appears (Bachman and Albert, 1985; Brozoski, Brown, Rosvold, et al., 1979). It is hypothesized that this neurotransmitter is important for relaying and integrating internal and external stimuli in the prefrontal system. Lesions in the ventral mesencephalic tegmental area of the dopamine frontal system cause disorders of attention (Simon, 1981). The dopamine frontal system appears important in self-stimulation, with the highest concentration of dopamine in those frontal areas thought to be most involved in the reward system of the brain (Goeders and Smith, 1983; Routtenberg, 1978). Finally, it has been postulated that the mesocortical and mesolimbic dopaminergic systems are significant in schizophrenia on the basis of frontal lobe control (Iverson, 1975; Snyder, Banerjee, Yamamura, et al., 1974).

A second major neurotransmitter, norepinephrine, innervates more widespread areas and within the frontal lobe has an even distribution (Coyle, 1982; Emson and Koob, 1978; Lindvall et al., 1978; Routtenberg, 1978). There also appear to be two norepinephrine systems (Moore, 1982). One system, originating from the locus ceruleus, is widespread, innervating all areas of the isocortex, as well as the cerebellum and thalamus. The second, a lateral tegmental system, appears to originate from the reticular formation and innervates the hypothalamus, brainstem, and spinal cord. Although widespread, with the highest concentration of norepinephrine in the somatosensory cortex, the norepinephrine system originating in the locus ceruleus enters frontally (Brown, Crane, and Goldman, 1979; Molliver, Grzanna, Lidov, et al., 1982). The norepinephrine system seems more related to behavioral arousal and regulation of autonomic and neuroendocrine systems (Moore, 1982). As such, it may play an important role in regulating other systems, including the more focal frontal dopaminergic system (see below).

Other neurotransmitters such as acetylcholine, glutamate, and gamma-aminobutyric acid (GABA) (Emson and Koob, 1978; Godukhin, Zharikoya, and Novoselov, 1980) have been found in the frontal cortex, but information on their distribution and potential functions remains scanty. Serotonin, emanating from the raphe nuclei, has a widespread cortical distribution, including frontal zones (Emson and Koob, 1978; Molliver et al., 1982). The pattern of distribution of serotonin is more uniform than that of norepinephrine with different terminations. A major serotonin metabolite, 5-hydroxyindoleacetic acid, is complementary to dopamine and has its lowest concentration in prefrontal and its highest in posterior regions (Brown et al., 1979). Future understanding of the neurotransmitter systems and their relationship to frontal lobe must consider the interaction among the various neurotransmitter systems and the various functional systems of the frontal lobe. At the present time, the interaction between dopamine and norepinephrine appears to be particularly important. As noted by Arnsten and Goldman-Rakic (1984, p. 15):

Present information suggests...that the NE- and serotonin-containing cells, which innervate widespread areas of cortex, receive a selective prefrontal cortical projection, whereas the dopamine-containing cells, which innervate a more restricted area of cortex, receive afferents from widespread regions of the cortical mantle.

The reciprocal interaction of neurotransmitters and anatomical areas indicates that future studies must consider not only structural damage and pathway disconnection but also more widespread effects that may be produced by very small frontal lobe lesions (Molliver et al., 1982; Morrison and Molliver, 1980).

DEVELOPMENTAL CHANGES

Accumulation of knowledge concerning postnatal maturation of the human brain has been complicated by several issues. First, there is a shortage of human specimens in the early stages. The animal model is clearly inappropriate as there is such a great difference in the amount of frontal cortex compared to the rest of the brain across various species [ranging from 3% for the cat, 15% for the chimpanzee, and up to 33% for man (Blinkov and Glaser, 1968; Goldman-Rakic, 1984b)], and performance on "frontal lobe" tests appears to be significantly correlated with the size of the prefrontal system (Masterton and Skeen, 1972). Second, the level of maturity varies with the specific anatomical aspect being studied. Finally, well-known individual differences are known to exist among humans, from both genetic and behavioral observations. Nevertheless, certain patterns of frontal lobe development appear to be relatively constant.

From a surface level, the presence of various cortical gyri appears to vary during prenatal development. At birth, however, almost all of the major gyri are present and distinguishable (Chi, Dooling, and Gilles, 1977). Shaping of the cortical surface by tertiary sulcation continues through life, but exact knowledge of patterns of this development is not available (Yakovlev, 1962).

Some specific information concerning morphological developmental changes is available. At birth the cell differentiation and division into sublayers in the frontal cortex is incomplete at best (Orzhekhovskaya, 1981). Even at age 4, division into sublayers is not yet finalized and prefrontal areas 9 and 10 lack complete pyramidalization. Morphological maturation of prefrontal cortex is first reached around the age of puberty, but quantitative and qualitative changes continue long into the human life span (Orzhekhovskaya, 1981; Yakovlev, 1962). Age-related changes in prefrontal neuronal RNA content followed a similar pattern of development to an adult level at age 9 years, relative constancy until age 66, and then a gradual decline until plateauing at approximately age 80 (Uemura and Hartmann, 1978).

Study of myelination provides a similar picture of maturation (Yakovlev, 1962; Yakovlev and Lecours, 1967). Three myeloarchitectonic zones are known. The paramedian or limbic zone (dorsal-medial thalamic nucleus, striatum, cingulate, hippocampus, amygdala, claustrum) begins myelination shortly after birth and is complete shortly before puberty. The median zone (median thalamus, hippocampus, hypothalamus) is intermediate in its myelination cycle time, finishing sometime after the first decade of life. The third, supralimbic, zone, composed of the frontal, parietal, and temporal association zones, has the longest myelination time. These association areas show a slow but continuing progressive myelination past the middle years. Progressive myelination occurs from within the primordial limbic zones outward to the terminal supralimbic zones of the prefrontal and parietal association areas, as well as from inner to outer cortical laminae (Yakovlev, 1962). A regression in the reverse order of myelination occurs with aging. The range and rate of change in width and cell density is greatest in prefrontal zones. In animals at least, there is a marked reduction in the number of normal cells (Stein and Firl, 1976). Yakovlev (1962) suggested that "the longer cycle of differentiation of the more plastic eulaminate supralimbic cortex [*might correlate*] with the slower exponential gain in the insight, understanding and maturity of judgement 'learned' from conscious experience through decades of later life" (p. 39). The frontal and temporal-parietal zones also appear to maintain a quasiembryonal plasticity. To state that these are morphological correlates of the late maturation of prefrontal cortex might be premature, however. Frontal association fibers have certain characteristics such as columnar organization that appear to mature earlier than similar organizations in the optic radiation fibers (Goldman and Nauta, 1977b; Goldman-Rakic, 1984a).

Knowledge is increasing concerning ontogenetic development of some of the specific neurotransmitters. For example, at all developmental stages studied, dorsal-lateral and orbital prefrontal cortex had higher concentrations of dopamine and norepinephrine than did the primary visual cortex (Brown and Goldman, 1977) with high dopamine levels in the adult prefrontal cortex. Developmental alterations in both dopamine and norepinephrine concentrations are specific to the neurotransmitters and to the brain areas studied (Brown and Goldman, 1977).

Understanding developmental changes could be beneficial in understanding specific behavioral changes throughout the life cycle. G. E. Alexander (1982), using cryogenic depression (hypothermia) causing local functional inactivation, demonstrated that prefrontal cortex does not participate in the classic "frontal" delayed response task until maturation is complete. Similar investigations may have practical application to human development in such areas as education.

SUMMARY

This brief synopsis of the anatomy of the frontal lobe provides a globe onto which knowledge of frontal lobe function may be mapped. The relative exactness of the basic structure is crucial, as related disciplines such as physiology and psychology are just beginning to evolve to the point of providing specific information about frontal functioning. There is need for a firm basis for interpretation of this newly produced information. This summary serves as an introduction to the ever-increasing knowledge of frontal organization and its relation to behavior, illustrated in a more detailed review (*Trends in Neuroscience*, 1984).

A major lesson to be learned from this study of frontal anatomy is that although a cytoarchitectonic specificity is lacking, different behavioral functions are related to the different regions, and it may be assumed that this activity is based on anatomical connections between the specific area of frontal cortex and other cortical and subcortical structures. Developments in biochemistry and anatomy suggest, however, that our present knowledge is still in its infancy, and that concomitant growth of knowledge in behavior, neuroanatomy, and neurochemistry of frontal lobes is essential.

Even more than with other areas of cortex, the functions of the frontal lobes are products of information gathered from many diverse areas of the nervous system. This position as final collection point for nervous activities represents one of the unique states of the frontal lobe. The massive growth of the human prefrontal cortex must be considered a major source of man's superior mental abilities; understanding the complex anatomical structure of the frontal lobe is essential to any attempt to interpret these abilities.

3

Clinical/Neuropathological Correlations

Despite their relatively large size, the frontal lobes are not often the site of clean focal pathology, a crucial point underlying the difficulty in characterizing frontal lobe functions. A number of factors explain the relative rarity of well-localized neuropathology in the frontal lobes.

Many disorders that alter frontal functions are truly widespread, simultaneously affecting multiple cerebral structures. Unlike the temporal lobes, which are separated by a considerable distance (and a good deal of important brain tissue), the frontal lobes of each hemisphere are in immediate juxtaposition. Pathology that affects one frontal area usually affects other areas, in both the same and the other hemisphere. In addition, the focal pathology that involves the frontal lobes often causes alterations in structure and/or function in other, more distant portions of the brain. For instance, tumors in the anterior fossa tend to become sizable before presenting with obvious neurological symptomatology. By this stage pressure alterations affect both contralateral and more posterior neuroanatomical structures, producing a mixed and variable group of clinical findings. To date, the best material for frontal behavioral/anatomical correlations has come from structural damage, particularly postsurgical states after removal of tumor, abscess, or seizure focus, or psychosurgical procedures. Such material from surgical approaches, however, is open to considerable criticism as evidence for clinical localization. For example, the presurgical problem may have produced changes in brain function or behavior that cannot be ascribed to the damaged surgical site alone.

The frontal lobes are both massive and neuroanatomically diverse. Their size predicates against generalizations; pathological involvement of different loci within the frontal lobes can be anticipated to produce quite different behavioral alterations. The uniqueness of the human prefrontal lobes removes the ability to use relatively clean animal studies for correlation; only human case material is valid. Thus the type of neuropathology and its relatively focal nature is of paramount importance to investigations of human frontal lobe functions.

Although there is a sizable and growing literature on frontal lobe malfunction (Damasio, 1979; Hécaen and Albert, 1975; *Trends in Neurosciences*, 1984), reliable correlations of the locus of neuropathology with behavioral alterations remain limited (Stuss and Benson, 1983b). This chapter reviews the types of neuropathology recognized as sources of frontal behavioral symptomatology. To expedite this review, the material is divided into two sections. The first groups pathological entities that are the basis of most studies of frontal behavior and which, at times, produce relatively well localized frontal damage. A second section mentions a sizable group of neuropathological entities that are known to involve the frontal lobes and can produce frontal behavioral symptomatology but are usually widespread in involvement and tend to produce a mixed clinical picture.

FOCAL FRONTAL CONDITIONS

Vascular Pathology

The frontal lobes are subserved by two major vascular networks. The medial aspects of the frontal lobes are fed by the anterior cerebral artery (ACA) and its branches, whereas much of the lateral convexity receives blood supply from the anterior branches of the middle cerebral artery (MCA) (see Chapter 2). Between these two lies an extensive but inconsistent border zone. Based on the comparatively extensive and separate systems, one would anticipate rather clearly defined vascular occlusion syndromes in the frontal lobe. This does not appear to be so. Collateral circulation between the right and left ACAs and between the anterior and middle cerebral arteries is sufficient that proximal occlusion of a single vessel, even a major artery, often fails to produce distal infarction. Conversely, the midline course of the ACA often produces bilateral infarction when occlusion is sufficient to produce symptomatology.

One of the more commonly recognized vascular problems of ACA circulation is aneurysm, usually arising at the anterior communicating artery. Bleeding from such an aneurysm may produce transient or permanent dysfunction based on ischemia to structures in the ACA, but the clinical picture is routinely clouded by symptomatology secondary to subarachnoid hemorrhage such as obtundation, obstructive hydrocephalus, decreased cerebral blood flow, meningismus, and so on, producing a confusing mixture of behavioral symptomatology (Adams and Victor, 1977/1981). By the time these findings have cleared, surgical procedures are often underway, further complicating the eventual clinical residua.

Critchley (1930) outlined the syndromes that could result from occlusion of branches of the ACA. Based on personal experience plus a review of the literature, he attempted to delineate the clinical pictures noted when specific ACA tributaries were occluded. A number of behavioral findings were recorded, but unfortunately many of the patients had evidence of additional areas of infarction, making precise behavioral/neuroanatomical correlations impossible.

More recent investigations (Perlmutter and Rhoton, 1978) suggested a somewhat different set of tributaries. Based on modern neuropathological studies and their own careful dissection of the anterior cerebral vessels, they presented an accurate anatomical/vascular correlation for the distribution area of each branch. They also demonstrated the considerable variation in branching patterns of the ACA; unfortunately, almost no clinical correlation data were provided. Thus despite a relatively long history and several good studies, this large and relatively isolated vascular tree does not appear to produce specific clinical syndromes with sufficient consistency to allow ready recognition. It also reflects our current state of ignorance concerning frontal lobe functions.

A number of anatomical/behavioral studies of ACA occlusion as defined by x-ray computed tomography (CT) provide better clinical information (Fig. 3-1). Rubens (1975), Alexander and Schmitt (1980), and others noted the occurrence of transcortical motor aphasia following infarction of the left ACA vascular bed, and Damasio and Van Hoesen (1983) reported akinetic mutism as a result of the same disorder. In none of these studies, however, was the anatomical localization exact, and whether the symptom pictures reflected damage to cingulate gyrus, supplementary motor area, frontal polar cortex, or major white matter connections is uncertain. Additional observations are necessary if the functions of these unique and specific frontal structures are to be delineated.

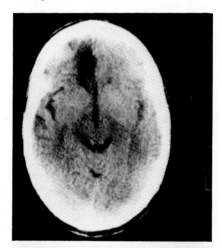

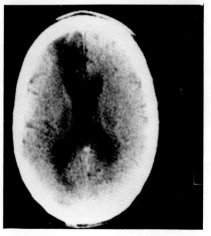

FIG. 3-1. X-ray CT views showing a lucency in the right anterior cerebral artery territory indicating infarction following vascular occlusion.

The situation concerning the contributions of the MCA to frontal function is every bit as confusing, but for a different reason. Rarely does MCA occlusion produce pure frontal infarction. Although occasionally seen, most frontal lobe infarctions following MCA occlusion are mixed with involvement of anterior parietal cortex, insular and other deep cerebral structures, or some combination. Some very specific language disturbances have been defined as frontal (Benson, 1979; Luria, 1966/1980) based at least partly on studies of MCA branch occlusions, although truly isolated frontal lobe syndromes based on infarction of MCA are uncommon. In particular, significant deep structure pathology is almost always present (Mohr, 1976). The anterior aphasias—Broca aphasia, aphemia, transcortical motor aphasia, and what some call supplementary motor area speech disturbance (see Chapter 11 for additional details)—almost invariably indicate left frontal lobe involvement, but more widespread abnormality is the rule not the exception (Mohr, Pessin, Finkelstein, et al., 1978). Specific syndromes based on damage to analogous areas of the nondominant (right) hemisphere have been suggested (Ross, 1981) but are not yet widely accepted (see Chapter 11 for additional review).

Other types of vascular pathology can involve the frontal lobe preferentially. One of the most focal is arteriovenous malformation (AVM). Unfortunately, AVMs almost invariably remain unrecognized until one or multiple intracranial bleeding episodes have occurred (Adams and Victor, 1977/1981). Following each hemorrhage from the AVM the area of damage is more widespread and the clinical picture becomes less focal so that even cases with small, tightly localized frontal lobe AVMs often present with nonfocal clinical residua.

Aneurysm formation is another well-demarcated focal abnormality that can affect frontal structures. Most aneurysms that involve the frontal lobe occur in the ACA circulation, almost always in the midline at the anterior communicating artery junction. As noted, although strikingly focal as neuropathological entities, most ACA aneurysms do not manifest until they bleed and then produce widespread clinical effects. MCA aneurysms are also fairly common but have an even greater tendency to present with nonfocal clinical findings. Thus vascular pathology, although not rare in the frontal area, has not provided a large body of clear-cut clinical/neuroanatomical correlations.

Neoplasms

Tumors, both primary and metastatic, not infrequently involve a single frontal lobe preferentially and, as such, can provide neuropathological localizing material. Major efforts in the outlining of frontal lobe-controlled behavior have been based on carefully studied tumor material (Botez, 1974; Brickner, 1936; Hebb and Penfield, 1940, Hécaen, 1964; Luria et al., 1964). Again, this material cannot be accepted without reservation. The frontal lobes tend to be relatively silent from a clinical viewpoint; because of the absence of elementary neurological abnormalities, patients with slow-growing frontal lobe neoplasms often have vague complaints and are misdiagnosed as having psychiatric problems for considerable periods. By the time the real problem is recognized, the tumor has often produced widespread effects, not only through infiltration into other portions of the brain or across the midline to the other hemisphere but, even more disturbing, through distant alterations secondary to asymmetrically increased intracranial pressure. The pressure may distort and alter tissues anywhere within the skull, thereby altering function at a distance from the neoplasm. In addition, pressure from a mass lesion can occlude branches of the anterior, middle, or posterior cerebral arteries and produce acute behavioral syndromes based on ischemia at a considerable distance from the site of the neoplasm. For instance, one common complication of increased intracranial pressure is tentorial herniation (Kernohan and Sayre, 1952), causing occlusion of the posterior cerebral artery as it arches over the tentorium. This can produce a posterior cerebral territory infarction with a striking clinical syndrome (homonymous hemianopsia) secondary to damage at a considerable distance from the site of the tumor. Despite such problems, some dramatic clinical syndromes have been recognized from the study of individuals with frontal lobe tumors.

One tumor commonly associated with abnormal behavior is the glioma. The glioma series is characterized by cerebral origin and spread through the brain tissues, often without greatly altering function as it spreads. Frontal glioblastomas often grow rapidly, causing headache, seizure, and behavioral alterations at a relatively early stage. Despite the rapid production of symptomatology, frontal glioblastomas can prove remarkably difficult to diagnose as they often fail to produce elementary neurological signs until well advanced (Blustein and Seeman, 1972; Remington and Rubert, 1962). If the onset is less rapid, behavioral alterations are routinely considered psychogenic and are often the only noteworthy findings (Broch and Wiesel, 1948; Donald, Still, and Pearson, 1972; Hobbs, 1963). Only with the occurrence of a seizure or the beginnings of unilateral paresis is the presence of a mass lesion suspected. The slower-growing gliomatous tumors—astrocytomas, oligodendrogliomas, and so on—may produce behavioral symptoms for many years before their presence is recognized (Holmes, 1931; Pool and Correll, 1958; Soniat, 1951). Most experienced psychiatrists have cared for patients who developed findings of a tumor after undergoing several years of psychotherapy aimed at relieving behavioral problems. It has been suggested, sarcastically, that it is virtually impossible to exorcise a glioma through psychotherapy (Pool and Correll, 1958), but it is just as difficult to diagnose a mass lesion until a pertinent picture develops. With increasing use of CT and magnetic resonance imaging (see Chapter 4), it can be anticipated that most patients with vague behavioral symptomatology will have a cerebral screening evaluation performed before entering long-term psychotherapy, leading to discovery of frontal tumor at an earlier stage.

If tumors are recognized at earlier stages, excellent frontal clinical/behavioral correlations should be demonstrable, but even this prospect has notable drawbacks. As noted, tumors of the glioma series tend to infiltrate rather than destroy; the tumor core may have little to do with the anatomical areas that produce specific behavioral symptomatology. The postoperative glioma, particularly if the surgeon has performed a decompression by removal of generous amounts of tumor material, has many characteristics of a focal vascular infarction. The lesion is focal, and the decompression has effectively destroyed the anatomical structures in the area. Localization of postoperative surgical material has not proved easy, however. The exact boundaries of the tumor decompression are routinely inexact. The surgeon sees only the surface, and the mass lesion often distorts cortical landmarks. X-ray CT has become a great aid to postoperative localization, but edema and distortion can compromise this approach. Although intracranial neoplasm can be accepted as a source of frontal clinical/anatomical correlations, use of this type of pathology produces serious difficulties and, to date, has not proved a valuable resource for precise localization.

Extracranial tumors often affect the frontal lobe, and studies of patients with these tumors have also played a role in the delineation of frontal lobe behavioral problems (Fig. 3-2). The most conspicuous example is the meningioma, a relatively common tumor in the anterior fossa. The parasagittal meningioma produces a striking clinical picture with important behavioral findings. Those located in the more posterior frontal parasagittal area eventually cause paresis involving the leg and shoulder (but not the arm, hand, or face), sensory loss in a similar location, a tendency toward hypophonia or mutism if the left side is preferentially involved, and vague behavioral alterations of an apathetic nature (Ausman, French, and Baker, 1974). Polar and convexity localizations of symptom-producing meningiomas are less common and often fail to produce clear-cut behavioral pictures. Instead, a neurasthenic behavior may persist for a long period before a diagnosis becomes evident. Meningiomas involving the orbital frontal surface often produce

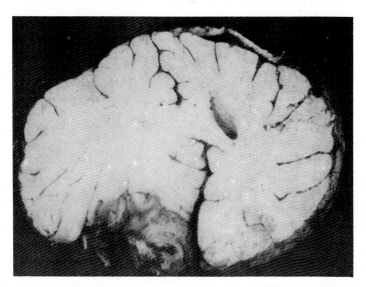

FIG. 3-2. Postmortem specimen illustrating a left frontal arachnoidal endothelioma with considerable depression and distortion of surrounding structures. (From Luria et al.: *Neuropsychologia*, 2:257–280, 1964, with permission.)

symptomatology referable to the visual system and diencephalon. Thus sphenoid ridge, olfactory groove, and suprasellar meningiomas can produce pressure effects on the chiasm and optic nerves, the hypothalamus, and the anterior third ventricle in addition to the frontal orbital and septal areas. They tend to produce a complex picture of behavioral and visceral alterations. Vague metabolic or hormonal syndromes are combined with equally vague behavioral changes to produce misleading clinical pictures. One striking finding is abulia, a decrease in drive giving an appearance of psychomotor retardation (Adams and Victor, 1977/1981) (Fig. 3-3), but hedonistic, antisocial, and even violent aggression can also be present. Misdiagnosis is common in the early stages.

A variety of other extracranial tumors can involve frontal structures, but most have not produced classic behavioral pictures. For instance, craniopharyngiomas, chordomas, suprasellar cysts, and so on often produce headaches, visual problems, and a great deal of visceral symptomatology of sufficient intensity to disguise the behavioral changes that occur.

Finally, metastatic cancer can involve the frontal lobes preferentially, may be either intracranial or extracranial, and at times produces dramatic behavioral symptomatology. Metastases tend to produce relatively acute symptom pictures, are often surrounded by considerable edema, and cause tissue distortion, thereby producing symptomatology at considerable distance from the actual site of metastasis. Nonetheless, an appropriately demarcated frontal metastasis can provide useful clinical localizing correlation data. In most instances, however, the findings are clouded by the systemic disorder caused by the primary tumor, by seeding to other body organs, and by treatment with radiation, chemotherapy, and so on. The behavioral picture in such cases is routinely complex. Also, until the advent of x-ray CT,

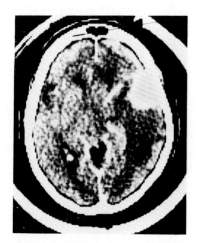 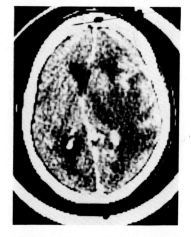

FIG. 3-3. X-ray CT scan showing a right sphenoid ridge meningioma with surrounding edema distorting the frontal structures. (From Benson: *Psychiatr. Ann.*, 14:192–197, 1984, with permission.)

metastases could rarely be localized until postmortem examination, by which time multiple metastases, pressure distortions, infarctions at a distance, and many additional pathologies obscured exact clinical correlations. Even with CT evidence of only a single metastasis, multiple tumors must be suspected. The resolution of x-ray CT is not adequate to delineate many symptom-producing metastatic lesions. To date, metastatic cancer has not proved a significant tool for clinical/pathological correlations.

Trauma

The frontal lobes are particularly susceptible to major damage from trauma, and many important studies of frontal function emanate from such incidents. The description of Phineas Gage (Harlow, 1868) and the many studies of behavioral malfunction following brain injury in the two world wars of the twentieth century rank high among the sources of clinical/pathological correlations of frontal function.

Two variations of brain injury deserve separate consideration; open and closed head injuries have some similarities, but the differences are notable. Much of the early work concerning frontal behavioral function came from studies of open head injuries caused by military combat (shrapnel, high- and low-velocity missiles). Feuchtwanger (1923), Kleist (1934a,b), Marie and Foix (1917), and many others studied individuals injured in the battlefields of World War I and produced excellent descriptions of altered behavior. Similar studies were carried out following World War II (Lishman, 1966; Luria, 1970b; Russell, 1951; Walker and Jablon, 1959), and additional reports have emanated from the military actions of subsequent years (Black, 1976; Grafman, Weingartner, Salazar, et al., 1984; Teuber, 1964). Open head injuries are relatively unusual except in military medicine, but they have provided a major focus for the study of localized cortical functions and behavior. In fact, Critchley, in a preface to the English translation of Luria's *Traumatic Aphasia* (1970b), stated bluntly that brain injury from a gunshot wound represented the cleanest and most accurate means of determining cortical localization. This statement was an exaggeration then and is certainly not true at present, but such reports have been of considerable influence in neurobehavioral studies.

Cerebral localization from open head injury is comparatively simple, almost on a point-to-point basis. Most studies accept that the area of skull damaged overlies the portion of the cortex damaged. This is frequently untrue, however (Courville, 1937); in fact, short of a full postmortem study, it is extremely difficult to determine the exact pathway traversed by a missile after it enters the skull. Deflection of the missile by bone and dura, plus rotation (spinning) of the foreign object, can produce a totally unpredictable trajectory. If the missile is multiple or breaks into fragments, the area of brain involved is even less exact. In general, only the portion of the lateral convexity first injured has been defined from the site of open brain injury, although some comparatively good data from orbital disturbances have been reported. Midline, sagittal, and deep pathology cannot be accurately determined. Even with the use of x-ray CT scans, the path of a missile trajectory through deep cerebral structures remains unrecognized unless the area of damage is huge.

Closed head injury, far more common in civilian practice, is even more difficult to use for localizing purposes. Nonetheless, closed head injury is common and can, on occasion, provide information for clinical/anatomical correlation (Fig. 3-4). Now that brain imaging techniques can provide definitive localization of brain injury in the living patient with closed head injury, considerable information for correlation studies should become available. The location of both intracerebral hematoma and destroyed brain structures can be visualized. If x-ray CT is accomplished during the acute stage, both contusion and laceration can be clearly seen (Fig. 3-5), whereas later investigation may reveal areas affected by the trauma and its concomitants (Fig. 3-6).

Studies of closed head injuries also have many drawbacks. Injury sufficient to contuse or lacerate one area of brain invariably indicates widespread effects within the skull. Passage of pressure waves, producing both coup and contrecoup injuries, are well recognized, and it is difficult to state that the entire brain is not, to a greater or lesser degree, affected by closed head trauma directed at a single point. A very susceptible brain region for closed head injury appears to be the upper mesencephalon, possibly based on shearing or tearing of pathways (Stritch, 1969), producing a state of unconsciousness which improves to a state of decreased

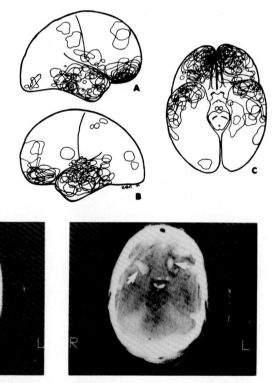

FIG. 3-4. This drawing of contusions after traumatic brain injury based on 40 consecutive cases clearly depicts the tendency for maximum pathology in the orbital frontal and temporal regions. (From Courville: *Pathology of the Central Nervous System.* Pacific Publishers, Mountain View, California, 1937, with permission.)

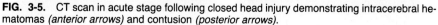

FIG. 3-5. CT scan in acute stage following closed head injury demonstrating intracerebral hematomas *(anterior arrows)* and contusion *(posterior arrows).*

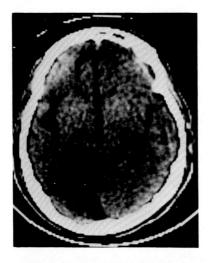

FIG. 3-6. X-ray CT scan in chronic posttraumatic brain injury state. Note the lucency at the frontal tips bilaterally (site of trauma) and the large left posterior cerebral artery territory lucency, a product of left posterior cerebral artery occlusion caused by tentorial herniation.

vigilance and attention (M. P. Alexander, 1982). Alterations of the conscious state seriously hamper correlations of behavior with frontal lobe closed head injury.

Two other areas of the brain very frequently affected by closed head trauma are the medial-inferior surface of the temporal lobes and the inferior (orbital) and polar surfaces of the frontal lobes (Courville, 1937) (Fig. 3-4). Injury to the medial-temporal structures is almost invariably associated with posttraumatic amnesia, a finding that complicates correlation of observed behavior with the location of head trauma. It is generally agreed that frontal lobe injury produces a poorly motivated, apathetic, and disinhibited behavior; this correlation is based more on preconceived notions of frontal lobe behavior than on firm localizing evidence, however. In fact, the possibility of widely spread, consistently different areas of brain suffering injury following closed head trauma is so great that behavioral-anatomical correlations from this source must always be suspect.

Thus although trauma to the frontal lobes is frequent and has provided a major source of accepted behavioral information, considerable question must be raised concerning its accuracy in any individual case.

Postsurgical State

Two major surgical approaches have proved useful for frontal lobe localization: (1) from postoperative status following neurosurgical treatment of brain disorders; and (2) from the planned surgical lesions performed in an attempt to control psychiatric disease. Each appears to have considerable potential for neuroanatomical/clinical correlation purposes, but each has defects as well.

Some important information concerning frontal behavioral abnormalities has been derived from follow-up studies of frontal lobe surgery. Most notable is the monograph by Brickner (1936) detailing the behavior of an individual who underwent bilateral frontal lobectomy in a successful attempt to remove a parasagittal meningioma. Brickner's excellent description provides one of the basic definitions of frontal lobe behavioral problems. Others have also carefully studied frontal lobe surgical cases (Penfield and Evans, 1935) to produce a picture of the behavior that follows massive frontal lobe removal.

Use of postsurgical material has rather obvious drawbacks, however. As noted earlier, tumors tend to grow large in the frontal lobes before meriting clinical attention, and detection of an AVM or aneurysm usually follows a bleed; observed behavioral abnormalities may not be related to the focal disorder. Although surgery in the frontal lobes is frequently unilateral and one could anticipate clear evidence of differences between right and left frontal lobe damage, such data are not common. Part of the problem is that increased pressure affects both hemispheres preoperatively, a problem that may remain in the postoperative state. Yet another problem is that anatomical landmarks are routinely distorted in the surgical field; the neurosurgeon is challenged to locate accurately the site of the lesion or even the exact anatomical area of the surgical procedure. In addition, the surgeon must keep the safety of his patient in mind; deep-lying pathology may never be exposed but may be a source of behavioral disturbance. Despite these shortcomings, post-surgical material can be valuable for frontal lobe behavioral correlations, particularly with postsurgical imaging by x-ray CT or radiopaque material placed in the surgical cavity. Both techniques localize the surgical site with fair accuracy.

When frontal lobe surgery was being performed on a wholesale basis as a treatment for psychiatric disease, it was anticipated that considerable psychological information would be derived from study of these cases. Time has demonstrated that this was not true; very few careful studies of the psychological residua of the frontal surgical procedures, particularly during long-term follow-up, are in existence. A number of reasons for this limitation deserve discussion.

One major difficulty in studying postpsychosurgical clinical correlations concerns the patient population studied. These procedures were performed primarily, if not exclusively, in mental health settings to treat psychologically abnormal individuals. The preoperative psychiatric disorder must be acknowledged as a major factor in any postsurgical anatomical/behavioral correlation. Schizophrenia, major affective disorder, major personality disorder, obsessive-compulsive disturbance, severe anxiety states, and so on were the prime targets for psychosurgery. These psychic disturbances affect many aspects of behavior and almost routinely cloud the postoperative status.

A second major problem hindering use of the psychosurgical material for brain research concerns the surgeon's inexact knowledge of the area attacked. Most of the psychosurgical procedures were performed blindly; even with the open procedures, the surgeon often knew only the general area of the brain destroyed by the leukotomy. Variability of anatomical landmarks on the surface of the brain has long been recognized, and although many surgeons attempted to be precise in lesion placement, postmortem studies demonstrated a considerable variation in the cortical and white matter structures destroyed (Eie, 1954; Meyer and Beck, 1954). Lesion size was inexact; although variable size and hemispheric asymmetry occurred, it could not be recognized in life until CT imaging was introduced (Fig. 3-7) (Naeser et al., 1981).

Another complicating factor concerns the many types of surgical procedure performed. The original, broadly destructive frontal lobotomy gave way to a variety of frontal leukotomies aimed at cutting frontal-thalamic pathways. Some of these procedures were done from a superior position (Fig. 3-8) (Poppen, 1948), others from a lateral approach (Freeman and Watts, 1950), and yet others through the roof of the orbit (Freeman, 1949). Later variations of frontal psychosurgery in-

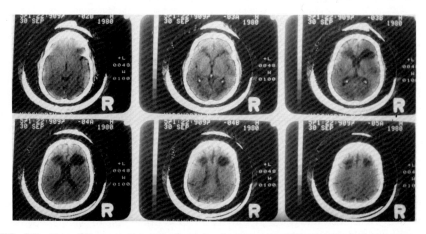

FIG. 3-7. X-ray CT scans demonstrating laterally placed frontal leukotomy lesions in one patient. There was no psychiatric recovery. Upper left is the lowest, lower right is the highest cut on the scan.

FIG. 3-8. Frontal leukotomy procedure. (From Poppen: *J. Neurosurg.*, 5:514–520, 1948, with permission.)

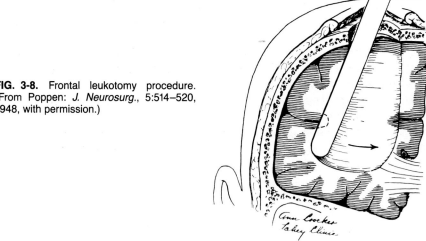

cluded orbital undercutting, either by leukotomy or placement of radioactive yttrium pellets in the orbital tissues (Knight, 1964; Scoville, 1949), cingulomotomy (Ballantine, Cassidy, Flanagan, and Marino, 1967), stereotactic destruction of various areas of the frontal lobe (Spiegel, Wycis, Freed, and Lee, 1948), and topectomy— the ablation of selected areas of frontal lobe cortex (Pool, Heath, and Weber, 1949). It has been stated, with only moderate exaggeration, that there were about as many neurosurgical approaches to psychosurgery as there were neurosurgeons who practiced psychosurgery (Hirose, 1965). Frontal psychosurgical lesions have proved extremely difficult to use for behavioral correlation studies.

A variation, questionably grouped with the psychosurgical procedures, is surgical removal of an epileptic focus. Although it most commonly involves the temporal lobe (leading to a number of excellent behavioral correlations), some frontal cortical ablations have been performed with pre- and postoperative behavioral studies (e.g., Milner, 1964, 1982; Penfield and Evans, 1935). On the surface, ablation of a portion of frontal cortex appears perfect for behavioral studies. Unfortunately, there are many problems. First, this procedure has not been done frequently; second, the area ablated has been inconsistent; third, the area ablated is abnormal and has abnormal connections; finally, the seizures themselves may well have produced both nearby and distant effects. Again, an observed behavior cannot be warranted to result from the area ablated.

Finally, another procedure that can be considered a form of psychosurgery, section of the corpus callosum, may affect the frontal lobes. The effects of this procedure have been intensely studied and deserve discussion (Bogen, 1969; Geschwind, 1965; Sperry and Gazzaniga, 1967). Split brain studies have produced valuable insights into differences in the functions of the two hemispheres (Gazzaniga, 1970; Gazzaniga, Smylie, Baynes, et al., 1984; Gazzaniga and Sperry, 1967; Zaidel, 1976), including some information concerning the two frontal lobes (Geschwind and Kaplan, 1962). Most studies following corpus callosum section probed elementary sensory-motor activities, but some reports document behavioral alterations (Bogen, 1969; Lishman, 1969). Behavioral observations on callosally sectioned subjects are also limited, however, as the procedure is never performed on normal individuals.

In summary, study of postsurgical cases had been used to determine frontal lobe function in the past and will continue to be a useful tool in the future. Such studies offer information of value, and their usefulness will increase in the future as better instruments for localizing the site of pathology in the living patient become available. For instance, modern stereotactic techniques allow placement of instruments in the brain with considerable anatomical precision. Nonetheless, the use of surgical pathology has significant defects, and considerable caution must be observed when interpreting data from this source.

MISCELLANEOUS CONDITIONS

A sizable variety of disorders that involve the nervous system can produce behavioral patterns considered to have frontal features. In general, however, these disorders produce widespread pathology and a variety of clinical findings; they are not sufficiently focal to be useful for frontal clinical/anatomical correlation.

Multiple Sclerosis

One common neurological disorder that often produces behavioral symptoms suggested to be frontal is multiple sclerosis (MS) (Vowels and Gates, 1984). Late in the course of the disease many MS patients develop a mixture of euphoria and apathy, an almost inert, unconcerned acceptance of the disorder; these findings are often construed as evidence of frontal disconnection (Adams and Victor, 1977/1981). In actuality, most plaques of MS involve the periventricular structures (Fog, 1965; Mastaglia and Cala, 1980), and although they may involve some frontal systems, including connections between frontal and more posterior structures, the areas of demyelination are too widespread for precise localization purposes. MS routinely produces lesions elsewhere in the white matter of the central nervous system (CNS) (brainstem, cerebellum, spinal cord), further clouding interpretation of observed behavior as a frontal disturbance.

Movement Disorders

The dementia of Huntington's disease (HD) is often considered a frontal disturbance, supported by the significant frontal "atrophy" present in some HD patients studied at postmortem (McMenemey, 1958). HD dementia has features suggesting frontal abnormality (Caine, Hunt, Weingartner, et al., 1978). These include slowness of thinking, forgetfulness, deterioration of cognitive functioning, and a placid acceptance of the disease process (including an apparent lack of motivation and drive). When these behavioral findings are correlated with frontal atrophy, the dementia of HD appears to be a frontal disturbance (Davenport and Muncey, 1916). More careful observation, however, suggests that the frontal "atrophy" is more apparent than real; there is no specific neuropathological picture of HD that involves cortical material (Corsellis, 1976; Cummings and Benson, 1983), and the mental impairment of HD has been called a variety of subcortical dementia (McHugh and Folstein, 1975). The primary pathology involves the caudate nucleus, and much of the gross appearance of atrophy of the frontal lobe results from loss of substance beneath the frontal structures. Nonetheless, the degenerated subcortical structures have major connections to frontal cortical structures, and the HD behavioral patterns may truly represent a frontal-systems disturbance.

Two other movement disorders with subcortical localization of brain degeneration—Parkinson's disease (PD) and progressive supranuclear palsy (PSP)—produce striking behavioral changes that also have a frontal lobe flavor (Albert, Feldman, and Willis, 1974; Teuber and Proctor, 1964). Psychomotor slowness, forgetfulness, deteriorated cognition, and bradykinesia, an apparent decrease in drive, suggest frontal lobe involvement, but pathological studies fail to demonstrate any consistent frontal lobe abnormality (Cummings and Benson, 1983). Again, multiple connecting pathways exist, and the term frontal system dysfunction may be an accurate description.

Degenerative Dementia

Behavioral alterations in the two best studied forms of degenerative dementia— Alzheimer disease and Pick disease—have suggested frontal lobe involvement. Pathological studies of both disorders show significant changes in the frontal cortical tissues, but in both disorders similar pathological changes affect other cortical areas making specific behavioral/anatomical correlations questionable. Alzheimer neuropathological changes not only affect frontal association cortices bilaterally but are found in parietal-temporal association cortex and hippocampal tissues (Cummings, 1982). Certain clinical features, particularly ideomotor apraxia and the characteristic unconcerned attitudes, are often considered evidence of frontal lobe involvement, but the widespread pathological changes do not allow proof of correlation.

Even more of a problem is Pick disease. Pathological studies demonstrate that two areas are particularly prone to degeneration in this disorder: the anterior and middle portions of the temporal lobes and the inferior and polar aspects of the frontal lobes (Malamud, 1957). General opinion links the behavioral aspects of Pick disease, particularly the early loss of social graces, with the frontal degeneration, but proof of this correlation remains uncertain because of the consistent involvement of other cortical areas.

Infectious Disorders

A disorder often said to be primarily frontal in nature is general paresis of the insane (GPI), the psychotic disturbance of tertiary syphilis. A predilection of the spirochetes for the frontal structures has been demonstrated (Greenfield, 1958; Noguchi and Moore, 1913), and it can be suggested that some of the mental disturbances of early GPI, e.g., forgetfulness, poor concentration, and altered emotional control, represent frontal malfunction. The grandiosity, the "simple" dementia, and the tendency for depression commonly reported in neurosyphilis have also been linked to frontal disturbance. The relatively intact memory function in a patient with a distinct dementia (Lishman, 1978) also suggests frontal lobe disturbance. Spirochete invasion of the cerebral tissues is never truly focal, however, and the wide variation in the symptom picture of GPI (Bruetsch, 1975) shows that neurosyphilis cannot be accepted as a purely frontal lobe disorder.

Other types of infection may involve frontal structures and, in some instances, appear focal. The focal disorders are usually a surgical problem, a mass lesion. Thus cysticercosis can produce a single cystic lesion involving one of the frontal lobes and produce focal findings. Epilepsy and headache are usually the major symptoms (Lishman, 1978), but behavioral changes in this state could be considered primarily due to frontal lobe involvement. As with most infections, cysticercosis tends to involve more than one area of the brain, and caution must be taken in accepting behavioral patterns in this disorder as due to a single focus.

Similarly, bacterial abscess can produce a true frontal focus, and abscesses emanating from the frontal sinuses often involve the frontal lobe (Greenfield, 1958). In the acute stage, abscesses are swollen and edematous, producing a mass lesion with a headache, increased intracranial pressure, and so on. If chronic, particularly if treated surgically, a focal abscess in the frontal lobe may provide good clinical/anatomical correlation material.

In general, however, most infectious disorders of the CNS are not specific for the frontal lobe, tend to produce generalized findings, and cannot be used as indicators of focal disturbance.

Aging

Studies in recent years suggest that some of the behavioral impairments of advanced age are based on frontal lobe deterioration. There is some suggestion of selective decrease in blood flow over frontal and prefrontal areas with aging (Dupui, Guell, Bessoles, et al., 1984) although this finding has been disputed (Duara, Grady, Haxby, et al., 1984). There are alterations that appear to be frontal lobe based including a general slowing, forgetfulness, deteriorated cognitive function, and a notable decrease in drive. Moscovitch and Winocur (1983) suggested that the memory alterations in at least some elderly people might be considered a frontal lobe system disorder. On the basis of selective neuropsychological test deficiencies, Albert and Kaplan (1980) suggested that right frontal abnormality was disproportionately greater with advancing age. The general behavioral changes with advancing age noted above more closely resemble the alterations reported with subcortical movement disorders (HD, PD, and PSP) suggesting that a frontal system (rather than truly frontal) disorder underlies the mental impairment of advancing age (Cummings and Benson, 1983).

Other Disorders

Finally, a number of other disorders are thought to involve the frontal lobes preferentially. Schizophrenia has been considered a frontal lobe disturbance by some (Buchsbaum, Ingvar, Kessler, et al., 1982; Franzen and Ingvar, 1975a,b; Ingvar, 1980; Levin, 1984a,b; Seidman, 1983), but the lack of demonstrated pathology and the apparent involvement of subcortical neurotransmitter systems weakens this approach (McGeer and McGeer, 1977). Hyperactivity (Mattes, 1980; Stamm and Kreder, 1979), delinquency (Pontius and Yudowitz, 1980), and depression (Phelps, Mazziotta, Baxter, et al., 1984; Robinson, Kubos, Starr, et al., 1984) have been reported to be associated with frontal lobe abnormality. Similarly, some complications of alcoholism such as Marchiafava-Bignami disease (Leventhal, Baringer, Arnason, et al., 1965), the degeneration of the dorsal medial nucleus of the thalamus (Victor, Adams, and Collins, 1971), and the predominantly frontal atrophy (Butters, 1984) indicate frontal lobe disturbance (Moscovitch, 1982; Squire,

1982), but again the disorders are not focal and correlations of observed behavioral abnormalities are suspect. In many of these disorders consideration should be given to frontal system abnormality rather than focal frontal disturbance.

SUMMARY

From this review of the disorders that can involve the frontal lobes pathologically and their potential usefulness for clinical/anatomical correlation, it can be seen that many difficulties exist. There is a strong tendency for frontal neuropathology to be either bilateral or to have a bilateral effect through edema, distortion of anatomical structures, compression of vessels, and so on. There is also a strong tendency for major frontal neuropathology to affect areas other than the frontal lobe, particularly the anterior parietal lobe, the temporal lobe, or structures deep in the medullary portion of the hemispheres or even in the brainstem.

Good correlations between frontal neuropathological abnormality and specific behavioral alterations have been difficult, although some individual instances, such as the Phineas Gage case, have provided dramatic information. The ability of x-ray CT and magnetic resonance imaging to demonstrate focal lesions in a patient who is alive and can be tested may change this status radically; the future offers improved opportunities to correlate focal frontal pathology with behavioral abnormalities.

4

Laboratory Assessment of the Frontal Lobe

One major problem curtailing efforts to determine behavioral functions of the frontal lobes has been a paucity of precise localizing information, as noted in Chapter 3. Studies must come from investigation of human cases as both the behavior and the anatomy of the frontal lobes of animals, even the highest apes, are far different. Correlation of behavior with focal pathology in humans is needed, but to date the diagnostic techniques capable of providing information on localization within the frontal lobes, particularly in the living, behaving human have remained limited.

Until recent years, techniques for localizing within the brain had a significant morbidity and could be used only in special circumstances. Most of the laboratory measures have been, at best, indirect, and much of the data reported on frontal function have had to be viewed with skepticism because of the inadequacies of the available localizing techniques. Nonetheless, careful study of selected individuals using these techniques provided most of the data on human frontal function currently available. During the past several decades many new laboratory techniques have been introduced and have provided additional information. A number of techniques, both old and new, are reviewed along with discussion of their respective strengths and weaknesses as research vehicles for probing frontal function.

NEUROLOGICAL EXAMINATION

Vast areas of the frontal lobes are considered "silent" to the routine neurological examination. A number of findings can point to frontal involvement, however, and when present can be useful as localizing correlates with behavior. Four parts of the neurological behavior examination are most suggestive of frontal involvement: motor impairment, anterior (motor) aphasia, unilateral inattention, and the so-called frontal release signs.

The most readily noted findings from the neurological examination that indicate frontal lobe abnormality come from the motor examination, and several basic principles deserve comment. Damage to the motor strip (Brodmann area 4) and/or the motor association cortex (area 6) is associated with degrees of paralysis and spasticity; consequently, the presence of either hemiplegia or hemiparesis suggests frontal damage. It has long been stated, although with little proof, that lesions involving area 4 produce weakness with little or no spasticity, whereas area 6 pathology produces both weakness and spasticity (Denny-Brown, 1951). Cortical damage rarely produces total hemiplegia; different areas of the motor homunculus are too distant from each other over the surface of the cortex to be involved simultaneously. Total hemiplegia more often indicates a deep (internal) capsule or adjacent motor pathways) problem, whereas a more restricted weakness can indicate focal cortical damage. Thus paralysis of the leg and shoulder of one side but with retained arm, hand, and face movements suggests medial sagittal damage, usually from involvement of the anterior cerebral artery; major paralysis of the face and arm with relative sparing of the leg is more likely with convexity damage. In contrast, the so/called predilection weakness (relatively greater residual motor strength in the antigravity limb musculature) is more common with deep destruction than with cortical damage. Rarely is an isolated limb weakness a manifestation of cortical damage; monoparesis is more often the result of a small lacunar lesion deep in the white matter (Fisher, 1965). A mixed picture of paresis and sensory loss suggests either a subcortical locus (internal capsule), involvement of both the frontal and parietal convexities, or a combination of both. Thus demonstration of paresis and spasticity, particularly in specific combinations, can suggest but does not prove the presence of frontal lobe injury. Motor perseveration has been reported as a frontal finding (Luria, 1965), but perseveration can also occur with pathology located elsewhere in the brain. Some of the motor findings secondary to frontal damage are discussed at greater length in Chapter 5.

Aphasia is a second finding of the neurological examination that can point to frontal lobe involvement. As discussed in Chapter 11, specific major types of speech and language disturbance and a number of related abnormalities are traditionally linked to frontal lobe involvement. Demonstration of one of the anterior language syndromes (Broca, aphemia) strongly suggests pathology in the posterior inferior aspect of the dominant (usually left) frontal lobe, a valuable localizing finding (Benson, 1979). Transcortical motor aphasia indicates frontal damage or disconnection (Freedman, Alexander, and Naeser, 1984). Supplementary motor area pathology affects language output (Alexander and Schmitt, 1980). Speech abnormalities, on the other hand, usually suggest deeper motor system involvement; in some instances, however, focal frontal damage may cause an articulatory disturbance. Although of tremendous lateralizing and considerable localizing value, the anterior speech and language syndromes tend to overlap with the motor findings. Neither the motor nor the language abnormalities are found after damage to most portions of the frontal lobes. Extensive frontal lobe damage may cause neither motor nor verbal output disturbance.

Certain oculomotor abnormalities, particularly conjugate deviation and gaze paresis, may point to frontal lobe damage. Damage to the frontal eye fields (Brodmann area 8) can produce a forced deviation of the eyes toward the side of the lesion (ictal involvement of the same area causes deviation to the side opposite). With effort the gaze can be brought to a central position, but the eyes fail to move toward the opposite side. Conjugate deviation is transient, usually lasting only a matter of days with consistent decrease in the absoluteness of the deviation. Even so, a residual paresis of gaze to the side opposite frontal eye field involvement may remain for months or even permanently (Holmes, 1918). Although clearly seen with frontal eye field damage, conjugate deviation is not an absolute frontal sign (Adams and Victor, 1977/1981; DeRenzi, Colombo, Faglioni, et al., 1982). A similar clinical picture occurs with parietal-occipital eye field (Crosby et al., 1962) and pontine damage (DeJong, 1979). Unilateral eye movement problems can offer excellent frontal localization information, but only if combined with other data.

A common finding on routine neurological examination—unilateral inattention (see Chapter 7)—is considerably more difficult to localize but, at least in some instances, can arise from acute damage to frontal association cortex (areas 6 or 8) (Damasio, Damasio, and Chui, 1980; Heilman, 1979b; Kennard, 1939; Stein and Volpe, 1983; Welch and Stuteville, 1958). Frontal inattention can involve motor activities (unilateral akinesis), somesthesis (unilateral sensory loss), or vision (pseudohemianopsia) and is characteristically temporary. Although easily produced in animals, the disorder is not frequently reported in the human (Heilman and Valenstein, 1972) and unilateral inattention is not exclusively a product of frontal damage. Heilman (1979b) and Watson, Valenstein, and Heilman (1981) have suggested a disorder in a complex limbic-reticulo-frontal network, an attention-response problem, whereas Denny-Brown and colleagues (1952, 1954) suggested amorphosynthesis—a discrepancy in hemispheric sensory sensitivity—a receptive disturbance. Although unilateral inattention cannot be confidently ascribed to frontal pathology without other localizing evidence such as one of the frontal aphasias, CT scan evidence of focal frontal damage, and so on, it does occur and can represent an important frontal finding.

Finally, a group of clinical findings usually called primitive reflexes or frontal release signs have long been accepted by neurologists as demonstrations of frontal abnormality. The most powerful of these, the grasp reflex (Denny-Brown, 1958), is most commonly associated with midline frontal abnormality but can also be seen with deeper hemispheric pathology and some drug and metabolic problems. Of the remainder, rooting, sucking, and snout occur most often with brainstem-diencephalic dysfunction, possibly indicating frontal system disturbance. The palmomental reflex appears to have almost no reliable localizing capability and certainly not a strict frontal relationship. All of the frontal release signs may be absent in the face of major structural pathology of the frontal lobes (Benson and Stuss, 1982). Complex motor tasks, particularly those demanding sequential actions, may be used as demonstrations of frontal abnormality, but they demand formal examination and are more appropriately discussed as neuropsychological tests (see Chapter 5).

In summary, despite the relatively immense size and unquestioned importance of the frontal lobes, focal abnormality is not easily demonstrated by the routine neurological examination. Massive areas of the frontal lobes may be damaged and yet be silent to the neurologist's routine evaluation (Brickner, 1936; Hebb and Penfield, 1940).

PSYCHIATRIC EXAMINATION

Traditionally, psychiatrists have not been as concerned with the area of the brain underlying the symptomatology they study; many do recognize, however, that certain behavioral findings suggest frontal abnormality. Many of these "indicators" of frontal involvement on psychiatric interview are evaluated in detail in later chapters, and only a synopsis of the suggestive findings is presented here.

A radical alteration of personality, particularly if it appears over a short period of time, always raises the possibility of a central nervous system (CNS) problem. Certain personality changes are traditionally identified with frontal disease. Apathy, disinterest, and loss of motivation, when producing a state of psychomotor retardation, are particularly suggestive, but affective disorder also produces these findings. If a patient suffers psychomotor retardation, but a depressed mood is absent and there is no history of psychiatrically significant depression, frontal lobe pathology can be suspected. Disinhibition, particularly social misbehavior by someone previously well mannered, also suggests frontal disturbance. The presence of inappropriate humor and wisecracking, poor judgment, grandiosity, unconcern, and an apparent lack of insight also suggests frontal problems. However, these findings are also present in other psychiatric disorders, e.g., mania and hypomania, sociopathy, and schizophrenia, producing difficult diagnostic problems for the psychiatrist. Not infrequently, patients with frontal lobe tumors or other frontal organic pathology develop interpersonal problems in a setting that offers a plausible psychodynamic explanation for the abnormal behavior. The psychiatrist can recognize these psychosocial problems as important sources of symptomatology, but psychotherapeutic intervention does not help if frontal damage is the source of the symptom complex. The psychiatric phenomenology of frontal disorder is presented in greater detail throughout this book, particularly in the discussion of personality and emotion (see Chapter 8).

NEUROPSYCHOLOGICAL TESTING

Most neuropsychological tests were evolved from clinical psychological tests and hence were not designed to be localizing techniques; nonetheless, they can provide considerable information and in competent hands offer good localizing data. The results of neuropsychological tests can be correlated with findings from the clinical examinations and thus provide confirmation of suspected frontal lobe pathology. Taken by themselves, indicators of focal frontal abnormality from psychological tests demand expert interpretation; the experience and caution of the clinical neuropsychologist is a major factor. Nonetheless, the paucity of laboratory techniques capable of localizing frontal abnormality in the living human has promoted neuropsychological testing to a major position as a tool for demonstration of frontal pathology. Much of the information presented in this book is derived from correlations of neuropsychological tests with clinically localized frontal pathology. A number of these tests are specialized, research-level tests not found in routine clinical psychological batteries and are discussed in context elsewhere in this volume. Some are more standard, and discussion of these neuropsychological techniques for demonstrating and/or interpreting frontal lobe abnormality is warranted. Three approaches to neuropsychological testing are currently in wide use: the Wechsler/Boston tests plus a series of augmenting tests, the Halstead-Reitan battery, and variations of Luria's neuropsychological test procedures. The primary purpose of each is to provide a general assessment of brain functioning, and none is specifically designed for assessment of frontal lobe disturbances. Nonetheless, data from each have been used to suggest frontal lobe malfunction with greater or less specificity. Although there are differences in localizing ability, depending on the tests used, the ultimate competency of each approach lies in the expertise of the neuropsychologist. Clinicians familiar with the syndromes of frontal lobe dysfunction and expert in the principles of test interpretation such as double dissociation of abilities (cf., Lezak, 1976/1983; Teuber, 1955, 1959) may use data from these batteries to interpret frontal lobe malfunction.

The Wechsler Adult Intelligence Scale (WAIS) (1955) and the Wechsler Memory Scale (WMS) (1945) have been used widely for many years, are well standardized, and have been administered to many individuals with frontal pathology. Many subtests of these two batteries may reflect frontal lobe malfunction (see Chapters 10,13, and 14), but the Wechsler tests were not designed to provide specific and reliable information for separating frontal lobe from more widespread disturbance. Frontal disturbance can be suspected from the quality of response in both the verbal and nonverbal aspects of both test batteries. In addition to a degree of carelessness and sloppiness, some specific qualitative responses have been interpreted as reflecting focal frontal lobe pathology (Goodglass and Kaplan, 1979; McFie and Thompson, 1972); these observations cannot be accepted as diagnostic. The tests used in association with the Wechsler tests to seek frontal malfunction vary among neuropsychologists. Most use some test of aphasia, as certain aphasic syndromes have definite correlation with the frontal lobes (see Chapter 11). Some psychological tests have been suggested as more specific to the frontal lobes. For example, the Wisconsin Card Sorting Test (Grant and Berg, 1948; Milner, 1963), the Stroop (1935; Perret, 1974), word fluency tests such as the F-A-S (Milner, 1964; Ramier and Hécaen, 1970; Spreen and Benton, 1969), the Porteus Maze test (Porteus, 1950; Smith, 1960), and certain of Luria's tests (Drewe, 1975a) such as the "go/no-go" tasks have proved to be at least partially successful at demonstrating frontal lobe disorder. Unfortunately, each of these tests, to a greater or lesser degree, is sensitive to generalized brain disturbance, can be disturbed by focal pathology involving other parts of the brain, or can be impaired for reasons other than acquired brain disease.

In summary, the Wechsler tests and associated specialized techniques as suggested by the Boston group (Goodglass and Kaplan, 1979; Kaplan, 1983; Stuss, Kaplan, Benson, et al., 1981b) can indicate frontal disturbance but require analysis of the qualitative processes leading to the response (Kaplan, 1983). These indications can suggest involvement of frontal lobes, but they cannot be interpreted as absolute and independent evidence of localization. An extremely valuable aspect of this approach is an ever-continuing search for more specific measures of focal brain involvement. A negative aspect is the lack of accumulation of normative data because of test alterations.

The Halstead-Reitan battery (Halstead, 1947a,b; Reitan, 1955; Reitan and Davison, 1974; Russell, Neuringer and Goldstein, 1970) is a collection of psychological tests presented with rigid consistency of both test material and examining techniques. It consists of a core of tests designed to yield an "Impairment Index" ranging from 0.0 to 1.0 (Halstead, 1947a) or an Average Impairment Rating Scale with a larger range (Russell et al., 1970), plus a number of additional tests which may vary to a minor degree among psychologists (Swiercinsky, 1978; Trites, 1977).

The Halstead-Reitan approach has the advantage over other clinical psychological test batteries of being specifically designed to provide statistically significant differences between brain-damaged and nonbrain-damaged individuals. In its earliest conception, Halstead (1947a) considered the tests to be a nonpsychometric measure of biological intelligence, more closely reflecting the human nervous system than do clinical psychological tests and maximally represented in the frontal lobes. Although the general sensitivity of these tests to brain damage has been repeatedly confirmed (e.g., Stuss and Trites, 1977), their particular sensitivity to the frontal lobes is not obvious (Reitan, 1964). Of greater concern, the Halstead-Reitan battery was devised during the 1940s and underwent its last major revision during the 1950s. This has been beneficial in allowing an accumulation of knowledge, experience, and normative data as a base for inter- and intraindividual comparison. On the other hand, this has curtailed development of more specific measures of frontal lobe functioning. Experienced neuropsychologists using the Halstead-Reitan battery frequently supplement their standardized test procedures with other tests, depending on the hypotheses raised by the initial evaluation. As with the Wechsler approach, the Halstead-Reitan battery and ancillary tests, in expert and cautious hands, can provide strong suggestion of focal frontal lobe abnormality.

Finally, two new batteries of tests have been prepared from the lifetime experience of the great Russian neuropsychologist Luria. A selection of his tests has been translated into English by Christensen (1975), and a second, independent battery (Luria-Nebraska test battery) designed to conform to current American psychological practices has been developed (Golden, 1981). Theoretically, with the Luria approach comparatively subtle frontal lobe disturbance can be sought and isolated (Luria, 1966/1980, 1969, 1973a). In particular, subtests such as rhythm tapping, "go/no-go," alternating figures, and others are suggested as particularly sensitive to frontal lobe malfunction. Unfortunately, many individuals with gross frontal lobe damage perform these tests normally (Benson and Stuss, 1982), and, conversely, pathology in other parts of the brain can interfere with their performance. Only a battery of specific clinical procedures can separate frontal from nonfrontal lobe pathology.

Published reports suggest that precise anatomical localization of damage, including that to the frontal lobe, can be made with the Luria-Nebraska battery (Golden, 1981; Lewis, Golden, Moses, et al., 1979; McKay and Golden, 1979). However, there has been disagreement concerning the relationship of the Luria-Nebraska battery to Luria's test procedures, as well as questions of the validity of the findings (Adams, 1980a,b; Golden, 1980; Spiers, 1981). Expert interpretation is necessary if the Luria batteries are to be used for localizing purposes, and most practicing psychologists have neither the skill nor the clinical background of Professor Luria.

At best, material from the general neuropsychological batteries can be used only for general localization purposes. The enormous size and complex integrative functions of the frontal lobes tend to produce combinations of abnormalities that are poorly demonstrated by rigidly administered psychological test batteries. Although frontal malfunction can be suspected on the basis of test results, specific psychological functions of discrete portions of the frontal lobe cannot be demonstrated. Ongoing research activities, such as those described in the following chapters, suggest that finer differentiation is possible. The commonly used neuropsychological batteries are useful as screening tests but are not yet competent tools for detecting independent frontal lobe functions. Clinical neuropsychological test procedures will eventually incorporate these more experimental techniques.

TISSUE SPECIMEN EXAMINATIONS

Among the accepted techniques for localizing pathology within the frontal lobe, evaluations of the tissue itself, either through biopsy or by study of autopsy material, is of importance. Both techniques can provide valuable information but have drawbacks that limit their usefulness.

Biopsy of the frontal lobes has been performed for many years, particularly in cases with tumor, and surgical decompression of an intracerebral tumor provides one of the better examples of focal damage. In both situations the site of tissue removal can be recorded with fair accuracy, and the specimen provides information concerning brain pathology; the combination provides valuable information for anatomical/behavioral correlation. Biopsy is a comparatively easy technique but does have a recognized morbidity; surgical decompression of a tumor is a mutilating and risky procedure. Neither is performed without strong clinical indications. Unfortunately, in many instances both techniques fail to provide good localizing information. Biopsy has been used most often to demonstrate widespread disorders such as cortical degenerative disease (Sim, Turner, and Smith, 1966), viral encephalitis, and so on. With the exception of tumor, biopsy is almost never performed for disorders with pathology localized to one or both frontal lobes. Most tumors that are biopsied or surgically decompressed are focal; but, as discussed in Chapter 3, through distant spread, surrounding edema, distortion of vascular pathways, and so on, they often produce behavior based on distant effects. The mere presence of tumor in the frontal region cannot be accepted as proof that the symptomatology which led to the surgical procedure was based on frontal lobe disturbance. In fact, review of behavioral data from the case histories of patients who have undergone surgery for frontal lobe tumor almost routinely reveals that the tumor was relatively silent during growth in the frontal lobe and became symptomatic by reaching sufficient size to produce distant effects (Chambers, 1955; Waggoner and Bagchi, 1954).

Another tissue specimen examination, the autopsy, is usually considered the ultimate procedure for correlation of abnormal behavior and neuroanatomical locus of pathology. Much of modern medicine has evolved from correlations of behavioral abnormality with postmortem findings. Autopsy studies can provide important information concerning both the site and the type of pathology with anatomical exactness, so that specific cortical areas, pathways, and so on can be related to the demonstrated behavior. The autopsy is not without significant limitations, however, and interpretations made from autopsy material must also be viewed with caution.

One problem that plagues behavioral interpretation from postmortem material is that the autopsy is performed long after the demonstration of the specific behavioral findings. An individual with findings suggesting frontal lobe dysfunction may live for many months or years; and although abnormality may be demonstrated within the frontal lobe at the time of autopsy, pathology that involves other areas is likely. With the constantly improving techniques for the maintenance of life, the delay between behavioral evaluation and final autopsy correlation is increasing rather than decreasing. Another problem hindering autopsy correlations concerns availability of material. The rates of autopsy performance have decreased in recent years, reflecting at least in part the fact that a vast number (probably a majority) of elderly patients die in nursing homes and permission for pathological evaluation is not routinely requested. Failure to obtain postmortem confirmation of suspected pathology is discouragingly common.

Despite the noted limitations, a specific diagnosis and/or localization of a behavioral abnormality is possible from autopsy material. For instance, if a patient has had appropriate treatment (e.g., surgery) for a disorder that involves the frontal lobe, if the patient's behavior is carefully recorded, and if the patient later succumbs with a disease process affecting other areas, not only can the focal nature of the original pathology be demonstrated but with appropriate study the more recent effects can be distinguished. Although such instances are not frequent, they offer valuable information and continued, even increased, use of autopsy material appears to be indicated in frontal lobe investigations.

NEURORADIOLOGICAL STUDIES

Of the many laboratory techniques used to locate frontal abnormality, various x-ray studies are the most common. Techniques have evolved and improved over the years and deserve documentation.

For many years, x-ray studies of the skull were a major source of localization information for suspected frontal lobe behavioral abnormality. Specifically, for the evaluation of trauma, particularly gunshot wounds to the head, the location of the skull injury was often equated with the area of brain injured. Many major studies of brain activity have utilized the site of entrance of a missile as focal information for behavioral/anatomical correlations. For instance, in the studies of aphasia by Bonhoeffer (1934), Conrad (1954), Luria (1970b), Russell and Espir (1961), and Schiller (1947), the site of skull injuries was used for anatomical correlation (Fig. 4-1). These studies rank as major contributions, not so much because of the accuracy of the localization procedure but because no better techniques were available. Localization of frontal malfunction could be determined by noting the site of the defect on a plain x-ray of the skull; it appears logical to expect that the area of the brain immediately adjacent to the skull injury would also be injured.

As noted in Chapter 3, however, the site of damage to the skull and the site of major damage in the brain may be quite different. Despite flat statements declaring

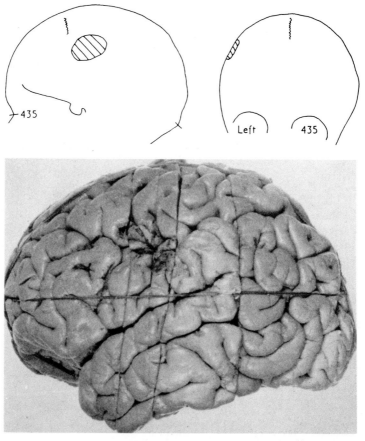

FIG. 4-1. Composite drawing showing **(top)** tracing of a skull x-ray following a gunshot wound to the left parietal area that resulted in a transient aphasia plus paresis and sensory disturbance of the right upper extremity and face; **(bottom)** postmortem appearance of brain showing location of brain injury. (From Russell and Espir, *Traumatic Aphasia*, with permission.)

that skull injuries provide the best material for localizing cerebral abnormalities currently available (Critchley, 1970), the technique presents many opportunities for error. Excellent frontal lobe behavioral anatomical correlation data have come from studies of patients with skull defects, but the data reflect more the skill and insight of the examiner than the precision of the procedure.

Radiological localization of the site of the brain affected by pathology has been advanced by special contrast techniques. Those techniques that use injected contrast materials include air encephalography, angiography, and the deposition of contrast material in a surgical decompression site. In general, these techniques provide improved visualization of intracranial foci. The air studies—pneumoencephalography (infusion of air through a lumbar or cervical puncture site) and ventriculography (infusion of air directly into the ventricle)—provide sharp outlines of the ventricular system and in most instances the subarachnoid spaces. These studies are particularly accurate for demonstrating the frontal horns of the lateral ventricles, the perichiasmal cisterns, the frontal sagittal subarachnoid space, and the orbital and dorsal convexity subarachnoid spaces (Peterson and Kieffer, 1970). At most, however, the air studies can offer only an indication of either a mass lesion or tissue loss through alteration of the normal ventricular pattern. Although anatomically sharp, the information from air studies is limited.

Angiography, the injection of contrast material into cerebral arteries by either direct carotid injection or femoral catheterization, can provide valuable information. The contrast material remains within the vessels, flowing with the blood, and interpretation is made from either distortion of the usual vessel pattern or the presence of abnormal vessels (Fig. 4-2). For localization purposes, the angiogram is most valuable in demonstrating great vessel occlusion or stenosis, arteriovenous malformations, or aneurysms but can also outline mass lesions and areas where

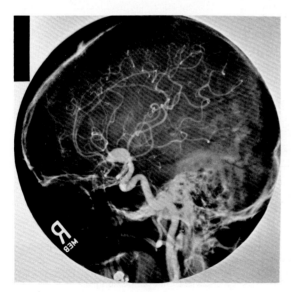

FIG. 4-2. Angiogram demonstrating large anterior communicating artery aneurysm in a patient with progressive headache and apathy. (Courtesy of John Bentson, M.D., UCLA School of Medicine.)

the blood supply has been lost (infarction). The latter cannot be interpreted literally, however. Occlusion of an intracranial vessel may not cause infarction in that vessel's territory (Taveras and Wood, 1976). Good collateral circulation is often available, and total occlusion of a vessel may produce little or no destruction of brain tissue. Angiography can provide useful localizing information, but because it is a difficult technique and is associated with some morbidity it is not extensively used at present.

On some occasions, surgeons have placed contrast material into a cerebral decompression site. Following tumor decompression, abscess drainage, or psycho-surgical procedures, the opaque material can provide a permanent record of the site of frontal damage for correlation with behavioral observations (Allen and Meacham, 1966). Some injected contrast material was thought to cause ongoing pathology, however, and with current improved radiological techniques this procedure is rarely used.

The x-ray procedure of greatest usefulness for localization purposes at present, one that has replaced most of the above procedures, is the x-ray computed tomogram (CT). This technique images tomographic slices of brain as degrees of density; major structures such as the skull, subarachnoid space, cerebral tissues, and ventricular system can be distinguished because of their different tissue densities (Oldendorf, 1980). Both plain x-ray CT and CT following enhancement with iodinated material demonstrate many intracranial abnormalities in the living patient without altering the patient's condition. Thus many tumors and most bleeding abnormalities such as hematomas are readily demonstrated, and with appropriate techniques the loss of tissue secondary to cerebral infarction or injury can often be demonstrated (see Chapter 3).

X-ray CT has greatly altered the practice of neurology by simply and accurately localizing many types of intracranial pathology. This very accuracy has had a negative effect, however. CT information is now accepted as absolute by many practitioners even though false-positive and false-negative results are widely recognized (Jacobson and Farmer, 1979). Abnormal behavior emanating from pathology invisible to the CT scan is now routinely missed or ignored if the same scan shows pathology involving some other site. Moreover, the best resolution presently possible (about 0.5 cm) excludes much purely cortical pathology, making interpretation of cortical area damage very difficult. As with all laboratory procedures, x-ray CT is best used to confirm a clinical impression and is open to errors of omission and commission when used for diagnosis.

Despite its wide use and many obvious advantages, to date comparatively few major advances in the study of frontal lobe function have stemmed from use of x-ray CT. Several reasons can be suggested. First, the pathology had often produced far-reaching effects before visualization by CT. Second, until recently, CT resolution has been relatively poor, permitting visualization of large lesions only. Even more significant, the x-ray CT visualizes only structural alterations; it has almost no ability to demonstrate problems based on functional alteration (metabolic, hypoxic, etc.). Major behavioral abnormality based on functional disturbance can be present in an individual whose x-ray CT scan is normal (Baker, Campbell,

Houser, et al., 1974). Nonetheless, intracranial localization has been greatly advanced by use of x-ray CT, and technical improvements are constantly increasing the technique's potential. X-ray CT offers considerable promise for future investigations of frontal lobe functions.

RADIOACTIVE NUCLIDE STUDIES

A number of techniques for investigating intracranial activity through use of radioactive isotopes have been developed during the past several decades (Oldendorf, 1980). Although all have some relevance for the localization of frontal pathology, none has added greatly to the body of information on the subject.

The first, and for a long time, the most widely used isotope study was radionuclide brain scanning. Following intravenous injection of a radioactive material, counts of radioactive emission were recorded over the lateral, anterior, and/or posterior portions of the skull by means of sensitive detectors. Areas of increased radioactivity, usually indicative of increased vascularity, could be outlined and imaged (Bull, 1965) (Fig. 4-3). Radioisotope scans were excellent for demonstrating highly vascular intracranial tumors, recent cerebrovascular infarctions, arteriovenous malformations (AVMs), and other disorders causing increased intracranial circulation. Unfortunately, the resolution of many scanning apparatuses, particularly the more modern units that rapidly produce images, is so poor that only the most gross anatomical information can be extracted. Although capable of locating brain abnormalities in the frontal lobes, the anatomical specificity is so limited that the radioactive brain scan has not played a major role in frontal lobe behavior investi-

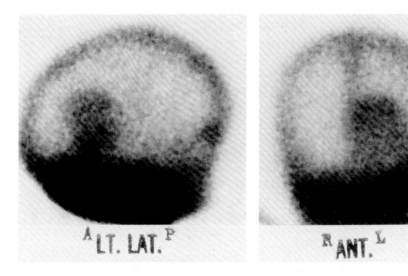

FIG. 4-3. Radioisotope brain scan of patients with left frontal lobe sarcoma. (Courtesy of David Kuhl, M.D., UCLA.)

gations. With the advent of the simpler x-ray CT, radioactive brain scans are infrequently performed.

A second technique which uses radioactive isotopes for brain investigation is isotope cisternography. A radioactive material is injected into the subarachnoid space through a routine lumbar or cisternal puncture (DiChiro, Reames, and Matthews, 1964); it rapidly diffuses through the cerebrospinal fluid (CSF) in the subarachnoid spaces and then flows with the CSF, providing a dynamic record of CSF circulation. If hydrocephalus is present, the isotope retrofluxes into the ventricular system, and with proper counting units an outline of the ventricles is produced. Enlarged frontal horns (Benson, Lemay, Pattern, et al., 1970) and cerebral cysts communicating with the ventricles (Silverberg, Castellino, and Goodwin, 1969) are the two most specific frontal lesions demonstrated by isotope cisternography. The resolution is relatively poor, limiting the information for localization purposes.

A more recent addition to the group of techniques using isotope activity for brain studies is positron emission tomography (PET) (Kuhl, Metter, Riege, et al., 1982a; Phelps, Huang, Hoffman, et al., 1979; Reivich, Kuhl, Wolf, et al., 1979). In this technique a specific compound (e.g., oxygen, carbon dioxide, deoxyglucose) tagged with a radioisotope that emits positrons is injected intravenously. As the compound circulates, appropriate counting studies can provide accurate estimates of cerebral circulation (Frackowiak, Pozzilli, Legg, et al., 1981) and, conversely, can indicate areas of decreased cerebral blood flow. Cell metabolism can also be studied with PET. For instance, one current technique uses deoxyglucose tagged with radioactive fluorine (FDG). FDG is metabolized as glucose, but cerebral cells lack sufficient quantities of the enzyme necessary to break down one of the metabolic products of deoxyglucose and the product accumulates in brain cells. Appropriate counting techniques provide data indicating the cellular metabolic rate in a given area, data that can be handled as counts of radioactivity in a region of interest or as a tomographic image. PET data from cerebral circulation and/or metabolic studies can indicate frontal lobe function and/or malfunction (Fig. 4-4). Unlike most other localizing data, the PET studies evaluate functional alterations (metabolic abnormalities), not structural changes, and are complementary to the structural information from the x-ray CT scan (Metter, Riege, Hanson, et al., 1984a).

PET is a new technique demanding highly specialized equipment. Currently it is used primarily as a research technique, and comparatively little specific information concerning frontal lobe function has been gathered. Several PET studies of cerebral blood flow during mental tasks suggest that frontal lobe metabolism is not as active during cognitive tasks in chronic schizophrenic patients as in normals (Buchsbaum et al., 1982; Franzen and Ingvar, 1975b; Ingvar and Franzen, 1974). Several types of progressive dementia (Alzheimer disease, Pick disease) appear to involve the frontal cortex (Benson, Kuhl, Hawkins, et al., 1983a), whereas others (normal-pressure hydrocephalus, Huntington disease) do not (Kuhl, Phelps, Markham, et al., 1982b). Studies of a variety of functions including language, memory, musical skill, cognition, and so on are being conducted in normal subjects with

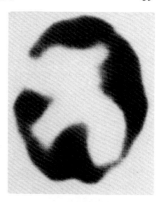

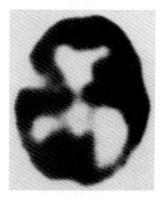

FIG. 4-4. PET scan of patient with Broca aphasia secondary to vascular occlusive disease. (Courtesy of David Kuhl, M.D., UCLA.)

this new tool, and valuable information concerning the role of the frontal lobes in a number of high level activities can be anticipated. Such studies have revealed a functional heterogeneity in frontal regions, different areas being recruited for different tasks (Roland, 1984). The PET scan, particularly its ability to study metabolism during normal physiological activities, offers a totally new avenue for investigating brain functions, many of which involve the frontal lobes.

A variation of PET, single photon emission computed tomography (SPECT), has been introduced for widespread use. To date, the resolution of pertinent features is considerably less than with PET, and only blood flow studies have been performed; however, the compounds are considerably more stable so the procedure can be carried out as a routine hospital diagnostic procedure. It is anticipated that PET will remain a valuable research tool but that SPECT will develop as a clinical resource of value. Both approaches should prove useful for investigation of the frontal lobes.

MAGNETIC RESONANCE IMAGING

Another recently introduced brain imaging technique, originally called nuclear magnetic resonance (NMR) but now known as magnetic resonance imaging (MRI), is neither isotopic nor radiological and holds considerable promise for future brain localization studies (Oldendorf, 1980). The procedure uses high-power magnetism to alter the polarity of selected intracranial cells; through monitoring the altered polarity and CT imaging of these data, brain structures can be outlined. MRI offers a somewhat different view than that available from x-ray CT; it is less obscured by osseus material and therefore provides better images in the posterior fossa and at the base of the brain (Fig. 4-5). Multiple sclerosis plaques are far better imaged by MRI, but some other types of pathology are not as well visualized. It appears that both procedures will have usefulness in the future. When fully developed, MRI will provide a highly useful and accurate means of imaging brain structures. In addition, current studies suggest that the technique may be modified to allow study of selected metabolites in the brain structures, providing useful functional information.

ELECTROPHYSIOLOGICAL STUDIES

The electroencephalogram (EEG) has been widely used for brain study and represents an entirely different approach. The EEG demonstrates alterations of normal brain physiology by recording changes in the basic electrical activity as monitored over the surface of the skull. The presence of focal slowing or epileptic foci emanating from the frontal regions can provide localizing information (Rasmussen, 1963). A number of behavioral changes occur in patients with frontal lobe epileptic foci and can be correlated with the location and type of frontal discharge (Penfield and Kristiansen, 1951; Quesney, Krieger, Leitner, et al., 1984). Most such recordings evaluate cortical surface only, a limiting factor, and it must be acknowledged that seizure activity is abnormal so the behavior observed may not represent true frontal lobe function. Nonetheless, EEG and behavioral correlations can provide useful localizing information on frontal lobe function. Correlation of EEG activity from different electrode sites during the performance of a task has been used experimentally to indicate frontal lobe functioning (Luria, 1973a).

A new electrophysiological technique, stimulus-evoked responses, has also been introduced. In this procedure, a simple or minimally complex stimulus (auditory,

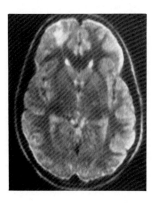

FIG. 4-5. MR scan of patient with low grade astrocytoma in the right prefrontal area. This lesion did not visualize or enhance on CT study. (Courtesy of Gabriel Wilson, M.D., UCLA.)

somesthetic, or visual) is repeated multiple times while the consequent changes in EEG pattern are recorded (Picton and Hink, 1974). When the recorded electrical responses are superimposed by computer techniques, background electrical activity tends to be subtracted, whereas the wave forms produced in response to the stimulus are magnified. A consistent and predictable wave pattern is produced. Correlation of alterations in the normal timing of this wave pattern with well-localized peripheral and central nervous system disorders has provided information about the part of the nervous system responsible for various portions of this waveform (Desmedt and Noel, 1973). Based on such studies, considerable information concerning the timing and transmission of sensory impulses through various sections of the CNS has been recorded. Unfortunately, comparatively little information relative to frontal lobe functions has been produced with sensory stimulus-evoked potentials, probably because the frontal lobe is involved in the late stages of sensory processing, and the technique appears best for demonstrating the early transmission and processing of sensory stimuli.

Of greater interest are the later scalp recorded event-related potentials (ERPs), which vary more with the psychological significance of the stimulus. Walter and colleagues (Walter, 1973; Walter, Cooper, Aldridge, et al., 1964) suggested that such brain potentials, in particular the Contingent Negative Variation (CNV), could be useful in addressing frontal lobe function. At least one such slow negative wave has been considered frontal in origin (Borda, 1970; Järvilehto and Fruhstorfer, 1970); comparison with animal research suggests a neuronal source (Fuster, 1984). Other waveforms theoretically associated with frontal lobes and the function of attention have been: (1) the "Nd" in the latency range of 100 msec, obtained when the ERPs to ignored stimuli are subtracted from the ERPs to attended stimuli (Hansen and Hillyard, 1980; Hillyard and Kutas, 1983); (2) the "processing negativity," a negative waveform in the latency range 100 to 250 msec which occurs during attention to incoming stimuli (Näätänen, 1982); and (3) one component of the ERP labeled the N2, reported to reflect frontal attentional involvement (Fitzgerald and Picton, 1983). Patients with frontal lobe lesions show a smaller negativity in the latency range 100 to 250 msec than do normal subjects (Knight, Hillyard, Woods, et al., 1981). Finally, a negative waveform in the latency range of 400 msec, the frontal N400, has been postulated to reflect a more generalized function, perhaps the initiation and supervision of higher levels of perceptual processing controlled by the frontal lobes (Delisle, Stuss, and Picton, 1985; Stuss, Sarazin, Leech, and Picton, 1983).

Although animal electrophysiological research, particularly with single cell recording, appears to be more advanced (Fuster, 1984), the use of electrophysiological techniques to assess specific psychological functions in humans remains in its infancy. Although some findings suggest that specific waveforms reflect frontal lobe abilities, current results must be considered only speculative. Further research, particularly with frontally damaged patients performing specific tasks, is necessary.

SUMMARY

As noted, studies for correlating behavioral abnormality with frontal disorder are, at best, rather limited. Although a number of improved techniques have become available during the past several decades, they remain indirect and nonspecific. To make use of future technical advances, the investigator needs better techniques for documenting the clinical manifestations of frontal lobe function and malfunction. Information from a wide variety of tests and a wide group of pathologies must be correlated to demonstrate frontal lobe functions. With this information as a base, later generations can use advanced techniques to corroborate both static and dynamic aspects of frontal functions that underlie frontal behavioral abnormalities. Such precision is important considering the specificity and functional heterogeneity now hypothesized for the frontal lobes (Milner and Petrides, 1984; Oscar-Berman, 1975, 1978; Roland, 1984; Rosenkilde, 1979).

5

Frontal Motor Functions

The control of motor response is the most evident of all frontal lobe functions. Frontal control of motor activity was first reported in 1691 by Robert Boyle, who observed a patient with unilateral paralysis of the arm and leg subsequent to a depressed frontal skull fracture (Henneman, 1980b). Hughlings Jackson (1864) suggested an organized motor area representing specific body zones, a concept subsequently confirmed and refined by electrical stimulation of the frontal lobes of various animals (Ferrier, 1875; Fritsch and Hitzig, 1870). The frontal lobe was thought not only to initiate the "final common pathway" for brain response but also to modulate the final response by integrating information from other cortical areas (Bianchi, 1895).

Frontal lobe motor activities are complex and must be subdivided for analysis. The motor functions of the precentral (and premotor) areas have been studied extensively during the twentieth century; they are well described in current neuroanatomy and physiology texts and need not be detailed here (for reviews see Henneman, 1980a,b; Ruch and Fetz, 1979). On the other hand, motor activities derived from prefrontal cortex and integrated with motor functions of the premotor association cortex are far more complex and have received less documentation (see Fuster, 1981). Nevertheless, the well-documented efferent connections from prefrontal cortex to motor areas, including the basal ganglia, mesencephalic and pontine tegmental areas, preoptic zones, pulvinar, tectum, and premotor cortex, suggest that prefrontal cortex is important in motor control and motor programming (Fuster, 1981; Stamm, 1979).

In this chapter the motor functions associated with these frontal areas are reviewed under a number of categories including neurological and behavioral signs, motor impersistence, and the classification of Luria. Psychological tests designed to elicit motor deficits, although usually not accepted as indices of prefrontal cortex activity, are then summarized. A final section reviews the role of the frontal lobes in the sensory-motor disturbances called apraxia.

MOTOR DEFICITS
Frontal Neurological Signs

The so-called frontal release signs, including the grasp, rooting, sucking, snout, and palmomental reflexes, plus Brun's ataxia and relative hyperactivity of the jaw jerk, are often attributed to frontal lobe pathology. In addition, impaired control or awareness of micturition and defecation may follow frontal damage, especially bifrontal lesions (Adams and Victor, 1977/1981). If lesions affect the more anterior frontal regions, an indifference may be superimposed. All may reflect frontal motor abnormality, but specific correlation of these findings with frontal lobe pathology has not been definitively established.

The *grasp reflex*, an involuntary, mandatory clasping of the thumb and index finger into a gripping of the examiner's finger (or other object) following light stimulation of the first dorsal interosseus space, is strongly suggestive of midline frontal abnormality. This is particularly true if the grasp reflex is unilateral, indicating contralateral medial frontal dysfunction. Bilateral self-grasping has been reported as secondary to symmetrical destructive frontal lesions in the absence of hemiparesis (Ropper, 1982). The other "frontal" signs—*rooting* (a lateral movement of the lips toward the side of the mouth stimulated), *sucking* (an involuntary pursing of the lips when an object is brought toward them), and *snout* (a pursing of the lips on tapping of the skin between the nostrils and the lips)—are present in infants but disappear with brain maturation and have been called primitive reflexes. Although the latter three most often reflect pathology in the diencephalon or upper brainstem, they have long been designated as frontal release signs; none of the three occur commonly with frontal cortex involvement. The *palmomental sign* (a contraction of the ipsilateral malar skin on scratching of the palm) is even more difficult to localize but most often reflects brainstem dysfunction.

The frontal release signs can be seen with diffuse cerebral dysfunction such as advanced Alzheimer disease or metabolic encephalopathy. As noted, brainstem and diencephalic pathology can produce "frontal" release signs, particularly when there is depression of the state of awareness. Even more important, patients with demonstrable frontal lobe damage may have no or few frontal neurological signs or motor deficits (Ackerly and Benton, 1947). A controlled study of the frontal release signs in patients with clearly documented, well-demarcated bilateral orbital frontal primary white matter lesions secondary to prefrontal leukotomy revealed no deficits in any of the patients (Benson and Stuss, 1982). The absence of impaired "frontal" neurological motor signs does not exclude frontal lobe pathology, and the frontal release signs are not reliable indicators of frontal pathology; nevertheless, they do occur in some patients with frontal dysfunction.

Motor Aspects of Frontal Behavior

Despite the lack of consistent, reliable frontal neurological signs, overt motor changes can appear subsequent to frontal lobe damage. Descriptions of these behaviors appear to be paradoxical and incongruous, ranging from hyperactivity, restlessness, euphoria, impulsivity, and facetiousness (Blumer and Benson, 1975; Greenblatt, Arnot, and Solomon, 1950; Greenblatt and Solomon, 1966) to apathy, lethargy, laziness, abulia, lack of initiative, loss of spontaneity, slowness, and dullness (Goldstein, 1944; Greenblatt and Solomon, 1966; Victor and Adams, 1977/

1981). The two extremes of motor disability following prefrontal pathology can be categorized as different behavior patterns that can be correlated with different localizations of pathology (Kleist, 1934b). The puerile, restless, and apparently more vigorous type of patient has been labeled "pseudopsychopathic" (Blumer and Benson, 1975) and usually suffers major pathology involving orbital frontal areas. In the most severe states, these patients burst into action, respond briefly but appropriately, and then return to an underlying multidirected inappropriate restlessness. In lesser degrees, a behavior characterized by immediate gratification without concern for social propriety leads to impulsive antisocial acts that may include sexual excesses, stealing, biting, crude humor (both self- and other-directed), and unreliability. The subject knows, and can relate, what is correct but apparently cannot control immediately gratifying actions. This produces a state resembling the sociopathic personality and has been clearly seen following orbital frontal brain damage.

The other variation, the hypokinetic, abulic frontal lobe patient, has been labeled "pseudodepressed" (Blumer and Benson, 1975) and is well recognized as occurring after frontal lobe damage (Goldstein, 1944; Kleist, 1934b; Lishman, 1978; Walch, 1956). Lesion location in this group has been said to be maximal in the dorsal-lateral frontal convexity (Blumer and Benson, 1975). Others have suggested a different localization for this abulia. Luria (1973a) suggested that the "apathetico-akinetico-abulic" syndrome is most typical of massive frontal lobe damage. The most severe form of this type of motor alteration is true akinetic mutism and can result from bilateral posterior-medial orbital frontal damage. Some have suggested that the disturbance results from severance of frontal-thalamic connections (Adams and Victor, 1977/1981), and others have suggested a disconnection of fibers connecting the reticular activating system to the prefrontal cortex (Benson and Geschwind, 1975; Ross and Stewart, 1981). The most striking finding in these individuals is a lack of drive, an inability to act as expected, coupled with an apparent helpless unconcern. Observations suggest a medial frontal localization for control of drive functions (Benson, 1985) (see Chapter 8). The inert, uncaring state resembles the psychomotor retardation of depression—hence the terms pseudodepression and pseudoretardation—but the mood does not appear to be that of depression, and as with the pseudopsychopathic disorder these individuals often have fully normal general intelligence. They fail to act on their knowledge.

Although both types of abnormal frontal lobe activity have been described frequently, the causative pathology is usually not well localized, and pure examples are not common. The general behavior of the leukotomized patients with maximum destruction in the orbital frontal regions more closely resembled the hyperkinetic type (Benson and Stuss, 1982). They also showed apathy, however, in that they acted little until commanded (Stuss and Benson, 1983a). Although they tended to confirm the localization/gross behavioral correlations described, without a comparative sample of dorsal-lateral frontal lobe patients this hypothesis remains unconfirmed. (See Chapter 8 for a detailed discussion of frontal personality disturbances.)

Motor Impersistence

Although recognized earlier, the first detailed investigations of motor impersistence were presented during the 1950s (Berlin, 1955; Fisher, 1956). Two basic phenomena have been described. The first is an inability to initiate a movement on command. Much more commonly, the deficit was considered an inability to maintain an initiated voluntary movement (which could be briefly performed normally), an interference with sustained control of the motor act, also described as a type of distractibility (Fisher, 1956).

The following deficits of maintenance have been described (Fisher, 1956): eyelid closure (peeking); tongue protrusion; mouth opening; central fixation of eyes; maintenance of conjugate gaze in any direction when looking at an object; steady hand-grip pressure; holding a deep breath; prolonged "ah." Formalized neuropsychological administration of tests of motor impersistence have been reported (Benton, Hamsher, Varney, and Spreen, 1983; Joynt, Benton, and Fogel, 1962). Not all signs are equally reported, with eyelid closure, mouth opening, and tongue protrusion most regularly noted (Berlin, 1955; Fisher, 1956). Whether this reflects an actual incidence of abnormality or the mere predominance of reporting is uncertain. Although normally transient, motor impersistence can persist (Fisher, 1956). It is frequently found after infarction and often associated with motor and sensory findings as well as some "mental impairment." Severity of the impersistence correlated with several factors but apparently was not reducible to them: age, general mental impairment, level of education, and extent of brain damage (Ben-Yishay, Diller, Gerstman et al., 1968; Hier, Mondlock, and Caplan, 1983; Joynt et al., 1962; Levin, 1973).

The possible relevance of motor impersistence to frontal lobe functioning is suggested by lesion location and theory. The most persistent suggestion of focal brain localization suggests that motor impersistence is secondary to nondominant pathology (Berlin, 1955; Fisher, 1956; Joynt et al., 1962). Earlier reports had also implicated frontal lobes (Fisher, 1956; Pinéas, 1924; Schilder, 1924). However, motor impersistence is frequently found with diffuse or bilateral brain damage, and it has been stated that it represents an index of brain damage without hemisphere differences (Ben-Yishay, Haas, and Diller, 1967; Joynt et al., 1962; Levin, 1973).

Motor impersistence (at least specific aspects) has been described as an apraxia (Atack and Suranyi, 1975; Lewandowsky, 1907) or as an inability to overcome the primitive vigilance attitude of eye opening (Berlin, 1955). More commonly, it has been implicated with deficits in initiation, persistence, and attention. Inattentiveness and lack of persistence in all assigned activities including motor functions have been described after frontal lobe impairment (Adams and Victor, 1977/1981; Arnot, 1952). Correlation of motor impersistence with disorders in attention have been reported (Ben-Yishay et al., 1967, 1968; Fisher, 1956). This correlation is reflected in such descriptive terms as "distractibility" and "inability to maintain," as well as in the general description of the phenomena. Hier et al. (1983) noted that impersistence was commonly grouped with signs of inattention such as denial of illness and extinction on double simultaneous stimulation, suggesting that motor impersistence implies pathology in an attentional brain system. When pathology is focal, right central and right frontal lesions appear to be predominant (Kertesz, Nicholson, Cancelliere, et al., 1985).

Luria's Classification

Luria based a classification of frontal motor disturbance on his theory that four separate conditions, dependent on four different cortical zones, were necessary for normal movement. Although the entire theory is beyond the intended scope of this chapter, in brief it can be stated that two of the four conditions reflected frontal cortical activity involving the premotor and prefrontal areas, respectively. Discussion of the effects of pathology in these two zones presupposes intactness of the other two conditions—afferent feedback and visual-spatial abilities—and provides insight into the function of the frontal motor areas in complex motor activity.

Function of the Premotor Zone

In Luria's theory, the premotor area is not responsible for independent human movements. Rather, this frontal area subserves the rapid and smooth transition of one component of a complex movement to the next, i.e., plays an essential role in learned, skilled movements. This requires denervation of a completed action and a facile change to the next stage, a learned activity. Any learned movement is originally made up of independent, isolated impulses. Practice results in a synthesis and fusion of the isolated impulses into a single integral component, sometimes called a "kinetic melody." With long practice this complex movement becomes automatic. Instead of individual pulses initiating each section of a movement, one impulse is sufficient to trigger the entire complex. The attaining of an athletic or musical skill illustrates one postulated function of the premotor zone.

A lesion in the premotor cortex (area 6) of the frontal lobe does not result in persistent paralysis or paresis of the contralateral limb (Luria, 1973a; Rizzolatti, Matelli, and Pavesi, 1983). Moreover, the intention to perform the movement and the general plan of execution are unimpaired (Luria, 1973a). However, speed, smoothness, and automaticity are disturbed; the individual components of an action again require separate impulses or initiation. The impairment is most obviously elicited with requests to perform complex movements demanding a rapid and smooth transition. Thus for the typist, the speed and almost instinctual knowledge of the keyboard is replaced by a necessity for letter by letter control.

Luria described several neuropsychological tests that he considered particularly sensitive to pathology in the premotor cortex. Complex rhythm tapping, requiring changes in number or intensity of beats, becomes discontinuous and fragmented and may be replaced by a stereotyped response. Even the rhythmical repetition of simple tapping may be disrupted. If required to alternate between square and triangle-topped figures, the program breaks down, replaced by a perseveration of one of the two responses, the "inertia of motor responses" (Fig. 5-1A).

FIG. 5-1. Four examples of frontal motor disturbances as described by Luria. **A:** Premotor area lesions disrupt the kinetic organization of the movement, impairing the smooth transition from one impulse to another. **B:** Extension of a premotor lesion to the basal ganglia or its connections with premotor cortex causes gross perseveration of movement. The patient does not stop an action once initiated. **C:** The patient is required to squeeze slowly to a short signal and quickly to a long signal [signals illustrated on bottom (downward deflection indicating length of signal), hand response on top]. Section A demonstrates how a patient with left parietal-occipital pathology can overcome the conflicting signal to respond correctly, whereas the left frontal lobe damaged patient (section B) cannot; he mimics the signal even though correctly verbalizing task demands. (From Luria: *Higher Cortical Functions in Man.* Consultant Bureaus, New York 1966/1980, with permission.)

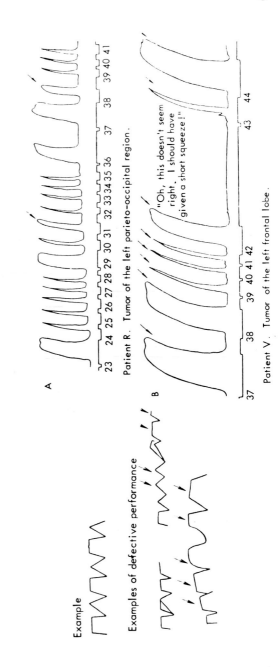

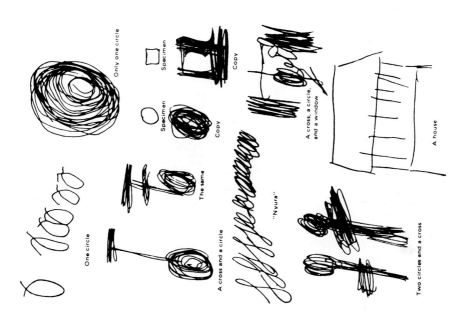

One circle

Only one circle

Specimen

Copy

Specimen

Copy

The same

A cross and a circle

A cross, a circle,
and a window

"Nyura"

A house

Two circles and a cross

B

Localization of premotor dysfunction is possible to a limited degree. The impairment is maximal contralateral to the affected hemisphere, although dominant hemisphere premotor pathology can result in bilateral deficit. Moreover, within the dominant hemisphere, there is a difference along the vertical axis of the premotor area. According to Luria, pathology in the lower premotor area results in a disorder of speech in which isolated speech sounds are normal but polysyllabic words result in perseverative repetition of the first syllable of the spoken or written word, or a deficit in smooth transition from syllable to syllable (Luria, 1970b, 1973a).

The basal ganglia are intimately connected with the frontal premotor zone and exert considerable inhibitory and modulatory influence. If premotor pathology extends deep (involving the basal ganglia or their connections to the frontal cortex), a loss of control results and additional symptoms occur. An individual movement, once begun, cannot be inhibited, resulting in elementary motor perseveration. If required to draw a circle, the patient continues to repeat the same movement over and over (Fig. 5-1B).

Prefrontal Cortex

Luria suggested that the prefrontal cortex has two major roles that affect motor activity: (1) the maintenance and control of cortical tone; (2) the regulation of higher forms of organized, conscious activity. Massive damage to the prefrontal cortex produces the apathetico-akinetico-abulic behavior described above. Pathology in this area may also result in the disorganization of active, voluntary, conscious movement. Whereas elementary activity is not impaired, the organization of conscious activity is disturbed. In some respects, the premotor and prefrontal deficits are similar, both resulting in "pathological inertia of existing stereotypes." For the premotor lesion, this inertia is primarily reflected in the effector aspect of the action   efrontal pathology, on the other hand, disrupts the scheme, or program, of the action itself.

The prefrontal disorder may be subdivided into four basic characteristics. The first concerns the intention to perform the motor task as well as attention to the command. For example, Luria noted that prefrontally damaged patients fail to answer a direct question but may respond when a question is directed to another patient. Extreme distractibility makes it difficult for them to initiate or complete any task.

Second, the prefrontal cortex is important for regulation of complex actions. With prefrontal dysfunction a verbal command remains firm in memory but loses its controlling influence (Fig. 5-1C). Luria described a frontal lobe patient discharged from the hospital who, on the way home, stopped in a town where a companion lived and remained there, even though his original goal was to return home. Although the patient recalled his original intention, it no longer directed his behavior; an immediate influence dominated. Tests for this disorganization of regulation utilize conflicting instructions. Such patients have no difficulty mimicking motor movements (echopraxia), indicating that inactivity cannot be accepted as the only cause of the problem. However, if given a verbal command that conflicts in some manner with the perceived signal, requiring that the patient not respond to what is apparent but to obey the verbal command and recode the observed connotation, these patients fall into echopractic movement. For instance, if told to tap twice when the examiner taps once, or vice versa, these patients soon do what the examiner is doing, even though they can still correctly verbalize the requirements of the task (Luria et al., 1964). In contrast, patients with premotor pathology tend to tap perseveratively, failing even to imitate correctly. "Go/no-go" tasks are another sensitive index of this disturbance, patients with prefrontal pathology being unable to inhibit responses to the "no-go" signal.

> A 56-year-old female who had a 5-year history of headache and occasional syncopal episodes rather suddenly became dull and lacked initiative. Examination revealed bilateral papilledema, ataxia, bilateral positive Babinski reflexes, bilateral grasp reflex, and bilateral anosmia. Neuropsychological testing revealed, in addition to marked slowness, a strong tendency for echopraxia and perseveration. Thus when asked to perform two movements in succession, she was unable to switch from one to the other and continued to fail even when verbal instructions were given. She was unable to imitate a simple rhythm (two beats—three beats—two beats, etc.), perseverating on one or the other of the group of beats. When asked to draw she correctly copied a circle but then perseverated by using this response for many other drawings, in response to verbal request and to copy. Electroencephalography (EEG) and arteriography both suggested a large mass lesion involving the frontal lobes bilaterally, greater on the left than the right. A huge tumor involving posterior portions of both frontal lobes at the midline was eventually demonstrated (Luria, 1965).

Luria's third characteristic of prefrontal motor disability concerns the unfolding of the motor program. Complex activities may dissolve into simpler behaviors or inert stereotypes. Thus if a frontal lobe patient is requested to raise his hand when the hand is under the bed covers, he cannot perform the task until the request is divided into two steps. New actions may be replaced by old stereotypic programs. Striking a match and lighting a candle is performed correctly, but the candle is then held like a cigarette. When requested to raise the right hand to one signal and the left hand to the second signal, the subject alternates correctly until the signals become irregular, at which time a stereotypic motor movement is used. When asked to draw two circles and a cross, the patient may continue by writing the number 2. The deficit in the general form of action is unlike the motor disinhibition and perseveration secondary to basal ganglia lesions described earlier and indicates prefrontal involvement.

The fourth condition under control of the prefrontal cortex is the guidance system required for monitoring and correcting voluntary conscious movements in which actual behavior is compared with the intended movement. Frontally damaged patients cannot compare the movement with the original intention and therefore fail to notice their errors. They can see errors in others, indicating that the problem is not conceptual.

There is need for additional research on the prefrontal motor signs proposed by Luria and colleagues. Validation in patients with sharply localized frontal lobe lesions is required. The frontal motor impairments described by Luria (1966/1980, 1973a) were most often the result of massive frontal damage with a strong probability of additional, distant defects (Hécaen and Albert, 1978). Localization of motor impairment in patients with more focal frontal lesions is not yet fully defined (see Chapter 15); moreover, demonstration of specificity of a "frontal" motor dysfunction requires careful control to exclude a "false-positive" diagnosis. Chronic schizophrenic patients without known focal pathology were seen to be significantly impaired on many frontal motor tests (Benson and Stuss, 1982). A model of motor control resembling in many respects Luria's conceptualization has been proposed (Paillard, 1982).

Psychological Tests of Motor Deficits

Neuropsychological assessment procedures utilize a number of tests of motor deficits. Many are derived from the Halstead-Reitan and Wisconsin motor batteries (Boll, 1981; Reitan and Davison, 1974). The most commonly used tests can be described in general terms, but the specific criteria for administration, scoring, and interpretation demand study of specific texts and manuals (Golden, Osmon, Moses, et al., 1981; Lezak, 1976/1983; Reitan and Davison, 1974; Russell et al., 1970; Swiercinsky, 1978; Trites, 1977). As a general rule, each test (except 10, below) is administered independently for both right and left sides.

1. *Hand-grip strength:* A hand dynamometer with adjustable grip provides a measure of lateral strength of grip.

2. *Finger-tapping speed (finger oscillation):* The patient is required to tap as quickly as possible with the index finger for a defined period of time on a manual or electric key that triggers a counter. Relative motor speed of the dominant and nondominant hands are compared.

3. *Foot-tapping speed:* This test is identical to finger oscillation, except for use of the foot.

4. *Static steadiness:* An electric stylus is held for a defined period in each of nine holes ranging in decreasing diameter from 12 to 3 mm. A score is derived from the number of times the stylus contacts the sides as well as from the duration of contact.

5. *Resting steadiness:* With the arm resting comfortably on a table, the stylus is placed in the sixth of the nine holes for a defined period of time.

6. *Vertical and horizontal groove steadiness:* A stylus is carefully moved through (up and down or back and forth) a groove of specified width and length. This test adds movement to the measurement of steadiness.

7. *Maze coordination:* The subject must move a stylus in a groove, horizontally and vertically, to trace a maze.

8. *Grooved pegboard test:* The subject is requested to place metal pegs rapidly into holes in the peg tray. To get the peg into the hole, the subject turns the peg to match a groove on the peg with a groove in the hole. Twenty-five holes are arranged in a 5×5 pattern. This test requires motor dextcrity plus hand–eye coordination.

9. *Purdue pegboard:* Using each hand separately and then both simultaneously (30 sec per condition), the subject places pegs in holes arranged vertically. Possible variations include rapid assembly of washers, pegs, and cuffs.

10. *Trail-making test:* This test consists of two sections. In part A, the subject traces a line between numbers from 1 to 25 placed in random and scattered order on a page. In part B, the line is drawn in alternating sequential manner between numbers and letters arranged randomly on a page (1–A–2–B–3–C...). Visual-motor coordination, symbol mediation, and sustained attention are demanded.

Many other tests with a motor component have been reported, but the above 10 tests are the most frequently used. They have proved to be relatively sensitive measures of lateralized brain damage as well as of brain damage in general (e.g., Costa, Vaughan, Levita, et al., 1963; Lezak, 1976/1983). They are not specific measures of isolated frontal lobe function, however. Impaired function may result from pathology in many areas of the brain (cerebellum, basal ganglia, pre- and/or postcentral gyrus, parietal-occipital area) as well as peripheral deficits or the influence of various pharmacological agents such as neuroleptics (Golden et al., 1981; Swiercinsky, 1978). Interpretation of the involvement of frontal areas in contrast to other brain areas usually requires comparison of the motor tests with other behaviors. Moreover, the relationship of defective performance to focal pathology has yet to be clarified. Kolb and Whishaw (1980), reviewing a series of psychological motor tests, divided them into two major categories: (1) tests that do not demand bilateral impairment for abnormal results, usually reflecting unilateral brain involvement (i.e., of paralysis and paresis); and (2) tests that demand bilateral impairment for abnormal results, considered tests for apraxia, not motor ability. Included in the latter category were the stylus maze and pegboard tests. Tasks requiring greater sensory-motor interaction are more susceptible to the effects of brain damage regardless of lateralization (Haaland and Delaney, 1981).

Although the psychological tests of motor functioning appear to be sensitive to the effects of brain damage, they must be interpreted in light of associated neurological findings. They cannot be used as evidence of frontal focus without corroborating evidence. If the frontal lobe is implicated, experience suggests a primarily precentral gyrus involvement. Patients with left hemisphere pathology have more difficulty with specific motor movements than those with right hemisphere brain damage (Kimura, 1977). Within the left hemisphere, there appears to be an anterior and posterior difference, most specific with single movements, the left frontal lesions controlling oral movements and the left parietal lesions controlling hand movements (Kimura, 1982). Although the frontal and parietal areas both appear to be necessary for the selection of correct movements, Kimura (1982) hypothesized that the left frontal region was involved with specific motor control systems, whereas the parietal region was involved with more general programming of movements. This concept appears to be similar to Heilman's (1979a) proposal of visuokinesthetic (parietal) and motor (frontal) engrams.

Although evidence using experimental procedures is accumulating, with progress in animal research (Evarts et al., 1984; Fuster, 1984; Petrides, 1982; Wise and Strick, 1984), the precise role of various brain regions, particularly the frontal cortex, in motor control remains controversial (e.g., DeRenzi, Faglioni, Lodesani, et al., 1983; Kimura, 1982; Kolb and Milner, 1981). Current evidence suggests that a relationship between the individual portions of the motor tests and a focal deficit in the central nervous system (CNS) will be very difficult to establish. One promising procedure appears to be regional cerebral blood flow and metabolic studies (Roland, 1984).

APRAXIA

Apraxia has been defined as the "impairment of ability to carry out purposeful movements by an individual who has normal primary motor skills (strength, reflexes, coordination) and normal comprehension of the act to be carried out (no agnosia, no general intellectual impairment)" (Hécaen, 1981, p. 257); it is considered by some as the disconnection of a verbal command from motor output (Geschwind, 1965, 1967, 1975). The relevance of the frontal cortex as a location (center) for apraxia has long been debated. Hécaen (1972) specifically excluded frontal cortex involvement in both ideomotor and ideational apraxia, but others disagree (Geschwind, 1967, 1975). The debate has been fueled by inconsistencies in definition leading to the use of different terms for a single disturbance and vice versa. For this review, apraxia is subdivided into popularly used subcategories; definitions are given, examples provided, and relevant theories discussed, all with an emphasis on frontal lobe participation.

Limb-Kinetic Apraxia

Four varieties of apraxia associated with frontal lobe pathology are grouped under the general heading of limb-kinetic apraxia, as it can be contended that all four represent a similar malfunction. Although comparison of the patients and the localization of the lesions described by different authors is difficult, it appears that areas 4 and 6 are involved to a greater or lesser extent in all. The more recent postulates also describe deficits in drive, energizing, volition, and conscious intention. These combine to suggest that the impairment may not be an apraxia, as defined in the narrow sense.

Limb-Kinetic Apraxia Proper

Limb-kinetic (melokinetic, glossokinetic, innervatory) apraxia is best described as a disturbance in the skill, speed, and delicacy of the performance of complex or serial movements. Whereas simple repetitive movements such as finger-tapping may be intact (Haaland, Porch, and Delaney, 1980), the limb-kinetic deficit appears to be an executive one, resulting in deficient linking or separation of the component movements required in complex or serial acts (Kleist, 1934b). This deficit would affect, for example, the skillful playing of a pianist or the rapid typing of a secretary without altering less complicated activities. A possible relationship of limb-kinetic apraxia with the kinetic organization of articulation is discussed in the section on apraxia of speech.

The site of a lesion necessary to produce limb-kinetic apraxia has been hypothesized as discrete pathology in the premotor area anterior to the motor cortex (DeAjuriaguerra and Tissot, 1969; Hécaen, 1981) or the anterior parietal lobe (Heilman, 1979a). Hécaen, as well as DeAjuriaguerra and Tissot, reported that a discrete lesion involving either premotor area can cause contralateral limb-kinetic apraxia. Heilman (1979a) suggested that the motor engrams required for skillful rapid movements are indeed contralateral and that lesions in either frontal lobe can cause contralateral inability to perform a movement skillfully to command. However, he also postulated the presence of separate visuokinesthetic motor programs that control the sequence of movements required to complete skillful acts (in contrast to the programs controlling specific muscle groups) which he localized in the dominant parietal lobe. Lesions in the left frontal area could disconnect these visuokinesthetic engrams to produce bilateral apraxia, whereas a right frontal lesion would promote only contralateral disturbance.

That the limb-kinetic disturbance is actually an apraxia has been questioned (DeAjuriaguerra and Tissot, 1969; Hécaen, 1981). Brodmann areas 6 and 4 are almost always involved (Fulton, 1934; Nielsen, 1936/1962), and many automatic movements may be clumsy (Ethelberg, 1951; Heilman, 1979a) as the result of pyramidal lesions (Lawrence and Kuypers, 1968), suggesting that the limb-kinetic deficit is a primary motor dysfunction rather than an apraxia.

Frontal or Magnetic Apraxia

Magnetic apraxia (often considered as either equivalent to or a subcomponent of kinetic apraxia) has been described as a compulsive exploration of the patient's immediate environment that is not related to conceptual ability (Denny-Brown, 1958). The most characteristic feature is a forced grasping with the hand (and less so by the foot) with difficulty relaxing the grasp unless the patient can "escape" from the stimulus (Goldberg, Mayer, and Toglia, 1981). Even when the hand is not in contact with an object, the use of the hand is clumsy. The disorder is perseverative in the sense that it persists in space even after contact has been broken. Not only is there a grasping reflex to somesthetic stimulation, but the patient may actively explore the environment and pursue a stimulus to grasp, even if commanded not to do so (Lhermitte, 1983). This phenomenon has been labeled utilization behavior and is never seen without involvement of frontal lobes (Lhermitte, 1983). If an object touches the lip, there is active pursuit with head-turning and sucking movements (rooting). Once contact is achieved, the limbs stiffen (*gegenhalten*, or negativism), making it appear that the limb and the object are glued together. If the patient attempts to walk, the leg may stiffen so the foot becomes "stuck" to the floor. With continued effort, this reflex is relaxed and the steps can become normal, suggesting that the disorder is an apraxia, not a motor disturbance (probably best termed as a frontal gait disturbance). When writing, the hand becomes fixed to the instrument, the so-called "apraxia of writing" (Denny-Brown, 1958). The severity varies greatly. Denny-Brown (1958) described an extreme case of a patient with thrombosis of the right anterior cerebral artery and a left magnetic apraxia who not only gathered any object on the bed with his left hand but used his right hand to put objects into the left.

The necessary lesion for magnetic apraxia appears to be prefrontal, mesial, and contralateral (DeAjuriaguerra and Tissot, 1969; Denny-Brown, 1958), although Lhermitte (1983) suggested that it indicates frontal lobe damage in general. Denny-Brown (1958) thought the deficit to be the result of a disturbance in the normal interaction of contact and prehension controlled by two cortical areas. The magnetic, exploratory tendency is a parietal lobe function, controlled (inhibited) by frontal (but also temporal) activity and released by appropriately placed lesions. The converse, a repellent, negative tendency, has been localized to premotor, cingulate, and hippocampal regions. The two tendencies normally work in synchrony. A lesion in one zone releases the other function. A lesion in the frontal area can cause perseveration of the parietal contactual, exploratory tendency and thereby produce a magnetic apraxia; in contrast, a parietal lesion releases the frontal withdrawal responses, resulting in a parietal or "repellent" apraxia. Bilateral prefrontal lesions can cause disturbance (apraxia) of bilateral movements—difficulty in initiating walking, sitting, or standing up despite the absence of spasticity.

Apraxia for Walking—Frontal Apraxia of Gait—Gait Apraxia—Frontal Ataxia

Gerstmann and Schilder (1926) originally described a disturbance of walking that appeared to fit the definition of a true apraxia (Van Bogaert and Martin, 1929). Although without paresis or other basic motor impairment, their patient with prefrontal lesions could not walk or imitate such actions as kicking, tracing symbols with the foot, or walking. Adams and Victor (1977/1981) described the difficulty as follows: feet separation greater than normal; slight postural flexion; short hesitant steps with some imbalance; feet "glued" to the floor resulting in difficulty in advancing; and turning executed by one foot fixed as a pivot, the other slowly advancing in a circle with uncertain steps. If pathology is advanced, the patient cannot sit or stand and the limbs have variable resistance when passively manipulated (*gegenhalten*). In more severe disturbance with extension into the basal ganglia (especially the globus pallidus), the patient curls to "cerebral paraplegia in flexion," unable to do anything.

The definitions of frontal gait disorders in the literature are not entirely clear. Brun's frontal lobe ataxia, described as a unilateral decomposition of gait and upright stance (Adams and Victor, 1977/1981), has an obvious similarity to the magnetic apraxia described above. It has been suggested that apraxia for walking is a bilateral magnetic apraxia (Mayer-Gross, 1936; Meyer and Barron, 1960) of the type described by Denny-Brown with bilateral frontal lobe lesions.

Supplementary Motor Area Disturbance

Abnormal motor functioning following involvement of the supplementary motor area (SMA), situated in the medial surface of the frontal lobe (Williams and Warwick, 1975), was suggested first by Foerster (1936a) and later by Penfield and Jasper (1954). Stimulation of SMA may produce speech arrest or vocalization, retardation or arrest of voluntary movements, or complex contralateral movements (Penfield and Roberts, 1959). Only recently have detailed animal neurophysiological studies or effects on motor functions of lesions in this area been described (Gelmers, 1983; Wise and Strick, 1984). Damasio and Van Hoesen (1980) reported global akinesia and neglect in four patients with localized SMA lesions. If the lesions were unilateral, the deficits eventually became lateralized. No true apraxia was seen. The impairment was interpreted as a dysfunction in the "energizer" or "drive" for the initiation or willing of movements rather than a disturbance in the actual execution. A somewhat similar theory, including participation in programming of motor subroutines, was proposed on the basis of blood flow studies (Orgogozo and Larsen, 1979; Roland, 1984; Roland, Larsen, and Lassen, 1980a; Roland, Skinhoj, and Lassen, 1980b). The SMA is considered a region where input representing external demands and internal needs meet to initiate established motor programs and establish new motor schemes.

A 59-year-old right-handed man with a history of severe, widespread vascular disease including known occlusive disease of the right carotid, left vertebral, left internal iliac, inferior mesenteric, and right superficial femoral arteries suddenly collapsed. On admission to a local hospital he showed right-sided paralysis and mutism. His ability to repeat improved considerably better than his spontaneous verbal output. By 6 weeks the paralysis was confined to his right lower extremity and right shoulder, with a strong grasp reflex on the right side. Similarly, the language disturbance had improved to meaningful but hesitant verbal output, contaminated by paraphasia. The latter disappeared completely with repetition which was normal.

Of major interest was a problem in control of the right hand, which consistently interrupted manual tasks. Thus when attempting to write with his left hand, the right hand would reach out and take the pen away. When attempting to do block designs, the right hand would steal the blocks from the left hand's successful activities. Often the right hand would reach out and grab nearby items. The patient could not control this except by use of the left hand to forcefully grab the right hand and change its position. The patient learned to sit on his right hand, and the nursing staff provided a post in the proper position on his wheelchair so that the right hand grasp reflex strongly held the post. This "alien hand syndrome" passed within a period of 3 to 4 weeks, and the patient was discharged home where he has been totally self-caring. X-ray CT scan (Fig. 5-2) demonstrated total infarction in the left anterior cerebral artery territory.

A role in "conscious intention" for the contralateral SMA has been proposed (Goldberg et al., 1981; Laplane, Talairach, Meininger, et al., 1977). Goldberg et al. reported two patients who suffered left medial frontal infarction and showed transcortical motor aphasia plus right arm motor disturbance (a strong grasp reflex, motor perseveration, and forced grasping). While walking, their right hands might reach out and impulsively grasp a door knob or push a buzzer; but when the action

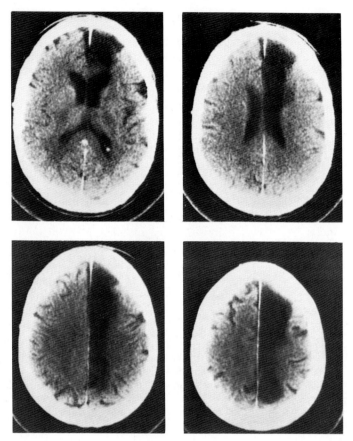

FIG. 5-2. Four x-ray CT scan views showing lucency in the territory of the left (left and right are reversed) anterior cerebral artery. This patient showed a marked "alien hand" syndrome at the time these scans were performed. (Courtesy of the Staff, Sepulveda (California) VA Medical Center.)

was completed it could not release the grip. The hand appeared to be "alien," as if the action was dissociated from conscious control. These patients learned to use the obedient left arm to control the alien hand, resulting in intermanual conflict (the Dr. Strangelove effect) (Bogen, 1979; Brion and Jedynak, 1972). One patient eventually learned to use verbal commands to control the problem (Goldberg et al., 1981). The authors suggested that similar observations with the left hand after pure callosal lesions (Bogen, 1979) might be secondary to right SMA damage caused during the callosal section operation. Patients with the alien hand syndrome have also been described by others (Mori and Yamadori, 1982). These movements, at least in some respects, resemble those of the magnetic apraxia described earlier. SMA pathology can produce significant motor disturbances without evidence of paresis.

Ideomotor Apraxia

This section describes a set of apractic syndromes in which the general symptoms are identical but their expression varies sufficiently in detail to allow separate identification and localization.

Bilateral Ideomotor Apraxia

Bilateral ideomotor apraxia is an impairment in the completion of voluntary movements in which the general intent or planning of an act is intact but the more elementary execution (but not speed or rhythm) is deficient (Hécaen, 1981; Heilman, 1979a). Asked to protrude the tongue (Jackson, 1878), whistle, make a fist, wave goodbye, and so on, the patient may fail totally or succeed only after an inordinate struggle (Brown, 1972; Goodglass and Kaplan, 1963; Hécaen, 1981). Similar difficulties may be seen in axial movements (stand up, walk backward), but these are often spared when both buccofacial and limb activities are failed. If asked to show how to brush teeth, the patient may use a finger as a toothbrush (body part for object) or rub the hand clumsily against the mouth. Movements may improve on imitation or with use of the actual object, but the gesture often remains impaired (Hécaen, 1981). Ideomotor apraxia has been defined as a dyskinesia of space centered on the body (DeAjuriaguerra and Tissot, 1969; Morlaas, 1928). According to this concept, the disorder is most obvious with central movements, such as making the sign of the cross or thumbing the nose. Others, however, report ideomotor apraxia occurring under a variety of other conditions, including movements away from the body, e.g., use of a hammer (Goodglass and Kaplan, 1963, 1979).

Lesions in individuals showing bilateral ideomotor apraxia are either bilateral or involve the dominant (left) hemisphere (Brown, 1972; DeAjuriaguerra and Tissot, 1969; DeRenzi, Motti, and Nichelli, 1980; Geschwind, 1967, 1975; Liepmann, 1905). Whether frontal cortical areas in the left hemisphere are involved has been debated. Many authors have suggested the parietal supramarginal areas or posterior perisylvian zones as most important (Brown, 1972; DeAjuriaguerra, Hécaen, and Angelergues, 1960; Geschwind, 1965; Liepmann, 1905). DeAjuriaguerra et al. (1960) also implicated the temporal lobe. Hécaen (1972, 1981) specifically excluded frontal involvement in ideomotor, ideational, or constructional apraxia. Haaland et al. (1980) reported that patients with ideomotor apraxia had additional motor problems. Those with left frontal lesions (apparently extending to premotor and prefrontal areas) had disruption of more complex movements that required inhibition of movement (i.e., static steadiness test) or sequencing of unique responses (i.e., grooved pegboard test). Frontal areas may be indirectly implicated in ideomotor apraxia with other motor deficits (Haaland et al., 1980). The absence of apraxia in patients with severe aphasia has been interpreted as involvement of right hemisphere parietal-frontal connections (Kertesz, Ferro, and Shewan, 1984).

Whether the frontal lobe is involved in ideomotor apraxia depends on theoretical/ anatomical concepts. Heilman and colleagues (Heilman, 1979a; Heilman, Rothi, and Valenstein, 1982) postulated at least two forms of ideomotor apraxia (Fig. 5-

3). Patients with lesions in the supramarginal gyrus cannot perform the required action correctly, nor can they discriminate clumsy from well-performed movements when they are demonstrated. They suggested that this defect is a consequence of pathological involvement in an area of visuokinesthetic engrams needed to carry out the complex movements. Lesions anterior to the supramarginal gyrus do not destroy these patterns but disconnect the visuokinesthetic engrams from the frontal motor areas that program and execute the actual movements. Although patients with lesions here fail to execute the movements correctly, they can discriminate quality of performance of the act. If this theory can be substantiated, frontal lobe lesions would cause a disconnection ideomotor apraxia. DeRenzi et al. (1983), however, noted that left frontal apraxia is not common and suggested that the pathway from left parietal motor planning areas does not necessarily run through

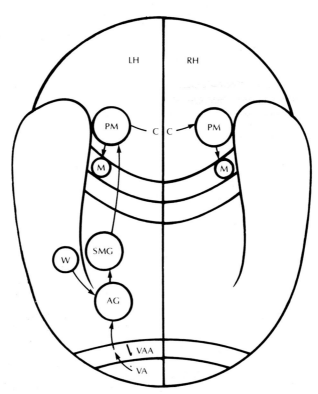

FIG. 5-3. This view from the top of the brain demonstrates Heilman's theoretical explanation of the pathways underlying apraxia. In comparison to Geschwind's schema (Fig. 5-4), two additional areas are specified: *AG*, angular gyrus; *SMG*, supramarginal gyrus. The latter is the center for visuokinesthetic engrams, the programs for sequences of movements for skilled acts. *VA*, primary visual area; *VAA*, visual association area; *W*, Wernicke's area; *PM*, motor association cortex (premotor area); *M*, motor cortex; *CC*, corpus callosum; *LH*, left hemisphere; *RH*, right hemisphere. (From Heilman: In: *Clinical Neuropsychology*, edited by Heilman and Valenstein. Oxford University Press, Oxford, 1979, with permission.)

left premotor areas; rather they proposed that the secondary pathway suggested by Kleist (1934b) via the parietal callosal connections is more common than considered.

Unilateral Apraxia (Sympathetic/Callosal)

The first documented case of unilateral apraxia was presented by Liepmann (1900, 1905), who reported a unilateral right-sided deficit in gesture (motor apraxia) in the Imperial civil servant Mr. T. On postmortem examination, lesions were present in the subcortical frontal rolandic region and the corpus callosum as well as in the left parietal area. On the basis of this and other findings, Liepmann and Maas (1907) postulated two types of unilateral apraxia: sympathetic and callosal. These concepts were later expanded by Geschwind (Geschwind, 1965, 1967, 1975; Geschwind and Kaplan, 1962), who postulated that for a right-handed individual to carry out an auditory command for movement of the left hand information must traverse the following left hemisphere pattern: auditory pathway–Heschl's gyrus–Wernicke's area–arcuate fasciculus–motor association cortex (area 6)–corpus callosum–right motor association cortex–right motor control region (area 4) for control of the left hand (Fig. 5-4). A lesion in the anterior corpus callosum could interrupt this mandatory pathway, producing unilateral left apraxia. Verbal information sent to the right hand would be intact, but verbal information necessary to control left hand movements could not cross from the left to the right motor association cortex

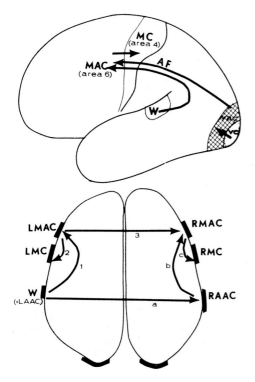

FIG. 5-4. Liepmann-Geschwind schema for apraxia. The top represents the lateral view, the bottom the horizontal section. *VC*, visual cortex; *VAC*, visual association cortex; *W*, Wernicke's area; *AF*, arcuate fasciculus; *MAC*, motor association cortex; *MC*, motor cortex; *L*, left; *R*, right. The arrows indicate major connections, and the numbers and letters indicate possible lesions. (From Geschwind: In: *Phenomenology of Will and Action*, edited by Strauss and Griffith. Duquesne University Press, Pittsburgh, 1967, with permission.)

because of the callosal lesion. Because callosal fibers connect cortical areas, the lesion could actually be in either the left or the right frontal subcortical tissues (i.e., white matter regions) (Geschwind, 1975).

A 42-year-old patient was discovered to have a glioblastoma involving the left frontal lobe. At surgery much of the left frontal lobe was found to be softened and cystic, and a frontal amputation was performed, revealing tumor throughout the resected lobe. During the procedure one branch of the anterior cerebral artery and some vessels on the medial surface of the frontal lobe were amputated. Postoperatively the patient had dense right hemiplegia and severe nonfluent aphasia, but this condition improved steadily and in 2 months he was capable of undergoing a series of neuropsychological tests. At that time the right leg remained severely paretic, but there was only a moderate weakness of the hand and arm; a strong grasp reflex was present in the right hand. He continued to improve and by the time of discharge only a mild weakness persisted in the right leg and right shoulder.

During this recovery a number of striking findings were demonstrated. For instance, although fully capable of carrying out actions to verbal command with his mildly paretic right hand, he would fail to perform these same actions with the left hand unless he could visualize right hand movement as a cue. Similarly, he failed to name objects placed in his left hand but succeeded with the right hand. He could, however, after-select with the left hand (i.e., when he failed to name an object placed in his left hand, that object could be placed in a sack with other objects and the left hand could select the appropriate object). He could write to dictation with his paretic right hand but was totally unable to write with his uninvolved left hand.

The patient eventually succumbed, and at postmortem examination both anterior cerebral arteries were found to be occluded with a resultant infarction that involved the entire anterior half of the corpus callosum (Geschwind and Kaplan, 1962).

Lesions that affect the left motor association cortex produce a "sympathetic" apraxia by destroying the left motor association origin of the callosal fibers, resulting in right hemiparesis and apraxia of the left hand plus (in most instances) Broca aphasia. If the patient was not hemiparetic, a right limb apraxia could be present as well.

Heilman (1979a; Watson and Heilman, 1983) followed the disconnection hypothesis but argued, based on the observation that most callosal patients are apractic to imitation and use of objects as well as to command, for disconnections of both language and visuokinesthetic engrams.

Hécaen and Gimeno (1960) described three major forms of unilateral apraxia, two with posterior lesions and one with mesial-frontal pathology. The latter, however, closely resembled Denny-Brown's magnetic apraxia and was more logically considered under the heading "melokinetic apraxia."

Buccolinguofacial (Oral) Apraxia

A 29-year-old right-handed male computer analyst suffered a left frontal cerebrovascular accident (CVA). CT x-ray scan revealed a lesion limited to Broca's area and underlying white matter. The patient was initially mute, with severe buccofacial apraxia, limb apraxia, and dysgraphia. Comprehension was preserved except for syntactical-relational material. The oral apraxia was dramatic; he was unable to perform complex acts to command (e.g., blowing out a match) and was clumsy with simple tasks (e.g., protruding the tongue). Spontaneously, these movements were performed normally. As he recovered, speech was slow and hesitant, but the linguistic qualities were correct except for minor tense agreement problems; he produced long and complete phrases and sentences. Limb apraxia disappeared. Six months after onset there was only minimal evidence of oral apraxia. His speech remained impaired, however, with increased difficulty in initiation and speed, as well as a dysprosody characterized by staccato-like verbalizations of multisyllabic words.

Oral apraxia is defined as the "inability to perform voluntary movements with the muscles of the larynx, pharynx, tongue, lips, and cheeks, although automatic movements of the same muscles are preserved" (DeRenzi, Pieczuro, and Vignolo, 1966, p. 50). The patient fails to perform nonverbal acts such as swallowing, moving the tongue, laughing, whistling, and blowing on command even though he can automatically chew food, smile, cough, blow out a match, and so on. It is difficult to distinguish oral apraxia from primary motor problems; in some instances the paralysis can be demonstrated to be unilateral whereas the buccolinguofacial apraxia is bilateral (Hécaen, 1981). The apraxia is more obvious in response to verbal commands than to imitation, although Poeck and Kirchensteiner (1975) argued that the way the information is presented is not relevant. The preserved ability to perform these tasks automatically probably reflects bilateral innervation of oral musculature.

The frontal localization of a lesion resulting in buccofacial lingual apraxia is usually said to be in the dominant anterior frontal operculum, i.e., the motor association cortex anterior to the face region of area 4 and very near Broca's area, including F1, F2, the base of F3, and the surrounding subcortical zones, anterior insula, and/or the deep internal capsule of either side (Alajouanine, Lhermitte, Cambier, et al., 1959; DeAjuriaguerra and Tissot, 1969; Geschwind, 1965, 1975; Hécaen, 1981; Tognola and Vignolo, 1980). Although the lesion usually involves the dominant hemisphere, Hécaen (1981) reported that right hemisphere lesions have been mentioned by some authors (Goldstein, 1909; Hartmann, 1907; Rose, 1908). Buccofacial apraxia has been reported, although less frequently, after posterior lesions (Benson, Sheremata, Bouchard, et al., 1973; Heilman, Rothi, and Kertesz, 1983a; Kertesz, 1979), perhaps of an ideomotor type (Kleist, 1934b). Multiple nonverbal oral movements in a series were less specifically localized within the left hemisphere (Mateer, 1978; Mateer and Kimura, 1977).

Verbal Apraxia; Apraxia of Speech

Closely allied with deficits in nonverbal gesture are problems in articulatory motor control. Although all articulatory motor problems are frequently labeled apraxia, this uncritical use of the term produces considerable controversy. Some have suggested that speech disturbances secondary to cortical pathology (cortical dysarthria) can be distinguished from the dysarthria of subcortical brain disturbance (Trost and Cantner, 1974). They suggested that cortical dysarthria tends to produce inconsistent articulation errors, substitutions of individual phonemes in contrast to distortions, no major vocal musculature paralysis, greater latency in speech production, and greater problems with initial than subsequent phonemes.

Two terms are commonly used by speech pathologists for the speech articulation disturbance that occurs with dominant hemisphere cortical damage: verbal apraxia and apraxia of speech. Many speech pathologists use verbal apraxia to represent the verbal output abnormalities characteristic of anterior language disorders (i.e., Broca aphasia). It consists of a sparse verbal output, produced with effort, poorly articulated, and showing short phase length and poor melody (Trost and Cantner, 1974). Apraxia of speech, as used by speech pathologists, is thought to be different and has been defined as "an articulatory disorder resulting from impairment, due to brain damage, of the capacity to program the positioning of speech musculature for the volitional production of phonemes and the sequencing of muscle movements for the production of words" (Darley, Aronson, and Brown, 1975, p. 255). Because damage in the general vicinity of Broca's area is the necessary lesion, there has been considerable controversy over the association or independence of Broca aphasia and these entities. Most accept verbal apraxia as similar or identical to the output problem of Broca aphasia. On the other hand, apraxia of speech is considered by some to be a fully independent disorder that might have Broca aphasia superimposed but can exist as a separate finding and is important to aphasia rehabilitation efforts (Darley et al., 1975).

Martin (1974), 1975) stated that there can be no speech–language dichotomy, as even the selection of phonemes is bound by linguistic parameters and is therefore a linguistic task. Disruption of the language system results in an aphasic phonological impairment, and in his opinion a pure apraxia of speech is not possible. Others, however, have suggested that apraxia and aphasia are distinctive phenomena (DeRenzi et al., 1980; Goodglass and Kaplan, 1963), and cases of apparently pure apraxia of speech have been reported (Benton and Joynt, 1960; Itoh, Sasanuma, and Ushijima, 1979). Mohr et al. (1978) reported that pathology involving only Broca's area produced mutism or speech disturbance but not Broca aphasia. A full Broca aphasia syndrome resulted from a large sylvian lesion involving operculum, insula, and surrounding white matter. Mohr et al.'s description of the pure Broca's area aphasia resembles the findings reported as aphemia (Bastian, 1898; Benson, 1979). This topic is discussed more fully in Chapter 11.

Within strict definitions apraxia of speech appears to be a pure speech disturbance, distinguishable from disturbance of language (aphasia) and based on frontal motor speech malfunction. Deficits in programming motor acts of the mouth have been reported after focal area 6 lesions in the monkey (Rizzolatti et al., 1983). Such a cortical motor speech problem should co-occur with buccolingual apraxia. Some (Geschwind, 1965; Hécaen, 1981) have insisted that problems in phonemic articulation and nonverbal oral movements can be dissociated. De Renzi et al. (1966), on the other hand, proposed that both verbal and nonverbal intentional oral movements are controlled by one keyboard. A single lesion affects both, and any differential recovery is dependent on the complexity of the movement, nonverbal being less complex.

LURIA'S CLASSIFICATION OF APRAXIA

Luria (1973a, 1966/1980) defined apraxia as the inability to manipulate objects in specific ways, the defect dependent on the movement observed. To understand Luria's views of apraxia it is necessary to review his theories of motor control. He postulated that voluntary movement is normally performed by four neuroanatomically separate functional zones, fully interrelated but with each zone performing an identifiable role: (1) kinesthetic afferentiation, i.e., the gathering of information concerning the present state of muscle tone, body position, oral-pharyngeal status, and so on is a function of the postcentral association cortex. A synthesis of (2) visual-spatial afferentiation is provided by the parietal-occipital tertiary zones and provides knowledge of movement in space. The kinetic organization of movement, (3) kinetic afferentiation, is dependent on combined activity of the basal ganglia and premotor areas. These three areas produce a chain of consecutive, integrated actions that result in appropriate movements. The fourth area, the prefrontal cortex, responds to (4) goal-directed movement at two levels: (a) instinctive, where the goals are innate programs, and (b) complex, conscious intention, where the goals are formed with the close participation of verbal regulation.

In Luria's view a specific type of apraxia is associated with lesions involving each of the four areas. Two are associated with the posterior sensory functions, but the other two are specifically relevant to the frontal lobes. Lesions in the basal ganglia–premotor areas can result in what he called kinetic apraxia, the disorganization of the smooth, consecutive transition of single movements. Lesions in prefrontal regions result in the "inability of the patient to subordinate his movements to the intention expressed in speech, the disintegration of organized programmes, and the replacement of a rational, goal-directed action by the echopraxic repetition of the patient's movements or by inert stereotypes which have lost their rational, goal-directed character" (Luria, 1973a, p. 37). Both of these frontal system motor control disturbances were described in some detail in the preceding sections.

MISCELLANEOUS CATEGORIES

Many other disturbances are called "apraxias." These include such diverse activities as constructional deficits, unilateral neglect and dressing disturbances, ocular palsies, and speech dysfluencies. As a general rule, frontal lobe involvement is not present in most of these problems (Hécaen, 1981). In fact, a number of investigators believe that apraxia is an inaccurate term for these problems (Benson and Geschwind, 1971). The possible role of frontal lobe in construction and neglect is described in later chapters.

CONCLUSIONS

Disorders of motor execution are the most obvious of the frontal lobe functions. Clinical observations and research allow the following summary to be made.

1. "Frontal" neurological signs, excluding paresis or paralysis, are not reliable indicators of the presence or absence of focal frontal lobe damage.

2. Disorders of general motor activity are frequent after frontal lobe insult, ranging from a "pseudopsychopathic" restless, hyperactive state to a "pseudodepressed" hypokinetic abulia.

3. Motor impersistence appears to be related to disorders of attention and in this sense may suggest frontal damage. Correlation, however, has not been consistently specific.

4. Frontal lobe damage may cause apraxia. In particular, bilateral or unilateral ideomotor apraxia may be caused by intra- or interhemisphere disconnection. Other hypothesized frontal apraxias are magnetic apraxia, frontal apraxia of gait, and the "alien hand syndrome."

5. Pathology in the premotor frontal zone results in a disturbance of rapid and smooth transition of individual movements. Differences have been reported according to locations of the lesion along the vertical axis. Pathology in the motor association cortex anterior to the face area of the motor cortex, for example, results in "apraxia of speech" and nonverbal oral apraxia.

6. Extension of a frontal lesion into other areas, particularly subcortical, can result in specific motor disturbances. In particular, there can be a disturbance in inhibiting initiated movements.

7. Prefrontal damage results in disturbance of organization and control of motor movements.

Motor functions of the frontal cortex are a model of the diversity of frontal lobe function. Within the frontal lobes there appears to be a gross caudal-rostral differentiation in function, with the prefrontal cortex having a superordinate role of controlling and monitoring in relation to the more automatic functions of the motor system. Further differentiation of the role of the frontal lobes in motor activities and motor disturbances is likely—and necessary. In particular, the contribution of a general theoretical model to which neurophysiological and blood flow studies could be applied appears to be important for the accumulation of knowledge of the role of specific brain areas in motor movements (Fuster, 1984; Luria, 1973a; Paillard, 1982; Roland, 1984).

6

Attention

Although "everyone knows what attention is" (James, 1980), there is no universal acceptance or clarity of definitions. Attention can define the mental state, reflect a mental resource, or depict a mental process (Picton, Stuss, and Marshall, 1986). Mental state refers to the level of arousal, anticipation of specific information, and preparation to respond. Mental resource refers to the allocation of mental processes but also reveals the limited capacity of the organism to respond adequately when faced with multiple stimuli. Finally, attention is "a control process that enables the individual to select, from a number of alternatives, the tasks he will perform, or the stimulus he will process, and the cognitive strategy he will adopt to carry out these operations" (Moscovitch, 1979, p. 422). Directivity and selectivity of mental processes, whether involuntary or voluntary, have been considered to be the underlying, fundamental criteria of attention (Luria, 1973a).

In addition to the definition of the function, related areas require clarification. First, some definitions of attention allow relatively good correlation with neuroanatomical systems; others are more psychological and correlate poorly with recognized neuroanatomical substrates. Second, attention may be defined solely in terms of the tests used. Third, attentional disorders may indirectly cause impaired performance in other functions (e.g., memory). Conversely, attention is closely related to other functions described independently, in particular the phenomenon of inattention (see Chapters 7 and 9) and the concept of the executive system (see Chapter 14). Finally, additional deficits have been described with psychiatric disorders and as secondary to both focal and diffuse brain damage. Specific correlation with frontal lobe dysfunction is difficult.

Despite significant problems, the importance of attention as a facet of frontal lobe function demands a specific review. A brief outline of related animal studies is followed by the clinical observations and research studies of human frontal lobe patients.

ANIMAL STUDIES

Early research on monkeys with bilateral frontal lobe lesions suggested a deficit of memory (Jacobsen, 1936), but subsequent work suggested that the deficit was more parsimoniously interpreted as an attentional disorder (see Chapter 12). The frontal lobes appeared to be most important in maintaining attention over time, organizing information into workable chunks, and preventing distraction (Brody and Pribram, 1978; Finan, 1942; Fuster, 1980; Fuster and Bauer, 1974; Kojima and Goldman-Rakic, 1982; Malmo, 1942; Pribram and Tubbs, 1967; Suzuki and Azuma, 1977; Wade, 1947).

The specificity of these concepts to the frontal lobe may be questioned. The brainstem nucleus locus ceruleus seems to be important in habituation to irrelevant stimuli (Mason, 1981). This specific finding is not universally accepted (Pisa and Fibiger, 1983). Disorders of attention are caused by lesions in the ventral mesencephalic tegmental area of the frontal dopamine system (Simon, 1981). The hippocampus also appears to serve attentional functions. In cats, for example, hippocampal theta rhythm is strongly correlated with attention to environmental stimuli (Bennett, 1975). Hippocampal lesions reduce the orienting response in cats and rats (Hendrickson, Kimble, and Kimble, 1969; Rogozea and Ungher, 1968; Senba and Iwahara, 1974), particularly if the animal was involved in some other activity. Parietal lobe involvement in visual fixation may also be related to selective attention (Mountcastle, 1978; Mountcastle, Andersen, and Motter, 1981). In toto, a number of other brain areas apparently act in attention processes, and the interrelationship of these areas to results in various tests of frontal function is crucial. One possible model is the neuroanatomical theory of inattention (Watson et al., 1981).

CLINICAL OBSERVATIONS

"From the first examination of the *[frontal lobe]* patient, the disorder of attention is noticeable; it is necessary to repeat questions and orders several times to obtain a response" (Hécaen and Albert, 1978, p. 368). This description of an attentional problem following frontal lobe damage is common. Frontal tumors depress arousal and alertness, resulting in confusion and impaired attention (Hécaen, 1964); trauma (Goldstein, 1936b, 1944; Lishman, 1978; Stuss, Alexander, Lieberman, and Levine, 1978) and frontal lobectomy (Angelergues, Hécaen, and DeAjuriaguerra, 1955; Greenblatt and Solomon, 1966; Hamlin, 1970; Rylander, 1939) may do the same.

Human disorders of consciousness and attention are usually described as deficits in either arousal or attending. Arousal is the ability to be awakened, to maintain wakefulness, and to follow signals and commands; unconscious states (coma, stupor, lethargy) often indicate pathology in the mesencephalic reticular formation (French, 1952; Plum and Posner, 1980). Akinetic mutism, intact sleep–wake cycles but little observable cognitive or motor functioning, is a striking example of an attentional arousal disorder. The akinetic-mute patient is inert and speechless, with limited responsiveness despite apparently normal sensory-motor mechanisms (Bricolo, Turazzi, and Feriotti, 1980). Two types of akinetic mutism have been described based on lesion location (Benson and Geschwind, 1975; Segarra, 1970). Pathology in the mesencephalic-diencephalic region results in *somnolent mutism.* The patient is immobile and unresponsive, with eyes closed, suggesting somnolence. Strong stimulation elicits only a limited response. Posteromedial-inferior frontal and/or hypothalamic damage, on the other hand, produces *coma vigil.* The patient is immobile and silent but follows visual stimuli with eye movements, suggesting vigilance.

Clinical attentional disorders, generally described as the impairment in direction of concentration and effort to specific demands for a defined period of time, can be conceptualized along a tripartite neuroanatomical division along the frontal-diencephalic-brainstem system (Stuss and Benson, 1984).

First, focal pathology in the brainstem reticular activating system may result in "drifting attention" (Benson and Geschwind, 1975). If phasic (transient) attention is intact the patient can attend for brief periods of time, but the disorder in tonic (ongoing) alertness results in a return to the somnolent state. In this state the disorder has been called *stupor* (Plum and Posner, 1980). A somewhat higher level of arousal, where responsiveness is consistent but slow, is called *obtundation*. At the lowest level of arousal, nonresponsiveness, the disorder is called *coma*.

A second type, "wandering attention," is the converse of drifting attention (Benson and Geschwind, 1975). The patient is alert and cooperative but easily distracted, suggesting a defect in the phasic component of attention. Focal pathology, if present, affects the diffuse thalamic projection system. The disorder is more common with metabolic or toxic brain dysfunction and is comparable to the delirium described by Plum and Posner (1980). Stupor and delirium (drifting and wandering attention) represent poles of a continuum of attention. In one attention is not sustained, in the other it cannot be directed. The two states have also been described as hypoactive and hyperactive delirium, differentiated by reduced or heightened arousal levels (Lipowski, 1980).

Finally, a third clinical attentional disorder can cause a deficit in conscious, directed attentive behavior. Pathology would produce disorders of complex behaviors that demand planning, selection, and monitoring of performance (Stuss and Benson, 1984). It has been postulated that this may represent a disorder of the frontal-thalamic gating system, controlling the ascending reticular activating system (RAS) and somatosensory fibers and the descending frontal cortex tracts (Scheibel, 1980).

Disorders of directed attention may occur with relatively focal frontal lobe disorders manifested at times by inflexibility and perseveration, and at other times by impulsivity, distractibility, and rapid alternation of attention. It has been hypothesized that attentional deficits can occur with an abnormality involving any portion of the tripartite neural axis including the RAS, thalamus, and the frontal lobes and their connections. The specific site of frontal lobe involvement has been difficult to demonstrate.

A 53-year-old man suffered a closed head injury that caused mild left hemiparesis, bilateral frontal slowing on electroencephalography (EEG), and a deep left frontal hypodensity on computed tomography (CT) scan (Fig. 6-1A). One month after the head injury, his behavior was characterized by distractibility and confabulation, with inclusion of extraneous information into ongoing conversation. Although seemingly normal on tests such as digit span (eight forward), he had obvious difficulty maintaining directed attention. After successfully completing the Wechsler Memory Scale counting by threes task (1–4–7–10 . . .), he failed serial sevens (100–93–86 . . .) by perseverating

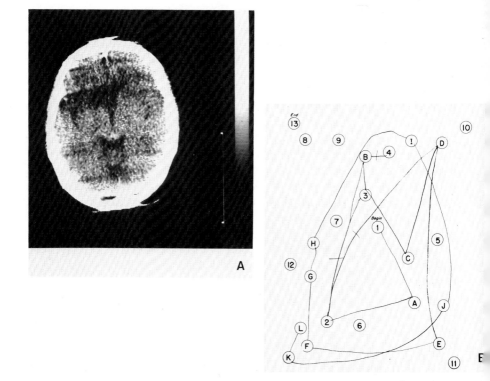

FIG. 6-1. Case study of a patient with a frontal lobe lesion. **A:** X-ray CT scan shows the deep infarct primarily in the left frontal lobe. **B:** On the Trail Making Test, Part B, the patient was unable to sustain the correct alternating response between numbers and letters. Crossed-out lines represent connecting lines that the patient was told were incorrect and was asked to redraw. The patient was not corrected after "C" in order to see if he could spontaneously alternate. (From Picton et al.: In: *The Brain, Cognition and Education*, edited by Friedman et al. Academic Press, New York, 1985, with permission.)

the subtraction by threes. He was aware of both the serial sevens task demands and his errors, saying, "Here I go with threes again." On the Trail Making Test, Part B, requiring alternation between numbers and letters (Fig. 6-1B), he merely joined the letters while verbalizing that he was forgetting to insert the numbers.

This case study illustrates impairment by perseveration and the inability to inhibit incorrect responses even though aware of the errors. The patient was alert and could maintain both tonic and phasic attention, but consciously directed behavior was severely impaired.

Confusional states represent a distinct classic entity, featuring an acute or subacute clouding of consciousness secondary to generalized brain dysfunction (Plum and Posner, 1980). At one level is mere clouding of consciousness; the patient is oriented but cannot think quickly and is easily distracted. At another level, the patient remains alert and can follow commands but is bewildered, distractible, and poorly oriented. Geschwind and colleagues (Geschwind, 1982; Mesulam, Waxman, Geschwind, et al., 1976) suggested a variant following focal right frontal or parietal lesions that disrupt the normal hierarchy of rules rather than alter arousal states. The major clinical features that have been described include: (1) loss of coherence with difficulty in selecting and maintaining attention; (2) paramnesias, including duplication of persons and places; (3) propagation of errors; (4) an elaborate verbal output that has been called occupational jargon (Weinstein and Kahn, 1955); (5) inattention to environmental stimuli; (6) pure agraphia (Chédru and Geschwind, 1972); (7) denial or unconcern about illness (Weinstein and Kahn, 1955); (8) playful and facetious behavior. Although often described as features of widespread, diffuse, or nonfrontal focal disorders, these findings appear to reflect either direct or indirect frontal lobe disturbance and resemble the case study described above (see also Chapters 7 and 8). Thus although confusion has been used to represent somewhat different states by different authorities, much of the symptomatology described appears to represent frontal dysfunction.

The basic disorder following acceleration–deceleration closed head injury (on which other disorders are often superimposed) appears to be an attentional deficit. After closed head injury, even when it is mild and after an apparently full recovery, problems may be demonstrated on multiple-choice reaction time tests (Van Zomeren, Brouwer, and Deelman, 1984); there may also be a slowness in adding pairs of successive numbers under time pressure (Gronwall and Sampson, 1974) and impaired maintenance of directed attention in the presence of interference (Stuss, Ely, Hugenholtz, et al., 1985). A disruption in the frontal-limbic-RAS control has been proposed as the underlying defect (Stuss et al., 1985; Van Zomeren et al., 1984).

A 49-year-old right-handed man was referred for neuropsychological examination because of poor performance at work. After 15 years on the job, he had never been promoted despite excellent performance on work assessment examinations. During the interview he spoke slowly, often failing to respond at all, or he presented a seemingly unrelated discourse after a question. It finally became apparent that he was responding to tiny details of the conversation rather than the general meaning. On examination, his performance on many tests was outstanding. His full-scale WAIS-R IQ was 136, Wechsler Memory Scale memory quotient was 135, and nonverbal Raven Standard Progressive Matrices was at the 99th percentile. Nonetheless, he had difficulty maintaining correct behavior, made many perseverative responses, was deficient in inhibiting interference in a memory task, and was slow in information-processing tasks. The history revealed that he had been involved in a serious motor vehicle accident 20 years earlier, with a combined coma-posttraumatic amnesia duration exceeding 4 months. Despite recovery of psychometric intellectual competence, his ability to process information rapidly and to direct responses was severely impaired.

This case offers a gross illustration of the disorder of selective attention that can follow closed head injury, a disorder poorly demonstrated by achievement tasks that primarily tap structured cognitive resources as did the IQ test. The demands of his job, however, even such simple tasks as sorting mail, elicited the deficit.

Disordered attention is also prominent in so-called functional states. Altered attention states represent one of the major psychological deficits of schizophrenia, not only in patients with active symptomatology, but also in subjects vulnerable to the disease (Asarnow, Steffy, MacCrimmon, et al., 1978; McGhie and Chapman, 1961; Zubin, 1975). Chapman's (1966) retrospective study of schizophrenics recovered from an acute psychotic break demonstrated serious attentional problems during the period prior to the actual psychotic episode. The disorder has been called hyperattention (McReynolds, 1960), narrowed attention (Venables, 1963), widened or overinclusive attention (Cameron, 1938; Shakow, 1963), and susceptibility to internal and external distractions (McGhie, Chapman, and Lawson, 1965). The most striking impairment occurs on tasks requiring planning and on sustaining behavior during distraction. These deficits resemble those described after frontal lobe injury (Seidman, 1983).

Decreased cerebral blood flow in the frontal lobes has been reported in chronic schizophrenia, suggesting decreased cellular metabolism (Franzen and Ingvar, 1975a; Ingvar and Franzen, 1974). Most cortical dopamine is present in the frontal lobes (Berger, 1981), and disordered dopamine regulation in the frontal cortex has been proposed as the underlying etiology of schizophrenic disorder (Joseph, Frith, and Waddington, 1979; Kety, 1980; Stevens, 1973). Major tranquilizers such as chlorpromazine used to treat schizophrenia have an ability to block dopamine activity in the brain (Carlsson, 1978). If a frontal abnormality underlies the schizophrenic attentional disorder, frontal leukotomy might improve the performance of schizophrenics on commonly used attentional tests, a finding suggested from postleukotomy testing (Stuss, Benson, Kaplan, et al., 1981a).

Attentional disorders have been implicated in childhood behavior and learning disorders to the degree that they are now called Attentional Deficit Disorders in *DSM-III* (1980). One variation combines an attentional disorder and impulsivity with increased motor activity; a second is a disorder of attention without hyperactivity. The behavioral similarity between some hyperactive children and frontal lobe patients (Stamm and Kreder, 1979) suggests that delayed frontal lobe maturation may underlie childhood attentional deficits. A similar hypothesis has been postulated to explain the impulsive acts and inability to learn from mistakes that characterize delinquent children (Pontius, 1972; Pontius and Yudowitz, 1980) (see Chapter 8). Circumstantial support for such a theory comes from experience with "self-instruction" or "self-taught" treatments for the attentional disorders of hyperactive schoolchildren (Meichenbaum and Goodman, 1971) and hospitalized schizophrenics (Meichenbaum and Cameron, 1973). A dissociation between what frontal patients say and what they do is commonly described (Luria and Homskaya, 1964). The self-taught procedure attempts to overcome similar problems in functional attentional disorders. Finally, the occasional effectiveness of medications that facilitate brain catecholamine actions (Barkley, 1977; Margolin, 1978) also suggests a relationship between attentional disorders and cerebral catecholamine systems.

In summary, study of human syndromes of disordered arousal and attention suggests involvement of the frontal-diencephalic-brainstem pathways. Some of the hypotheses generated from these observations, particularly those concerning the functional disorders, remain conjectural and must be viewed with caution.

NEUROPSYCHOLOGICAL RESULTS

The neuropsychological assessment of attention has serious deficiencies. Few tests are available, and these have not been carefully validated for different patient populations. The most frequently used tests are not derived from theories of attention, and improvement in the techniques for evaluation of attention, particularly for clinical use, has been limited. The ability to concentrate on a task without giving up or becoming distracted is most frequently evaluated (Lezak, 1976/1983). Vigilance tasks, the ability to focus attention, and the ability to perform divided attention tasks are less often assessed. None are truly specific.

Tests of Mental Control

Mental control tests assess the patient's ability to perform automatic tasks, to concentrate, and to complete a task without giving up or becoming distracted. Recital of the alphabet, counting backward by one or forward by three (Wechsler, 1945), and serial subtraction of sevens (Smith, 1967) are examples. Luria (1966/ 1980) described specific patterns of errors in frontal lobe patients on tests such as serial sevens (100–93–83–73 . . .), but other reports of test results have been inconclusive, with both patient and control groups making similar errors (Smith, 1967; Struckett, 1953; Stuss et al., 1981a). These tests have limited relevance unless performance is grossly impaired (Smith, 1967). Although the applicability of these tests for acute injury might remain valid (Ruesch and Moore, 1943; Struckett, 1953), there is little evidence for specificity to the frontal lobes. Patterns of errors may be a more useful indicator (Luria, 1966/1980) but of themselves are not diagnostic as both psychiatric patients and normal individuals make similar errors (Hayman, 1942; Smith, 1967).

Digit Span

The classic test of attention is the digit span (Heilbrun, 1958; Lezak, 1976/ 1983), a test considered highly vulnerable to brain damage (Black and Strub, 1978). Various measures have been considered most sensitive, including digits forward (Black and Strub, 1978), digits backward (Costa, 1975; Weinberg, Diller, Gerstman, and Schulman, 1972), or the forward-backward span discrepancy (Goodglass and Kaplan, 1979; Rudel and Denckla, 1974). Brain damage of different etiology and in different locations (Black and Strub, 1978; Costa, 1975; DeRenzi and Nichelli, 1975; McFie, 1969; Newcombe, 1969; Rudel and Denckla, 1974; Russell, 1972; Spreen and Benton, 1965; Warrington, Logue, and Pratt, 1971) including frontal lobe damage (Hamlin, 1970; Smith and Kinder, 1959) may cause impairment. The digit span, however, does not consistently show decline after brain damage (Rosvold, Mirsky, Sarason, et al., 1956; Sterne, 1969; Wheeler, Burke, and Reitan, 1963). In particular, many studies of frontal system disorders report normal digit span performance; these include patients with frontal gunshot wounds (Teuber, 1964), confabulators with frontal lesions (Stuss et al., 1978), trauma victims (Lezak, 1979), Korsakoff patients (Drachman and Arbit, 1966; Milner, 1962), and those who have had psychosurgical procedures (Mettler, 1949, 1952; Partridge, 1950; Petrie, 1952b; Stuss et al., 1981a). Similar negative results have been reported with visual presentations (Stuss et al., 1981a; Teuber, 1964). Regional location within the frontal lobes may have some bearing on results (Hamlin, 1970), and impairment might occur in the early stages after injury with subsequent return to normal (Lezak, 1979; Scherer, Klett, and Winne, 1957). In general, span tests have not proved particularly sensitive to frontal lobe pathology.

Digit Symbol

A performance subtest of the WAIS (Wechsler, 1955), digit symbol, is considered a good test of sustained attention, concentration, and speed of information-processing (as well as other factors) and a sensitive measure of brain pathology (Gonen, 1970; Hewson, 1949; Hunt, 1949; Smith, 1962; Wolff, 1960). Formal studies of digit symbol in frontal patients has not supported this finding, however (Mettler, 1949, 1952; Partridge, 1950; Petrie, 1952b; Hamlin, 1970; Stuss et al., 1981a), although it did distinguish operated from nonoperated psychiatric patients in early recovery stages (Lewis, Landis, and King, 1956; Mettler, 1949). As normally performed, the test may be too brief to demonstrate a decreased speed of processing; a slowdown that does not reach statistical significance has been noted in some frontal lobe and closed head injury patients (Stuss et al., 1981a, 1985).

Trail Making Test

One component of the Halstead-Reitan impairment index, the Trail Making Test, is also considered a good screening test for brain damage (Boll and Reitan, 1973; Spreen and Benton, 1965; Wheeler et al., 1963). When frontal patients are impaired on this test, the deficit is qualitatively striking (Fig. 6-1). Part B, requiring alternation between numbers and letters, is said to be particularly sensitive to frontal lobe damage (Reitan, 1958), but large bifrontal lesions may not cause impaired performance (Stuss et al., 1981a).

Stroop Test

The Stroop Test (Stroop, 1935) has an interference component requiring the subject to perform one response (name the color of ink in which a color name is printed) while inhibiting another (the reading of the word) and has been considered a measure of focused attention (Shiffrin and Schneider, 1977). Perret (1974) stressed the importance of the frontal lobes for inhibiting interfering stimuli and adapting behavior to unusual situations. Again, patients with large chronic bifrontal lesions have performed well on the Stroop Test (Stuss et al., 1981a). Whether this negative result reflected lesion localization or test insensitivity cannot be determined from the available data.

Miscellaneous Tests

Various other psychological tests have been used to assess the attentional disorder of frontal pathology. Patients with frontal epileptic foci performed normally on a measure of vigilance, the continuous performance test (Mirsky, Primac, Marsan, et al., 1960). Topectomy patients showed variable results on a similar task, impairment occurring only if the lesion involved areas 8, 9, and 46 (H. E. King, 1949). Orbital frontal lobe damaged patients were impaired on the consonant trigrams test of memory (Brown, 1958; Peterson and Peterson, 1959), a deficit interpreted as an inability to maintain directed attention to new information in the face of interference (Stuss, Kaplan, Benson, et al., 1982b). Sensitivity to interference after frontal lobe pathology had been reported earlier (Malmo, 1948; Malmo and Amsel, 1948). Finally, impaired performance of frontal lobe patients on many tests demanding multiple mental activities such as the Wisconsin Card Sorting Test could include a deficit in attention.

Event-Related Potentials

The effectiveness of event-related potentials as an index of attention in normal subjects (Picton et al., 1985; Schwent, Hillyard, and Galambos, 1976) suggested use of the technique to measure disordered attention in frontal lobe patients. A diminished negative waveform (processing negativity) in patients with lesions of the frontal lobe during a selective attention task suggested that the frontal lobes are important in the control of stimulus-set attention (Knight et al., 1980) but are not the primary generators of the attention-related negative waves (Näätänen, 1982). Although frontal lobe patients generated normal P300 complexes to expected target stimuli, electrophysiological responses to novel stimuli were deficient (Knight, 1984). The deficit was interpreted as an impairment in the control of attention and orientation systems.

In summary, the effect of frontal lobe damage on standard psychological tests for attention appears contradictory to the observed behavior. Subjectively, the frontal lobe patient shows impaired attention, but this is difficult to prove objectively, one cause for the "paradox of the frontal lobes." Close observation suggests that, in structured testing situations, the examiner acts as the frontal lobe for these patients, analogous to the use of external controls such as darkness in overcoming performance deficits in frontal lobe damaged monkeys (Isaac and DeVito, 1958; Malmo, 1942; Orbach and Fischer, 1959; Stuss et al., 1981a). Despite the consistently negative results of psychological testing, frontal lobe damage frequently interferes with attention. Inadequate control of factors such as age, etiology, chronicity, lesion size, and location cloud the picture. Moreover, commonly used psychological tests appear to be inadequate to test attention. The greatest problem, however, is the combination of inadequate definitions of attention and the use of inappropriate test batteries based on outmoded psychological theories. Attention deficit does occur in the frontal lobe patient but is not adequately probed by currently used psychological tests.

SUMMARY

Disorders of attention represent a frontier in contemporary neuropsychology (Geschwind, 1982). Although something is known about disorders of attention in frontal lobe damage, much more is to be discovered. Two important approaches are obvious. First, the determination of a precise theoretical definition of attention would allow development of directed neuropsychological tests. This would demand that attention be differentiated from other frontal disorders and that the relationship to phenomena such as inattention be clarified. The second approach would be to devise and validate attention tests on patients with both focal and diffuse brain disorders. Such investigations should be interdisciplinary, combining convergent evidence from different fields. It can be hypothesized that an integrated functional system will be revealed and that each cerebral zone involved with attention has a discrete role in the process with ultimate control of the attentional system being the domain of the frontal lobes.

7

Abnormal Awareness

Since Babinski's (1914) demonstration of total denial of hemiplegia, disturbed awareness of illness has been recognized and studied. Critchley (1953) reviewed this literature, presented a detailed classification of disturbances in the awareness of bodily ills, and described many cases from his own experience and from the literature. Weinstein and Kahn (1955) investigated and discussed the denial of illness, described a number of clinical findings that were seen with this disorder, and presented a theoretical explanation based in part on the psychodynamic postulations prevalent at the time. The denial of an obvious physical disturbance such as hemiplegia, blindness, or even amputation by the afflicted individual is dramatic and warrants behavioral investigation.

In agreement with many other investigators, Critchley (1953) suggested that parietal lobe dysfunction was a prime source of disturbed awareness. The investigations of Weinstein and Kahn (1955), however, clearly showed that parietal lobe abnormality, although often present, was not essential for clinical denial, and they postulated a more widespread malfunction. Although subsequent investigators have proposed explanations based on a variety of neural disorders, frontal lobe malfunction has not usually been considered a major factor. Nonetheless, some types of abnormal awareness have findings suggestive of frontal malfunction, and the most recent theories include frontal abnormality as a factor. This material is reviewed, syndromes featuring disordered awareness of bodily illness described, and the significance of frontal abnormality in unawareness syndromes probed.

DEFINITIONS

Many terms have come into use to describe disorders of awareness. A large number of terms were collected by Critchley (1953), and even more have been added subsequently, the totality making a significant contribution to the confusion surrounding this topic (Table 7-1). For brevity's sake only a relatively simple outline of the major varieties of disturbed awareness is utilized. A hierarchical progression of the difficulties of awareness (neglect, unawareness, unconcern, denial) is presented, but the division is descriptive only. Overlap of symptomatology is standard with alteration from one state to another based on physical condition (lethargy, fever, drug ingestion) commonly noted. Some additional terms currently in use are presented in context.

TABLE 7-1. *Terms describing disorders of awareness*[a]

Unilateral neglect
Anosodiaphoria: lack of concern about hemiparesis
Defective appreciation of hemiparesis, with rationalization
Anosognosia: unawareness of hemiparesis
Denial of hemiparesis
Denial of hemiparesis with confabulation
Hemidepersonalization ⎱ loss of awareness of one-half of body
Asomatognosia ⎰
Hyperschematia: undue heaviness or lifelessness of one-half of body
Phantom third limb
Misoplegia

[a]Adapted from Critchley: *The Parietal Lobes.* Hafner, New York, 1953.

Neglect

The most common disturbance of bodily awareness is neglect, a frequent finding in neurological evaluations. The disturbance is often called unilateral inattention, and the two terms, neglect and inattention, are used interchangeably. The modifier unilateral is not essential; inattention to nonlateralized disorders, although less commonly noted, do occur (e.g., pain asymbolia, Anton's syndrome). Unilateral neglect is commonly demonstrated in neurological practice by use of double simultaneous stimulation (DeJong, 1979). The patient is aware of somesthetic, auditory, or visual stimuli presented to either side, but when stimuli are presented to both sides of the body or space simultaneously, only that received on one side is recognized. The stimulus to the neglected side is said to be "extinguished." Careful study of this phenomenon demonstrates that increasing the degree (force) of stimulation so that the neglected side receives a considerably greater stimulation fosters recognition on both sides (Denny-Brown, Meyer, and Horenstein, 1952). Demonstrations of unilateral neglect are common in careful neurological examinations, and this focal attention deficit appears to be a key abnormality underlying the syndromes of unawareness. Several anatomically based explanations of unilateral inattention have been proposed and are discussed later.

Unawareness

A greater degree of inattention occurs in some patients and is best demonstrated by simple observations of routine activities. Again, the disorder may be unilateral or bilateral. These patients do not appear to be aware that they have a disability until the disorder is brought to their attention by another party. The degree of unawareness varies from mild (the patient who uses only one of the two limbs in most activities, although both are capable of movement) to severe (the patient who allows the hemiplegic side to be damaged by hot liquids, body pressure, etc.). A classic, easily observed demonstration of unilateral unawareness is the hemiplegic patient lying in a hospital bed who fails to acknowledge the presence of someone standing on the paralyzed side but immediately recognizes and associates with him when he moves to the nonparalyzed side. When asked about the condition, however, the patient with this degree of unilateral neglect recognizes, at least in verbal discussion, the presence of a significant disorder. Nonetheless, in many daily circumstances the degree of awareness of the problem is clearly deficient.

Unconcern

An additional problem present in many patients with the more severe degrees of unawareness described above is an attitude of unconcern. The patient acts blasé, appears apathetic, is not interested in his physical disability, and may provide lame excuses or rationalizations for unawareness of a portion of himself or his environment and for deficient physical performances. If confronted, the patient admits the problem but does not register appropriate concern (Critchley, 1957). A combination of unawareness and unconcern seriously interferes with rehabilitation measures and hinders recovery from brain damage.

A related but opposite disturbance of unilateral inattention has been called misoplegia (Critchley, 1953). In this state the hemiplegic patient, although manifesting unilateral inattention and often appearing unaware of the damaged side, displays a strong dislike for the affected limbs. Contempt of sufficient intensity to be called hatred is expressed; the good limb may be used to hit the paralyzed limbs, and the patient may bite or otherwise mutilate the paralyzed limbs.

A 63-year-old woman sustained two major cerebrovascular accidents (CVAs) over a period of 10 years, both involving the right hemisphere, leaving her with a severe left hemiplegia including flexion contractures of the upper extremity. Although the latter were painful and totally disabling, the patient often appeared unaware of her paralyzed side. At other times, particularly when both limbs were needed to carry out a project, she expressed disdain for the left side, stating that she hated it, wished it could be sawed off or given away, and at times was seen to both hit and bite her paralyzed left upper extremity.

Denial

The most dramatic and quite possibly the most easily recognized of the disturbances of bodily awareness, a total ignorance and denial of major, obvious disability, commonly has been called anosognosia by clinicians. First described by Babinski (1914) in several patients who had sustained left hemiplegia but denied any weakness, this extreme degree of denial has been demonstrated in a number of variations. In addition to the denial of hemiplegia, denial of blindness (Anton's syndrome) (see Chapter 9), headache, amnesia, amputation, and so on have been recorded. The patient with total denial may agree that the paralysis or blindness is present if the obvious defect is pointed out but within moments may again demonstrate total unawareness of the disturbance.

A hierarchy of disturbed awareness has been presented. Each disorder features some degree of inattention or neglect, with the ensuing entities aggravated by greater and greater degrees of cognitive disturbance. Although the degree of physical disturbance remains relatively fixed, alterations to the state of general awareness may totally change the patient's unawareness of the defects.

A 62-year-old man suffered a subarachnoid hemorrhage. A right middle cerebral artery aneurysm was demonstrated and successfully ligated, but the patient awoke with left hemiplegia. At first he adamantly denied the hemiplegia. At this time he was disoriented and had a retrograde amnesia covering at least 2 years prior to the surgery. When evaluated early one morning about 2 weeks postoperatively, he spontaneously described his paralysis, was oriented to both time and place, but had no memory of his cranial surgery. A full mental status evaluation was immediately undertaken; among other items, his digit span was six, and his conversation was coherent. After about 15 min of testing it was noted that he no longer responded in a coherent fashion; with retesting, his digit span had dropped to four. Specific questioning concerning his physical condition produced denial of any arm or leg weakness, similar to the earlier anosognosia. He was allowed to rest and by that afternoon was again aware of his hemiplegia. Over the next few days his general strength improved, and he never again denied the paralysis.

The disturbance of cognitive function in the above case probably represents dysfunction at the level of the reticular activating system, and, as such, widespread malfunction would be surmised. In addition to the change in memory function clearly demonstrated, there appeared to be alterations in a number of other cognitive functions. It is in the latter aspect, the associated cognitive disturbances, that frontal lobe malfunction appears to play a part in the syndromes of unawareness. To explore the effect of the frontal lobes on disturbances of awareness, a number of pertinent clinical syndromes are reviewed.

SYNDROMES OF UNAWARENESS

Anosognosia

Babinski's (1914) demonstration of ignorance and denial of hemiplegia was confirmed by others (Ehrenwald, 1931; Lhermitte, 1939), and the denial of hemiplegia was compared to other forms of denial of illness (Critchley, 1953; Weinstein and Kahn, 1955). For most clinicians, anosognosia is synonymous with the denial of left hemiplegia. By dictionary definition and for practical purposes, however, anosognosia is better defined as ignorance and denial of illness and can refer to any state in which the patient denies an obvious physical abnormality. Most reviews of anosognosia emphasize the presence of a physical disturbance plus some "clouding" of the conscious state (Sandifer, 1946; Spillane, 1942). The latter descriptions vary from a dream-like state (Hécaen and Albert, 1978) to flippancy and facetiousness (Weinstein and Kahn, 1950). The illness denied is most often left hemiplegia but denial of right hemiplegia is reported (Denny-Brown et al., 1952) and denial of blindness (Anton's syndrome) is a well-established entity (Anton, 1899). Three cases illustrate anosognosia.

A 57-year-old hypertensive man sustained an acute intracerebral hemorrhage involving the right putaminal area. On admission to hospital he was stuporous with profound left hemiplegia, left hemisensory loss, and left hemianopsia. Following a stormy course his condition stabilized, allowing behavioral observations. He was disoriented for time and place, could not remember his doctors' names, and actively denied any physical disability. When asked if he could walk or dance, he would immediately say yes; when asked to raise his arms or legs, he would raise the right limbs and insist that both arms or both legs had been raised. When his hemiplegia was demonstrated to him he would accept the obvious fact and repeat the examiner's statement concerning the cause of the disability but within minutes, if asked whether he had any disability, would adamantly deny hemiplegia. The denial state remained static for 3 weeks and then, over a period of approximately 1 week, disappeared concurrent with a demonstrable improvement in the state of amnesia. For several weeks following this recovery, however, he could easily be led into discussing his current activities as though he had no paresis.

A 68-year-old man with a history of angina and peripheral vascular disorder suddenly complained of severe dizziness and collapsed into a chair. He was hospitalized, and his condition stabilized, but it was noted that he did not appear to see. Formal tests of vision could demonstrate no evidence of visual acuity. Behaviorally, he was unconcerned, disoriented to time and place, and failed to learn new material such as the name of the hospital, although he easily discussed older information. His pupils reacted to light, but he was unable to describe objects placed in front of him, count fingers, and so on. When asked to perform such tasks the patient often confabulated, giving an incorrect number of fingers, descriptions of items different from those held in front of him, and so on. More often, however, he stated that he could not see the objects or the fingers clearly. He strongly denied any problem with his vision, excusing his failure by saying that the lights were dim, that it was the dark of night, that he was not wearing the correct pair of glasses, etc. X-ray computed tomography (CT) demonstrated bilateral posterior cerebral artery territory hypodensities. The behavioral disturbance, including both Anton's syndrome and amnesia, remained unchanged.

A 39-year-old male was brought to the emergency room in a comatose state with an obvious right parietal scalp contusion. His condition remained unstable for several weeks as his state of consciousness varied. Laboratory studies suggested contusion and swelling of the right parietal temporal cortex. There was, however, no paresis, significant hemisensory loss, or visual field disturbance. With improvement he manifested a striking inability to learn new material and adamantly denied the current hospitalization. When asked why he was in hospital he always replied that he was visiting; when shown that he was dressed in hospital garb he would say either that he was there to have his eyes checked or to have his feet evaluated. A retrograde amnesia obliterated approximately 4 years prior to the brain injury. Information from family members confirmed that the only times he had ever consulted a physician prior to the present illness was to have his eyes checked on one occasion and his feet evaluated on another. Approximately 10 weeks after the injury, the amnesia suddenly lifted, and over a period of several weeks the duration of the retrograde amnesia gradually shrunk. As soon as the amnesia lifted, however, the patient no longer denied the head injury (Benson and Geschwind, 1967)

As in each of these cases, almost all reported cases of active denial of illness have had some degree of either amnesia or confusional state (decreased ability to attend). These behavioral factors appear to be essential to the pathogenesis of anosognosia. The disturbed state of memory (amnesia or confusional state) appears to explain the patient's inability to remember the presence of a physical defect. Several features suggest that additional problems are present, however. The patient's inability to monitor the obvious falseness of his statements in the face of observed difficulties, the lack of attention to the disbelief of the attending staff, the crude unreality of proferred explanations, and so on appear to be important for the full syndrome of anosognosia. That the frontal lobe may be crucial to these monitoring activities deserves consideration.

Reduplicative Paramnesia

Originally described by Pick (1903), whose demented patient relocated the hospital to a place nearer her own home, reduplication of place has come to be called reduplicative paramnesia but is reported only infrequently. Paterson and Zangwill (1944) described two brain-injured soldiers who learned the name of the hospital in which they were recuperating but located the hospital in their own home towns. Weinstein and associates (Weinstein, 1969; Weinstein and Kahn, 1955; Weinstein, Kahn, and Sugarman, 1952) subsequently recorded a number of such cases. Reduplicative paramnesia has always been reported with coarse brain disease, and the syndrome is most frequently correlated with nondominant parietal injury (Benson, Gardner, and Meadows, 1976; Ruff and Volpe, 1981). Some investigators have noted that frontal lobe damage is common, and some suggest it may be mandatory for the development of reduplicative paramnesia.

A 29-year-old man sustained a head injury in a one-car traffic accident. He was unconscious for a period of several days and then had a stormy posttraumatic recovery period that included frightening visual hallucinations. There were no basic neurological deficits, but mental status testing showed a posttraumatic amnesia that slowly cleared. Over a period of 6 weeks he became oriented to time and place and learned the full details of the accident so that he could recite them correctly and with clarity. Nonetheless, he continuously misplaced the hospital (which he correctly named) to a distant army base where he had been stationed a few years earlier. The mandatory reduplication of the hospital persisted after he could learn new information despite many explanations of the true location of the hospital. Even after several weekend leaves to his home, he continued to name the hospital correctly but located it at the distant army base. Although the reduplication of place remained for approximately 6 weeks after clearing of the amnesia, the strength of the belief consistently decreased. When seen at follow-up several months later, there was no hint of reduplicative paramnesia (Benson et al., 1976).

A number of studies (Benson et al., 1976; Benson, Gardner and Meadows, 1976; Ruff and Volpe, 1981) have correlated the presence of reduplicative paramnesia with focal brain damage. All reported patients had evidence of right parietal damage, and most had obvious frontal lobe damage; in addition, it has been conjectured that the presence of amnesia in the early stage was evidence of temporal lobe or limbic dysfunction. In most reported cases, bifrontal structural damage was evident. One report (Ruff and Volpe, 1981) suggested that unilateral right frontal pathology (in addition to nondominant parietal damage) is sufficient to produce environmental reduplication. In addition, each individual with reduplicative paramnesia had undergone a notable alteration of emotional behavior that included an unconcerned attitude, a tendency toward apathy, some degree of euphoria, and inappropriate contentment with the current status. All authors postulated that a combination of cognitive disorders, including some impairment of memory function, some disturbance in topographical orientation, and some disturbance of awareness, was necessary to produce the syndrome. Reduplicative paramnesia appears to result from partial damage to a number of brain sites, one of which is frontal.

Capgras Syndrome

In contrast to reduplicative paramnesia, which has consistently been accepted as a neurological problem, another syndrome featuring reduplication, the Capgras syndrome, has always been discussed as a psychiatric problem (Enoch and Trethowan, 1979; Lehmann, 1975; Rudnik, 1982). Phenomenologically, the Capgras syndrome features reduplication of close relatives, well-known acquaintances, or personal possessions. The patient with the Capgras syndrome is convinced that a person, almost always a close relative, is an imposter who closely resembles but is not the original individual.

A 44-year-old man sustained a serious head injury including a large right frontal subdural hematoma when struck by a moving vehicle. There was a prolonged recovery with slowly improving amnesia; as clearing of the memory function was beginning, his wife arrived to take him home for a weekend visit in a new automobile. From that date on, the patient was convinced that the lady who had picked him up was not his wife but a second wife. The imposter resembled his first wife and had the same name and the same number of children, each of whom had the same names as his own children from his first wife, but they were each approximately 1 year older than his children. He believed that the house he visited was either his own house or a very similar house that had been built on the same property. He remained totally convinced that the lady who picked him up was not his true wife. He was satisfied with the situation, stating that his wife had probably got this friend to take her place and that there must be some important reason why his true wife was no longer able to visit him. The delusion remained fixed over a period of years despite constant arguments to the contrary. Localizing studies demonstrated bifrontal and right temporal lobe hypodensities consistent with old brain injuries (Fig. 7-1) (Alexander, Stuss and Benson, 1979).

The Capgras syndrome is only infrequently reported, usually as an unusual psychiatric syndrome. In fact, the delusion of reduplicated persons has often been accepted as prime evidence that the patient suffered from schizophrenia. Often, however, the only schizophrenic finding was the presence of the fixed delusion. Other evidence, such as family history, first rank symptoms, or other schizophrenic phenomenology, were often absent. More than half of the cases reviewed by Alexander et al. (1979) had evidence of some type of organic abnormality. Nonetheless, most cases of the Capgras syndrome recorded in the literature have no evidence of structural brain damage; the organic abnormality has far more often been nonfocal—disorders such as drug intoxication, degenerative dementias, metabolic encephalopathies, and so on. The relationship of the Capgras delusion to schizophrenia or other psychiatric disorder remains unsettled, although the simultaneous presence of both a psychosis and brain dysfunction has been proposed (Waziri, 1978).

In the Capgras syndrome, as with reduplicative paramnesia, the patient demonstrates an awareness of the correct data, such as the name and appearance of the family member, but cannot accept or act on these data as though they were real.

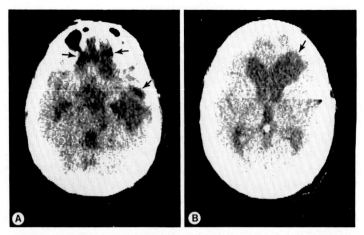

FIG. 7-1. Capgras syndrome. **A:** X-ray CT scan demonstrates bifrontal and right temporal hypodensity *(arrows).* **B:** There is moderate, diffuse ventricular enlargement with a particularly prominent right frontal horn *(arrow).* (From Alexander et al.: *Neurology (NY)*, 29:334–339, 1979, with permission.)

The delusions are firmly held, even in the face of absolute evidence of their falseness. The similarity between the Capgras syndrome and reduplicative paramnesia has been noted (Alexander et al., 1979), and the possibility that frontal malfunction plays a role in the Capgras syndrome, in a manner similar to that suggested for reduplicative paramnesia, appears rational.

Other Reduplicative Phenomena

Weinstein and Kahn (1955) listed three reduplicative phenomena (person, place, and time) observed in their extensive collection. In general, reduplicative phenomena are uncommon (Weinstein, 1969), and almost no pathological basis has been demonstrated. The resemblance of all reduplicative phenomenology to the cases of reduplicative paramnesia and the Capgras syndrome described suggest that all reduplicative phenomena may indicate frontal disturbance, an interference with the individual's ability to self-monitor and self-correct, but this has not been fully substantiated.

Confabulation

Confabulation, the production of false and bizarre responses to routine questions, is well recognized in both neurological and psychiatric literature, particularly in association with amnesia. In fact, the Korsakoff syndrome was once officially called the amnestic-confabulatory syndrome (American Psychiatric Association, 1952), emphasizing the importance of confabulation as a diagnostic feature. The incorrect information is most characteristically produced in response to a standard question but may be presented spontaneously. Confabulations range from a mild elaboration to a totally fantastic and wildly bizarre fabrication. Although discussed for many years (Berlyne, 1972; Bonhoeffer, 1904), most specifically as a distinctive feature of the Korsakoff syndrome (Victor et al., 1971), only in recent years have the mechanisms of confabulation been probed. Mercer, Wapner, Gardner, et al. (1977) demonstrated that in patients with amnesia the degree of confabulation did not correlate closely with either the severity of memory disturbance or the suggestibility of the individual. Instead, a close correlation was demonstrated between the presence of confabulation and the subject's ability to be self-corrective. As self-monitoring improved, confabulation decreased in quantity, even if the amnesia remained profound. The inability to be self-corrective suggested an abnormality of awareness, an inattention to the inappropriateness of the response being produced; it could be conjectured that this lack of critical control might indicate frontal malfunction. Although most individuals with an amnesic syndrome do not have evidence of frontal structural damage, the possibility that a functional disturbance affects frontal lobe monitoring activities deserves consideration.

To a different degree, several studies (Kapur and Coughlan, 1980; Stuss et al., 1978) have reported patients who spontaneously produced fantastic, bizarre confabulations. Each reported patient had evidence of significant frontal lobe structural damage. Kapur and Coughlan (1980) demonstrated that the quantity of confabulation decreased concomitant with improvement in the patient's performance on "frontal lobe tests." Shapiro, Alexander, Gardner, et al. (1981) verified the presence of confabulation in patients with frontal lobe damage and demonstrated that such patients had great difficulty examining the incongruities of their own verbalizations.

A 47-year-old man had suffered a ruptured anterior communicating artery. The aneurysm was successfully treated surgically, and there was no evidence of physical residua. The patient did not recover normal mental functions, however, and had to be institutionalized. When examined 5 years after the surgery he was disoriented for time and place and manifested severe problems in learning new material but showed no other cognitive deficit. His affect was generally euphoric, and he appeared inappropriately satisfied. Wild, bizarre confabulations would appear in the midst of a conversation that did not provide stimuli for the material in the confabulations. The occurrences described by the patient were fantastic, almost always sadistic and violent, usually including mutilation or death of members of his family. These were presented with a detached "Isn't that a strange thing that happened?" attitude. X-ray CT demonstrated marked ventricular enlargement, much greater in the frontal lobes than elsewhere (Fig. 7-2). Normal-pressure hydrocephalus was diagnosed, and a ventriculoperitoneal shunt was performed. Although the shunt decreased the size of the ventricles, it did not alter the patient's mental condition significantly (Stuss et al., 1978).

It appears that confabulation is a cognitive disorder that involves self-awareness and the ability to be self-corrective as well as some degree of disturbance in memory function. The full clinical picture manifests not only confabulation but a behavioral alteration featuring a general deficiency in reality testing that produces a strikingly abnormal relationship between the individual and environment. Actual damage to frontal structures is not reported in most patients who confabulate, but a number of patients who showed the severe, spontaneous confabulations reported

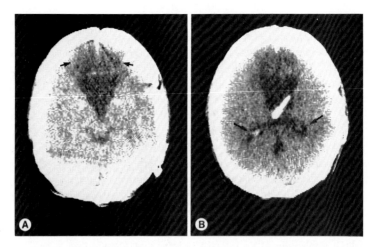

FIG. 7-2. X-ray CT of an individual manifesting spontaneous confabulation. **A:** There is an extensive decrease in density of both frontal lobes in the anterior cerebral artery distributions *(arrows)*, and both lateral ventricular horns are considerably dilated. **B:** At a higher level the ventricular shunt is seen in the anterior horn of the right lateral ventricle. The disproportionate enlargement of the anterior horns relative to the trigones *(arrows)* of the lateral ventricles is quite evident. (From Stuss et al.: *Neurology (NY)*, 28:1166–1172, 1978, with permission.)

above have had evidence of bifrontal structural pathology. Although not conclusive, this suggests that frontal malfunction may be an element, possibly a crucial element, in the pathogenesis of confabulation.

INATTENTION AND UNAWARENESS

Many investigators have suggested various localizations for inattention and abnormal awareness based on damage to a single or a precise combination of anatomical areas. In particular, the mandatory presence of right hemisphere disorder is included in many theories (Brain, 1941; Heilman and Van den Abell, 1980). The presence of thalamic (Watson and Heilman, 1979) or parietal (Critchley, 1953) lobe damage has also been popular. Complex theories have been presented, usually based on combinations of clinical observations and theoretical postulations. Although presented as separate and distinct, considerable overlap can be noted between the theories; several of these theories are presented.

Amorphosynthesis

Denny-Brown and colleagues (Denny-Brown, 1963; Denny-Brown and Banker, 1954; Denny-Brown et al., 1952) have proposed a cause of unilateral inattention based on damage to one hemisphere's perceptual system. They noted that each cerebral hemisphere is concerned with the opposite side of the body and of external space. Thus the right hemisphere processes information that arises from the left side of the body and from stimuli emanating from the left side of the individual's external space. Over the many years of an individual's existence the two hemispheres become extremely competent at gauging the relative degree of stimulation received. Thus when a weight held in one hand is transferred to the other hand, it is judged exactly the same by the two sensory systems. This type of judgment is practiced incessantly with similar observations made for the intensity of light, the intensity of sound, etc. coming to the two hemispheres (perceptual rivalry).

Amorphosynthesis is their term to suggest that damage to some aspect of one of the two sensory systems produces an inequality in this carefully balanced system; the hemisphere that now receives a decreased amount of stimulation needs a greater quantity of stimulation to reach a level of awareness of the stimulus equal to that of the undamaged side. Extinction on double simultaneous stimulation can be overcome by increasing the intensity of the stimulation on the damaged side. Thus unilateral neglect can be based on unilateral damage anywhere in the sensory system including the external sensory receptors (particularly somesthetic and proprioceptive receptors but also auditory or visual receptors), the sensory pathways of the spinal cord, brainstem, and/or appropriate diencephalic centers, or the sensory cortex. In fact, a sizable number of cases of unilateral inattention in clinical practice do show some degree of unilateral sensory disturbance, confirming the presence of amorphosynthesis. Although apparently real, amorphosynthesis alone does not appear to explain all features present in the varieties of unawareness described.

Frontal Inattention

Starting with the observations of the early neurophysiologists (Bianchi, 1895) and subsequent work by Kennard (1939) and Welch and Stuteville (1958), it has been recognized that damage to specific portions of the frontal lobe of animals could produce a transient disturbance of response to sensory stimuli. Although the anatomical ablations performed by Bianchi were crude, his observations of unilateral neglect were clearly correlated with damage to the frontal lobes. Kennard ablated portions of the arcuate sulcus of one hemisphere of a monkey, producing a complex behavioral syndrome including conjugate deviation of the eyes, forced circling (toward the side of the surgery), and a contralateral visual field defect, a "pseudohemianopsia." The visual field defect was total but transient, disappearing within 10 to 14 days. Kennard's work was replicated by Welch and Stuteville, who noted that the frontal lesion produced not only the transient hemianopic defect but also a transient loss of response to contralateral somesthetic and auditory stimuli. Thus monkeys lesioned in the arcuate sulcus of the frontal lobe unilaterally were temporarily unaware of all contralateral stimuli. For instance, when peanut butter was placed on the lips of a hungry monkey after arcuate sulcus ablation, the animal rapidly removed all food matter from the side of the mouth ipsilateral to the surgery but totally ignored that on the contralateral side. Welch and Stuteville did not believe that this represented a true sensory loss and suggested instead a severe unilateral inattention based on destruction of frontal lobe tissues. Frontal lobe neglect in the monkey may be secondary to dysfunction in distinct subcortical centers rather than the damaged cortical areas per se (Deuel and Collins, 1983, 1984).

In the human, Brodmann area 8 is considered roughly analogous to the superior lip of the arcuate sulcus in the monkey. Humans who suffer damage in Brodmann area 8 develop a conjugate deviation of the eyes toward the side of the pathology in a manner similar to that in the monkeys. Several cases with a unilateral inattention syndrome secondary to frontal abnormality have been described (Damasio et al., 1980; Heilman, 1979b; Heilman and Valenstein, 1972; Stein and Volpe, 1983). Unfortunately, these reports of human cases with precise localization of the caus-ative pathology have been rare, and the presence of an inattention syndrome in the human based on focal frontal damage must remain a question.

Reticulolimbic Inattention

As a follow-up on the frontal inattention animal work described above, Watson, Heilman, and colleagues (Heilman, 1979b; Watson, Heilman, Cauthen, and King, 1973; Watson, Heilman, Miller, et al., 1974) have lesioned various anatomical areas in monkeys unilaterally and observed syndromes similar to those described by Kennard and by Welch and Stuteville, but at least in some instances inattention has been permanent. One area lesioned was the cingulate gyrus and another the reticular substance of the mesencephalon; following unilateral damage in these areas the animal demonstrated unilateral inattention, neglecting the contralateral side in a manner similar to that following frontal ablation except for the persistence of the findings. To date, these experiments have been performed on few animals and have not been fully replicated, but the results agree with earlier observations. A specific circuit that includes reticulolimbic and frontal areas is hypothesized as essential for the maintenance of attention to the opposite side (Heilman and Van den Abell, 1980; Mesulam, 1981). According to this theory, damage to any of the noted structures or their connecting pathways can produce the syndrome of unilateral inattention (see Chapter 9).

Other Theories of Inattention

Clinically, some types of unilateral inattention are rather obvious and more readily correlated with clinical findings than others. This is particularly true of visual-spatial inattention; the tendency to neglect visualized objects has led to many theories concerning unilateral attention. Most observers have noted that left neglect is far more prevalent than right neglect, as demonstrated in drawings of clock faces and so on (Critchley, 1953), the ability to cross out lines (Albert, 1973), and omission of objects or facial features from appropriate tasks (Battersby, Bender, Pollack, et al., 1956; Gainotti, Messerli, and Tissot, 1972; Hécaen, 1962). Based on the frequency of left-sided neglect in clinical experience, many investigators (Benton, 1967; Hécaen, 1962) have postulated that the right hemisphere is dominant for visual-spatial activities. Mesulam (1981) thoroughly reviewed the literature on the suspected anatomical substrata of attention and emphasized the prevalence of right hemisphere disturbance in clinical observations and the importance of the right visual-spatial sensory pathways for attention. These observations come almost entirely, however, from constructional tasks, an activity in which the right hemisphere is conceded to be of major importance. Some have suggested that left inattention is an effect, not the source, of the constructional asymmetries (Arrigoni and DeRenzi, 1964). The frequency of right-sided extinction on double simultaneous stimulation to both somesthetic and visual stimuli in general neurological practice suggests that right hemisphere damage is not essential to produce focal inattention if the definition of inattention includes the extinction phenomenon.

Kinsbourne (1977b) has postulated an active, rather than a passive, explanation for unilateral inattention. Based on a combination of kinesthetic and sensory cues, he suggested that mutually inhibitory cortical control centers exist for right and left orientation, the rightward-orienting tendency being dominant. Unilateral pathology results in an imbalance, with excessive orienting to the side ipsilateral to the lesion. Right hemisphere pathology, for example, releases the potent and now uninhibited rightward-orienting tendency of the left hemisphere, resulting in a left inattention. The bias is not in relation to the personal visual field but to the end of the structured visual field defined by the presented stimulus.

Psychogenic Denial

Despite the anatomical explanations of neglect and inattention proposed in recent years, a strong underlying feeling remains that some or all of the denial of illness is based on psychodynamic factors. At least in part, this pervading feeling is derived from the unreality of the clinical situation. The patient in a hospital suffering an obvious neurological deficit who flatly denies the deficit and substitutes minimal problems or patently false explanations certainly appears to have a psychiatric problem. Many theories emphasizing psychogenic causes of denial have been proposed (Janet, 1920; Schilder, 1935, 1939), some utilizing classic Freudian defense mechanisms such as suppression, sublimation, and so on, others emphasizing psychosocial states, premorbid personality, and so on.

Weinstein and Cole (1963), in a retrospective study, compared individuals anosognosic for hemiplegia to patients with a similar but undenied hemiplegia and found that a higher number of the anosognosics had a history of denial. Thus they had tended to avoid medical care, to downplay personal problems, and were more rigid and work-oriented than the group who did not develop anosognosia. The differences between the two groups were not large, however, and there were many individual exceptions. It was difficult to state that anosognosia was clearly a product of a premorbid personality trait. More recent research which looks at the presence or absence of chronic pain following injury suggests a different picture. The pain-prone individual (Blumer, 1982) is described as rigid, compulsive, and hard-working; the injury breaks this habit pattern, and the maintenance of the pain syndrome allows permanent escape.

Several features of psychogenic denial deserve mention. Psychogenic (conversion, hysterical) unilateral neurological abnormality has been described frequently (Head, 1922; Weintraub, 1983). Most often the dysfunction involves the left side (Stern, 1977). Pertinent psychodynamic factors are frequently present in such subjects, but similar factors are so prevalent in the general population that it becomes difficult to accept that they cause a striking syndrome such as anosognosia in one individual but not in another. That psychogenic factors contribute to unilateral inattention or denial in some individuals can be hypothesized; that they are the major factor in most appears dubious.

SUMMARY

The descriptions of clinical disturbances of awareness and the proposed theories of abnormal awareness include a number of aspects that suggest frontal lobe involvement. Inattention (most often unilateral) apparently occurs with pathology involving a number of anatomical sites, one being the frontal eye field area. If there is a neural circuit underlying attention as suggested, the frontal cortex (and quite possibly anterior portions of the cingulate gyrus) appears to be important. Greater degrees of unawareness, such as unconcern, anosognosia, reduplication, confabulation, etc., probably demand simultaneous malfunction of several cerebral areas, with different degrees and combinations producing different syndromes. The specific behavioral abnormality (e.g., denial of blindness) may be dependent on a specific combination of brain abnormalities. Thus both nondominant parietal damage and frontal damage are reported in reduplicative paramnesia, and an anatomical study of Capgras syndrome showed nondominant temporal lobe plus bifrontal pathology. The few reports to date that support this conjecture are based on individual cases recovering from severe brain injury. Whether the frontal damage can be unilateral or must be bilateral to produce these syndromes remains totally unknown.

Although frontal structure damage has not been demonstrated in most reported disorders of awareness, the possibility of a functional disturbance involving frontal areas deserves consideration. Syndromes of disturbed awareness feature an inability to be self-monitoring or to self-correct (Mercer et al., 1977), and there is a growing belief that the almost uniquely human competency of self-awareness demands intact prefrontal function (see Chapter 17). It seems probable that some degree of frontal abnormality is necessary for all of the syndromes of disturbed awareness discussed in this chapter except for some cases of amorphosynthesis.

8

Personality and Emotion

Striking behavioral disturbances may occur after frontal lobe damage; these alterations are of sufficient magnitude to warrant clinical attention but sufficiently nonspecific that they have been difficult to characterize. "Frontal lobishness" is a term often used in referring to an association between the frontal lobes and certain alterations of emotion and personality. In this chapter we describe a number of the more common characteristics of the frontally damaged emotional state, discuss other disorders with superficially similar problems, and attempt to integrate and interpret this material.

A beautiful description of the altered personality following frontal damage is the classic case report of Phineas Gage given by Harlow (1868). Phineas Gage was an efficient and capable foreman of a railroad construction crew who sustained a severe frontal lobe injury when an iron tamping bar was blown upward into his left maxilla with the point exiting just to the left of the midline of the frontal skull (Fig. 8-1). Gage survived, and his physical recovery was essentially total; there was no paresis, aphasia, or other significant physical change. In contrast, his emotional behavior and personality were greatly altered. As described by Harlow (pp. 339–340):

> His physical health is good, and I am inclined to say that he is recovered .... The equilibrium or balance, so to speak, between his intellectual faculty and animal propensities, seems to have been destroyed. He is fitful, irreverent, indulging at times in the grossest profanity (which was not previously his custom), manifesting but little deference for his fellows, impatient of restraint or advice when it conflicts with his desires, at times pertinaciously obstinate, yet capricious and vacillating, devising many plans of future operation, which are no sooner arranged than they are abandoned in turn for others appearing more feasible. A child in his intellectual capacity and manifestations, he has the animal passions of a strong man. Previous to his injury, though untrained in the schools, he possessed a well-balanced mind, and was looked upon by those who knew him as a shrewd, smart businessman, very energetic and persistent in executing all his plans of operation. In this regard his mind was radically changed, so decidedly that his friends and acquaintances said he was "no longer Gage."

The correlation of localized brain pathology and behavioral alteration demonstrated in this case has been confirmed by additional observations in patients who had survived severe frontal lobe damage (e.g., Ackerly and Benton, 1947; Brickner, 1936). A variety of emotional disorders have been described, however, and the relationship of specific behavior patterns with the exact frontal locus of damage

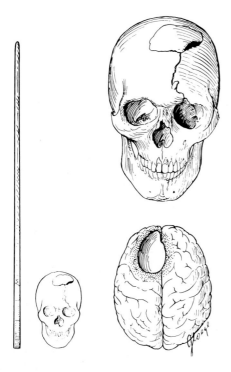

FIG. 8-1. Phineas Gage. On the left is the relationship of the size of the tamping bar to the size and location of the frontal skull lesion. On the right is an enlarged illustration of the skull defect *(top)* and an artistic rendering of the probable location of brain destruction. (From Stuss and Benson: In: *Neuropsychology of Human Emotion*, edited by Heilman and Satz. Guilford Press, New York, 1983, with permission.)

has proved difficult. Although a correlation between behavioral alteration and frontal lobe damage is widely accepted, the association of specific behaviors with specific areas of frontal lobe involvement has, with only a few exceptions, not been documented satisfactorily (Blumer and Benson, 1975; Damasio and Van Hoesen, 1983; Grafman, Vance, Weingartner, et al., 1985b).

Several reasons behind the limited correlation have already been outlined. First, precisely localized frontal lobe pathology is not common. Second, animal experimentation can provide only limited insight into the behavioral changes of humans following frontal damage. Third, the altered emotional state caused by frontal lobe damage may vary on the basis of premorbid emotional states.

Finally, but of crucial importance, orderly discussion of the emotional disorders caused by brain disorders of any locale has been hindered by a lack of consistent terminology. The terms that define aspects of emotion have not been used consistently. More than 1,000 words are currently used to describe various emotions. Conte (1975) selected 223 separate words used to represent various emotions in literary sources. Davitz (1969) asked a group of students to write brief descriptions of emotional experiences and compiled a list of 556 words and phrases used to denote emotion. In addition to these literary and "folk" uses, emotion has been described from the academic views of ethnology, psychoanalysis, psychophysiology, evolution, sociobiology, information processing, and a plethora of psychological theories. Each approach has produced a specialized and semi-idiosyncratic vocabulary. Hundreds of imprecise, overlapping terms are currently used to discuss emotion, a massive, ill-defined lexicon that seriously confuses the topic. A few major terms are defined here to serve as a guide for the following discussion.

Mood can be defined as a frame of mind or emotional state of a person [*Oxford English Dictionary (OED)*, 1979; *Stedman's Medical Dictionary (SMD)*, 1979], the internal expression of the subjective feeling tone (Hinsie and Campbell, 1970; *OED*, 1979). As such, mood may be specific (e.g., anger, joy) or may oscillate or swing (Hinsie and Campbell, 1970; *OED*, 1979; *SMD*, 1979). Mood is a relatively pervasive internal disposition, defined by or synonymous with the internal state of mind and often called "feeling tone." Mood does not signify the external behavioral manifestations that indicate emotion, however. Although often similar, mood refers only to the subjective, inner feeling.

Affect has a biphasic meaning in current terminology. It has been used to indicate a purely inward disposition, a mental state; in this sense the term "affect" is synonymous with mood, feelings, desires, and emotional tones; however, affect is used in this context almost exclusively as a contrast with reason (*OED*, 1979). Far more commonly, affect is defined as a set of physical aspects, the external manifestations, that reflect the feeling tone (*OED*, 1979; *SMD*, 1979; *New Webster's Dictionary*, 1975). Affect can thus be distinguished from mood in that it refers only to the external manifestations of feelings. In the use noted first, affect refers to a combination of the inner subjective feeling tone (mood) and the external manifestations (Hinsie and Campbell, 1970). Thus in one dictionary of psychology (Harriman, 1947), affect is defined as a general term describing emotion, feeling, mood and (usually) temperamental attributes. Affects are more pervasive and enduring than temporary emotional states, and are associated with drives and propensities. The contents of affects are vague and generalized. All definitions of affect emphasize the outward manifestations of the inner feeling with comparatively little association to reason or ideation. Although not common, an observed affect may not coincide with the individual's mood, as in the wild overflow of emotional expression of pseudobulbar palsy (Lieberman and Benson, 1977) or the observed euphoria of multiple sclerosis, which may disguise a significant depression (Trimble and Grant, 1982). Four clinically distinct affects have been described (Benson, 1985): mood relevant, verbal, nonverbal, and pseudobulbar.

Drive has been called a force that activates human impulses (*Dorland's Illustrated Medical Dictionary*, 1974), as an urgent, basic or instinctual need (*A Psychiatric Glossary*, 1980; *Webster's New Collegiate Dictionary*, 1979), or as an energy or strong motivating force that produces an organized effort (*New Webster's Dictionary*, 1975). Psychoanalysts consider drive a mental constituent, probably genetically determined, capable of producing a state of tension that impels the individual to act to alleviate the tension (Freedman, Kaplan, and Sadock, 1975; Hinsie and Campbell, 1970). Drive is separated from *instinct*, which is considered to be solely biologically oriented (*A Psychiatric Glossary*, 1980) as drive is also affected by learned incentives. Drive is thus defined as a force or need that energizes human activities.

Motivation is closely related to drive and is also considered a force that regulates, impels, or induces behavior by providing an incentive (*Dorland's Medical Dictionary*, 1974; Freedman et al., 1975; *New Webster's Dictionary*, 1975; *Webster's New Collegiate Dictionary*, 1979). Motivation is the source of energy that propels an organism to seek a goal or satisfy a need (Hinsie and Campbell, 1970). Although knowledge of the goal to be attained, forethought, planning, and anticipated gratification are more strongly emphasized in definitions of motivation, drive and motivation remain closely linked terms.

Emotion is a far more difficult term to define and, as suggested, is used both broadly and vaguely. The term may be used to suggest an agitated, excited mental state (emotional behavior). On the other hand, emotion is often given a more cognitive connotation than either mood or affect, although both of the latter are usually included within the scope of emotion. Emotion has been defined as "the affective state of consciousness in which joy, fear, fate and the like is experienced" (*New Webster's Dictionary*, 1975). Hinsie and Campbell (1970) suggested that: "In current usage, emotion and affect are used interchangeably, although some use *emotion* to refer primarily to the consciously perceived feelings and their objective manifestations, and *affect* to include also the drive energies that are presumed to generate both conscious and unconscious feelings" (p. 261). Benson (1984) defined emotion as a behavioral response, an admixture that includes the underlying mood, the effects on this of both verbal and nonverbal affect, and, in turn, the effects of both drive and cognitive control. Emotion is a broad term, encompassing a sizable number of behavioral responses that link bodily and mental activities to the underlying feeling tone. As such, emotion is a far more vague concept than either mood or affect and is difficult to use with precision.

Personality can be considered the sum of characteristics or qualities that make an individual a unique self and an intelligent being (*OED*, 1979; *SMD*, 1979; *New Webster's Dictionary*, 1975). As such, personality may be affected by a number of behavioral aspects including mood, affect, emotion, attention, memory, self-reflection, and so on. Personality encompasses the characteristic, and to some extent predictable, behavior-response patterns that each person evolves, consciously and unconsciously, as a style of life. It has been said to represent a compromise between inner drive and needs and the controls that limit or regulate the expression of these drives. Such controls are both internal (e.g., consciousness, superego) and external (reality demands). The personality functions to "maintain a stable reciprocal relationship between a person and his environment" (Hinsie and Campbell, 1970). Personality is even more vague than the terms previously presented but, in general, represents an amalgam of mood, affect, and emotion as described above with many cognitive, learned functions, the sum producing relatively consistent behavior patterns for an individual.

Alterations of mood, affect, drive, motivation, emotion, and personality have been used to describe the effects of frontal lobe damage on human behavior. The use of the terms has been vague, an understandable problem as the terms are difficult to define; unfortunately, review of the literature and presentation of data concerning the effects of frontal lobe damage on emotion have been significantly hindered by these imprecise definitions. Additional study will clarify the effects of frontal damage on emotional behavior only as the reactions can be defined specifically.

BACKGROUND

Emotional behavior is often obvious, and observations have been recorded since antiquity; theories concerning emotional behavior abound. The ancients described four humors—sanguine, choleric, phlegmatic, melancholic—intimating that emotional behavior at any given time was based on the prevalence of any one over the others (not unlike some current neurotransmitter theories). Other major postulations include evolutionary (Darwin, 1892/1965), physiological (Cannon, 1927; James, 1890), psychoanalytical (Freud, 1933), psychological (Chance, 1980), and anatomical (MacLean, 1949).

Most postulated schemes suffer limitations. On the basis of a few observations, a theory is hypothesized, supporting data are gathered, and the theory is presented as an explanation of emotion. Many investigations of emotional behavior evaluate only normal subjects, using external modifying factors as the main variable under study. Potential variations in response patterns among subjects has been largely ignored. Other investigators have utilized animal behavior, modified either physically or environmentally, and interpolated their observations to human emotions. Remarkably few reports of emotional alterations secondary to brain injury have attempted to dissect the behaviors. Both anatomical localization and psychological factors observed have been inadequately defined. Despite many current studies, the available knowledge of emotional behavior remains superficial.

The importance placed on the frontal lobe for emotional response varies. For some, the prime importance of the frontal lobes is accepted even though proof has been less than overwhelming. With a few exceptions, clinical observations have been only moderately helpful. Most current investigations of emotional behavior avoid correlation with localized brain dysfunction, and most of those that do avoid discussion of frontal lobe influences.

To discuss the position of the frontal lobes in emotional behavior, we review a mixture of animal experimentation and human observations.

ANIMAL EXPERIMENTATION

Because of their prominence, easy accessibility, and relatively good outlook following surgical ablation, experimentation on the frontal lobes of animals has always been popular. Bianchi (1895) and contemporaries suggested a crucial integrating function for the frontal lobes that affected all aspects of behavior. The neurophysiologists of the early twentieth century often observed behavior following frontal ablation (Fulton and Ingraham, 1929; Fulton and Jacobsen, 1935; Jacobsen and Nissen, 1937; Kennard, 1939), and their techniques were subsequently utilized by many psychologists to study frontal functions (Finan, 1942; Harlow and Settlage, 1948; Mishkin, 1964; Pribram, 1961). The correlation of primate observations with human emotional behavior remains largely conjectural, however. Emotion is difficult to define in animals, and the comparison of these observations with the far more complicated emotional reactions of humans is frustratingly inexact.

Butter and colleagues (Butter, Mishkin, and Mirsky, 1968; Butter and Snyder, 1972; Butter, Mishkin, and Rosvold, 1963; Butter, Snyder, and McDonald, 1970) suggested that orbital frontal cortical lesions produced a profound effect on emotional reactions in the monkey, whereas dorsal-lateral lesions had little or no effect. Sato (1971) also reported that the orbital and lateral cortices of cats were differentially involved in emotional adaptations to changes in environment. Rosenkilde (1979) further subdivided this correlation into five subregions of prefrontal cortex. The medial orbital area appeared to be most relevant for autonomic emotional reactions, whereas lesions in other areas resulted in behaviors resembling "frontal lobe personality." However, the premorbid emotional behavior of the animal appeared crucial. There is considerable agreement that, regardless of the species (cat, rat, monkey), frontal ablation does not drastically change the premorbid behavior; instead, the prior behavior becomes accentuated (Langworthy and Richter, 1939; Messimy, 1948; Richter and Hawkes, 1939; Sato, 1971). Sex and age are important variables in the emotional behavior resulting from frontal ablation in the animal (Pollitt, 1960; Tan, Marks, and Marset, 1971). In addition, no animal has a prefrontal cortex comparable to that in the human, and the observable emotional attributes of animals are far less complex than those of humans. At best, animal experimentation offers a limited approach to the effect of the frontal lobes on emotional behavior.

HUMAN CLINICAL OBSERVATIONS

Multiple observations on individuals suffering frontal pathology suggest characteristic changes in emotional behavior, but inconsistencies of the observed emotion are reported.

Frontal tumors have provided many observations on altered emotional status (Luria, 1965; Luria et al., 1964; Peterson, 1975). As early as 1884, Starr reported 23 cases with frontal lobe lesions and observed that the individuals lacked self-control and had a decreased ability to fix their attention. Kolodny (1929) described two frontal lobe behavioral alterations in patients with frontal lobe tumor. The first was a "psychic" change, defined as an altered mood, either exaltation or depression. The second was a change in "behavior" affecting social aspects, a decreased concern with social propriety. Holmes (1931) described three personality changes with frontal lesions: (1) apathy and indifference; (2) depression, automaticity, and incontinence; (3) restlessness, exuberance, euphoria, and "witzelsucht." These findings were confirmed by Stookey, Scarff, and Teitelbaum (1941), who noted that stupor and vesicle incontinence were also seen following frontal damage. The term "despontaneity" was suggested by Belyi (1979) as a major personality alteration in individuals with frontal lobe tumors. By this was meant a sharp decrease in initiative and spontaneous volition coupled with crude changes in emotional control and disorders of thinking. Belyi also suggested that alterations in behavior were dependent primarily on whether the tumor was unilateral or bilateral. Because of widespread effects, however, behavioral abnormalities noted with frontal mass lesions demand that symptomatology from other, more distant areas be considered.

A more voluminous group of reports concerned abnormal emotional status following traumatic injury, particularly gunshot wounds, to the frontal lobes (Faust, 1960; Feuchtwanger, 1923; Forster, 1919; Kleist, 1934a; Kretschmer, 1949; Lishman, 1966, 1968; Walch, 1956). Although terminology and emphasis varied, a consistent picture has evolved. Lishman (1968) summarized this and suggested a behavioral syndrome produced by frontal damage that included: "one or more of the following symptoms in severe degrees: lack of judgement, reliability or foresight; facetiousness, childish behavior, disinhibition and euphoria." Apathy would be added to Lishman's list by many. Geschwind (1977) suggested that three behavioral factors epitomized the frontal lobe injury: an unholy triad of apathy, euphoria, and irritability.

Depression, anxiety, aspontaneity, social withdrawal, and unawareness of the severity of cognitive deficit were reported following closed head injury (Levin and Grossman, 1978; Levin, Grossman, Rose, and Teasdale, 1979). Although this suggests frontal damage as a major factor, confirmation was not available. Roberts (1976) and Stuss and Richard (1982) described socially inappropriate behavior, outbursts or irritability, changes in attitude toward social mores, and a general lack of inhibition in long-term follow-up of patients with closed head injury. Again, frontal abnormality was implied. The prominence of frontal lobe contusion after closed head injury has been suggested as the reason for the frequency of personality changes after head injury (Bond, 1984; Teasdale and Mendelow, 1984).

Using examples of both mass lesion and brain trauma, Blumer and Benson (1975) suggested two distinct syndromes of frontal personality alteration. One, called pseudodepression, featured retardation of all activity as manifested by apathy, unconcern, lack of drive, and lack of emotional reactivity. This syndrome of frontal retardation occurred with pathology that involved either the anterior convexity, including the anterior poles, and/or the medial aspects of one or both hemispheres. In the second syndrome, called pseudopsychopathic, the major feature was disinhibition including facetiousness, sexual and personal hedonism, and a lack of concern for others. Orbital frontal pathology was present in the psychopathic variation. A distinction between possible emotional changes secondary to either dorsal-lateral or orbital/medial frontal areas has also been reported by others (Damasio and Van Hoesen, 1983; Grafman et al., 1985b). Orbital frontal cortex appears to be important in the regulation of mood states (Gray, 1981). These descriptions agree in general with Kleist's (1934a) review of World War I open head trauma cases.

It has long been surmised that the behavioral abnormalities of a number of chronic neurological conditions are based on frontal abnormality. A classic example is the "frontal" behavior of Huntington's disease, a disorder that primarily, if not exclusively, involves subcortical structures (Cummings and Benson, 1983). Alterations in frontal cortex are neither specific nor consistent in Huntington's disease, however, and a disturbance of frontal systems, a partial disconnection of prefrontal areas from subcortical structures, appears to be the prime disorder. Similarly, multiple sclerosis often produces euphoria, a behavioral abnormality common in frontal damage (Pratt, 1951); multiple sclerosis, however, has widespread pathology, and it is difficult to state that the behavioral disturbances are exclusively or even significantly based on frontal abnormality (Trimble and Grant, 1982).

Vascular infarctions focal to the frontal lobe are relatively rare; most cerebrovascular disease involves other parts of the brain, most particularly deep structures. In addition, with the exception of the relatively uncommon anterior cerebral artery occlusion, cerebrovascular disease of the middle cerebral territory involving frontal lobe tissue routinely affects parietal and/or temporal lobes also. Aneurysms and arteriovenous malformations that bleed into the frontal lobe often produce behavioral changes, but again widespread effects cannot be excluded. Central nervous system (CNS) syphilis was said to affect the frontal cortex more than many other areas, and the grandiosity, retarded depression, and other symptoms of tertiary lues have been ascribed to frontal malfunction (Wechsler, 1952). Once again, however, CNS lues is a generalized disorder with widespread cerebral involvement. Herpes simplex encephalitis appears to affect orbital frontal cortex, with extension to other limbic structures bilaterally (Damasio and Van Hoesen, 1983). Thus although some of the symptomatology of chronic neurological disorders resembles features seen in suspected frontal abnormalities, these disorders cannot be accepted as strictly frontal.

Patients who had undergone prefrontal psychosurgery (lobotomy, leukotomy, etc.) have been looked on as rich sources for behavioral observation, but these studies also suffer serious inadequacies. The early reports following frontal lobectomy described a number of personality alterations including inertia, lack of ambition, decrease in consecutive thinking, indifference to opinions of others, satisfaction with results of inferior quality, and poor judgment (Freeman and Watts, 1942). Rylander (1939) and Reitman (1946) noted extraversion, lack of restraint, increased motor activity (restlessness), and euphoria. Greenblatt and associates (1950) originally suggested that two major personality alterations followed more selective leukotomy: (1) lack of inhibition producing euphoria, restlessness, and purposelessness; (2) a slowness of thinking and acting producing a dullness, decreased emotional expression, and decreased interest and drive. Later, Greenblatt and Solomon (1966) reported four outcomes of "total bilateral frontal lobotomy": (1) decreased drive; (2) decreased self-concern; (3) depression of outwardly directed behavior and social sense; (4) shallow affective life. Some personality studies have described purely psychological alterations such as decreased neuroticism, depression, and intropunitiveness in the face of increased extraversion (Meyer, 1960;

Petrie, 1952a,b; Smith, Kiloh, Cochrane, and Kljajic, 1976). The type and severity of personality changes reflected the type of psychosurgery (Rees, 1973; Strom-Olsen and Carlisle, 1970; Tan et al., 1971), and the premorbid state, particularly psychiatric disease and seizures, clouded the picture. The localization of the psychosurgical lesion was poor, making reliable correlation difficult in all reported studies.

Not all reports agree that emotional change consistently results from frontal lobe damage. In a careful study, including a 6-year follow-up of four patients who had undergone excision of frontal lobe tissue, Hebb (1945) was unable to demonstrate any of the three mental changes suggested earlier by Holmes (1931) and suggested that the surgery had not yielded any interpretable evidence concerning normal frontal lobe functions. Also, many of the psychological tests used in early leukotomy studies proved inadequate. Both the Thematic Apperception Test (TAT) and Rorschach inkblot interpretations failed to reveal specific alterations (Scoville and Bettis, 1977). The Minnesota Multiphasic Personality Inventory (MMPI) was administered to many postleukotomy patients without conclusive results. Whether the inability of these formal tests to demonstrate personality alteration reflects an absence of behavioral alteration or inadequacy of the test has been argued; the latter appears most likely.

In summary, observations of humans after frontal lobe damage frequently reveal altered emotional behavior. These alterations have been described in a kaleidoscope of terms supported by a plethora of confusing data; nonetheless, some consistent features appear. The most common are decreased drive (apathy) and self-monitoring and a lack of control (disinhibition). The ultimate effect of frontal damage on emotional behavior is, to a considerable degree, dependent on premorbid personality. Correlation of behavioral changes with a specific anatomical locus has been, at best, crude. Drive and motivation appear to be most disturbed by pathology that involves the medial convexity and frontal polar structures, whereas disinhibition seems to be most pronounced following orbital frontal disturbance.

HUMAN CLINICAL INVESTIGATIONS

Relatively little formal investigation of the effect of frontal damage on emotional behavior has been reported. Few reliable tests of emotion and personality are recognized, and such studies can be performed only on humans. Luria (1966/1980; 1973a; Luria and Homskaya, 1964) has probably reported the most formal testing on individuals with frontal pathology but has emphasized a motor-cognitive approach. Luria's work provides a significant reservoir of information concerning the behavioral abnormalities following frontal damage but contains only classifications and interpretations of emotional change. Milner (1963, 1964, 1982) also studied patients who had undergone frontal and prefrontal ablation, but her testing was directed primarily at cognition. Emotional behavior was discussed by implication only.

Some investigations on the laterality of emotionality appear to offer insight concerning the position of the frontal lobes in emotional behavior even though not directed at frontal functions. Based on clinical observations, Gainotti (1972), Ross and colleagues (Ross, 1981; Ross, Harney, de Lacoste-Utamsing, et al., 1981; Ross and Mesulam, 1979; Ross and Rush, 1981), Bear (1983), and Geschwind (1977) suggested that the right hemisphere is of greater significance (dominant) for emotional behavior. Decreased emotional response (an anosognosic phenomenon) is more common following right hemisphere pathology, whereas depression and increased personal concern are seen more often with left hemisphere focal pathology (Gainotti, 1972). Ross and Mesulam (1979) noted that if a lesion involved the right frontal opercular area (the analog of Broca's area in the right hemisphere), the patient was unable to express emotion through either gesture or vocal melody. Other studies (Benton, 1977; Botez and Wertheim, 1959; Henschen, 1926; Ross, 1981) agreed that the right posterior, inferior frontal lobe was key to the expression of emotion. Tucker (1981) gathered clinical observations and research results to support the importance of the right hemisphere in emotion.

From a different approach, Robinson and colleagues (Robinson and Benson, 1981; Robinson and Price, 1982; Robinson, Starr, Kubos, and Price, 1983) have studied the occurrence of depression following cerebrovascular disease. Their findings agree with those of other observers (Gainotti, 1972) that depression is more common following left hemisphere damage; they also demonstrated that depression is far more common after left anterior (frontal) lesions than with left posterior lesions, with the severity of the depression significantly correlating with the proximity of the left anterior lesion to the frontal pole (Lipsey, Robinson, Pearlson, et al., 1983; Robinson et al., 1984; Robinson and Szetela, 1981) (Fig. 8-2). Robinson

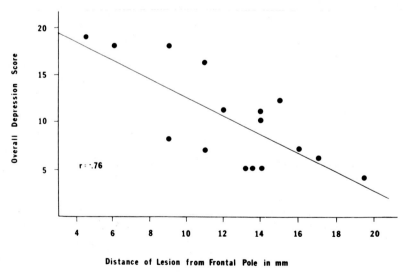

FIG. 8-2. Degree of depression with involvement of the frontal lobe by infarction. The further anterior the lesion is in the left frontal lobe, the greater is the degree of depression. (From Robinson and Szetela: *Ann. Neurol.*, 9:447–453, 1981, with permission.)

et al. suggested that the anterior-posterior dichotomy follows damage to noradrenergic pathways coursing from the mesencephalic-diencephalic junction to the frontal structures. The unexpected focal frontal abnormality underlying depressive behavior has been corroborated independently by metabolic studies using radioactive deoxyglucose and positron computed tomography. Phelps et al. (1984) used this technique to study patients with severe unipolar and bipolar depressive disease (Fig. 8-3). Asymmetry of metabolism was noted. The most marked hypometabolism was in the left hemisphere, and within the left hemisphere there was a gradient with the frontal structures more hypometabolic than more posterior structures. Successful treatment of the depression was followed by a return to normal rates of metabolic activity and hemispheric symmetry.

In an effort to investigate emotional responses of individuals with focal frontal lesions, Stuss and Benson (1983a) observed the emotional state and administered formal tests to 16 leukotomized patients and 10 nonleukotomized control subjects. The formal tests included selected portions of the TAT (Murray, 1943), a formal test of the ability to match facial expressions with verbal descriptions of emotion (Cicone, Wapner, and Gardner, 1980), and an Emotional Situations Test (specifically designed for use with these subjects) which probed the response to emotionally charged drawings (Fig. 8-4). Three major findings were noted. First, the emotional state proved difficult to assess by simple observation. The emotional reaction (affect) and the underlying mood were often hidden by the premorbid psychiatric problems. Although apathy and psychomotor retardation were often present, the subjects did not express depression and few mood swings were noted. The patients were poor at verbalizing their emotional state, and a lack of relationship between the patient's verbal response and the observed manifestations were suspected. All of the leukotomized patients had a history of schizophrenia, and many still showed

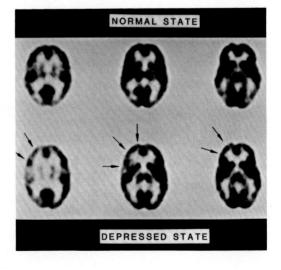

FIG. 8-3. Composite view of FDG PET scans of young patient during *(lower)* and after *(upper)* severe unipolar depressive episode. Note the asymmetric hypometabolism during the depression *(arrows)*, most pronounced in the left frontal area. (Reprinted from *Ann. Neurol.*, supplement to Volume 15, 1984 with permission.)

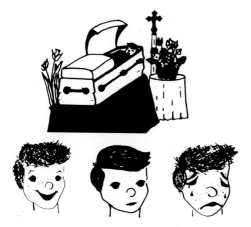

FIG. 8-4. Emotional Situations Test. Three possible types of emotional situation in pictorial form were presented to the subject: happy, sad, neutral. This example *(top)* depicts a sad situation. The facial expressions presented for matching to the emotional situation are shown in the lower half of the figure. (From Stuss and Benson: In: *Neuropsychology of Human Emotion*, edited by Heilman and Satz. Guilford Press, New York, 1983, with permission.)

active schizophrenic symptomatology. The emotional behavior of the leukotomized patients was too complex to be judged on a purely observational basis.

The leukotomized subjects, including those still seriously psychotic, gave responses to the TAT that were not significantly different from the nonleukotomized control subjects. The unstructured situation of the TAT, demanding projection of the subject's emotional responses, did not separate the effect of localized prefrontal damage from other states. In the second formal test, where facial expressions were matched, those leukotomized subjects with the largest orbital frontal leukotomy lesions did not perform as well as the normal subjects, but the difference did not reach significance; the other two leukotomy groups, those with lesser degrees of bilateral frontal pathology, scored as well as the normal controls. Bifrontal leukotomy lesions did not appear to cause disability in the matching of emotional facial expressions. This finding disagrees with an earlier report suggesting that the frontally damaged patients performed poorly in this task (Cicone et al., 1980). The latter study did not use matched controls, and the variations of age and severity of psychiatric disease in their subjects may account for the reported differences.

The third study, the Emotional Situations Test, did demonstrate significant group differences. Normal subjects performed considerably better than any of the frontally damaged patients or the schizophrenic control group. Although it could be assumed that the subjects still showing serious schizophrenia would perform more poorly than the normal subjects, a similar deterioration was noted in the relatively well-recovered subjects, those with the largest prefrontal leukotomy lesions. This result suggests that prefrontal damage may interfere with the analysis of the emotional aspects of a pictured situation.

Another finding of potential significance was noted. Only the normal control group presented abstract interpretations. Their response to the emotional situation might be correct or incorrect, but when challenged to support their answer they often produced metaphoric interpretations. Neither the leukotomized nor the nonleukotomized schizophrenic subjects did this. The nonleukotomized group often produced totally unrelated responses, often quite bizarre ("That's Bing Crosby, I think"; "That's what the pillar looks like unwrapped"; "Guilty of murder with a salad bowl"). In contrast, the leukotomized subjects noted similarities and relationships even when the interpretation was in error. Thus when a happy face was matched with a coffin scene, the subject's explanation was that the picture was happy because he, personally, was not in the coffin.

Stuss and Benson (1983a) suggested that the emotional abnormality of frontally damaged schizophrenics could be differentiated from that of the nonleukotomized schizophrenics, even though both groups performed poorly. The leukotomized subjects appeared to perceive emotion (Matching Facial Expressions Test) correctly but failed to associate the perception with a situation (Emotional Situations Test) correctly. Such a dissociation of perception and cognition could seriously affect personality, the individual with prefrontal damage being unable to translate his own mood or emotion into an appropriate behavior and, even more notable, responding inappropriately to emotion-laden situations. That these responses reflect the underlying psychosis appears reasonable, but their presence in the relatively well-recovered leukotomized subjects suggests some loss of self-monitoring.

PSYCHIATRIC CONSIDERATIONS

Although firm data demonstrating the exact effect of frontal pathology on emotional behavior are relatively scanty, few doubt that significant behavioral problems follow frontal damage. Against this background, the role of frontal malfunction has been postulated in a number of psychiatric disorders. Inasmuch as such considerations remain entirely conjectural, only a few of the more striking disorders are mentioned; even these discussions are based on hypotheses, not on proved correlations.

Delinquency, Sociopathy, and Episodic Dyscontrol

Among the most troublesome of all psychiatric problems are the antisocial personality disorders that may be called sociopathy in the adult and delinquency in the child. A multitude of explanations have been offered for these behaviors over the years (Glueck and Glueck, 1970; Hirschi, 1969), most of which emphasize deprived socioeconomic status or troubled interrelationships in the family, suggesting that the sociopathic personality develops in an individual estranged from family and society (Rutter, 1972). Inadequate familial discipline in the formative years appears to be significant (Robins, 1966), and heredity may be a factor but is difficult to separate from environmental factors (Schulsinger, 1972). Delinquent activity is prevalent in the adolescent and young adult, but the occurrence decreases sharply with advancing years (Robins, 1966), suggesting a factor of maturation, either physical or mental (Kiloh and Osselton, 1966). In addition, serious sociopathic aberrations are far more frequently noted in the male (Winokur and Crowe, 1975), reminiscent of other developmental problems such as stuttering and developmental dyslexia. The question of physical or emotional maturity can again be raised. In a phenomenologically similar condition called episodic dyscontrol, the individual recognizes the seriousness of his or her behavioral outbursts and expresses deep remorse for the misconduct but cannot control the actions during the episode (Monroe, 1970; Rickler, 1982).

The sociopathic individual recognizes what is right but fails to inhibit socially incorrect behavior, a description which resembles certain behavioral abnormalities that can follow frontal abnormality (Blumer and Benson, 1975). The sociopathic or delinquent individual may demonstrate full knowledge of what is considered right and wrong by society but acts in a hedonistic and therefore often asocial manner (Cleckley, 1964). This lack of cognitive control leading to an uninhibited hedonistic action is strikingly similar to behavior reported after frontal lobe damage (e.g., Phineas Gage, postleukotomy). The possibility that sociopathic behavior could be related to frontal malfunction has been recognized (Pontius, 1972). Several etiologies could be considered. Actual structural damage to frontal cortex and/or pathways can lead to uncontrolled behavior in the adult; similar damage during development may underlie the sociopathic behavior or episodic dyscontrol syndrome in some cases. Even more enticing is the possibility that a lag in the laying down of myelin (Yakovlev and Lecours, 1967) could be the source of frontal malfunction during the early years of physical maturation. Unfortunately, there is almost no real evidence to support either theory. In fact, only the characteristics of the behavior, the inability of the subject to act on knowledge, can be considered evidence to support a frontal abnormality theory at present.

Sensation Seeking

The behavioral characteristic of sensation or notoriety seeking also has the flavor of a frontal abnormality. The behavioral disinhibition reported as a consequence of some types of frontal abnormality (Blumer and Benson, 1975; Kleist, 1934a) could lead to this type of behavior. Here the response is not so much action without knowledge as disregard for the recognized social restrictions and/or an inability to disinhibit actions. Again, an explanation based on conjectural frontal behavioral abnormalities is enticing. It is easy to interpret the effect of frontal damage as a loss of the frontal lobes' inability to exert an inhibitory influence on cognitive, motor, or personality processes. In fact, some investigators call the syndrome of frontal damage the *disinhibition syndrome* (Hécaen, 1964; Lishman, 1968). Again, however, focal frontal abnormality has not been consistently demonstrated as the source of this behavior, and there is no real evidence that sensation seeking is based on frontal disturbance.

Extraversion/Introversion

Eysenck and colleagues (1947, 1952) developed a "personality" test demonstrating tendencies toward either outward action or inner response. A number of authors have stated that frontal damage leads to the main characteristics used to describe extraversion: disinhibition, euphoria, puerilism, and sensation seeking (Blakemore, 1967; Eysenck, 1967; Gray, 1970; Willett, 1960). Other investigators, however, either failed to support the frontal-extraversion correlation (Passingham, 1970) or suggest that other factors such as anxiety, depression, and neuroticism are the ones changed by frontal damage (Smith, Kiloh, and Boots, 1977). In contrast to extraversion, the introverted individual displays apathy, a dulled affect, decreased emotional display, weak initiative, restricted volition, and so on, behavioral traits that also suggest frontal lobe malfunction. Most of the formal psychological studies of extraversion/introversion have treated frontal damage as a single factor. The possibility that two diametrically opposed and anatomically distinct frontal functions were involved was not considered and may explain the failure of these studies to demonstrate conclusive alterations following frontal damage. Extraversion could more easily be linked with prior discussions of orbital frontal personality changes, whereas the introversion factors are consistent with descriptions of medial and anterior-polar frontal damage (Blumer and Benson, 1975; Kleist, 1934a). Again, although enticing, real proof that the traits demonstrated by the tests of Eysenck and colleagues actually emanate from or represent frontal abnormality remains weak.

DISCUSSION

Studies of the role of the frontal and prefrontal cortex in emotional behavior demonstrate several important facets. First, the investigation of emotional behavior is highly dependent on the definitions used; most current approaches are hindered and limited because they fail to define, with precision, the facet of emotion under study. Second, premorbid emotional behavior is a crucial element. The altered personality based on brain damage may be quite different in different individuals. With these caveats, an attempt can be made to integrate observations and investigations of emotional behavior with the neuroanatomy and the conjectured functions of frontal and prefrontal cortex.

The frontal lobe and its cortical-cortical connections appear to be significant for planning, initiating, and executing behavior as well as for monitoring the effect of actions on the external environment (Luria, 1966, 1973a; Nauta, 1971, 1972, 1973). The frontal-reticular activating system and frontal-thalamic connections appear to affect selective arousal and selective gating of information (Luria, 1973a; Scheibel, 1980). Damage to these systems seems to produce apathy and inappropriate behavior. Frontal-limbic connections also appear to be important for emotional control. Livingston (1969, 1977) described two separate but parallel circuits of frontal-limbic-hypothalamic-midbrain pathways (Fig. 8-5). Both the medial frontal-cingulate-hippocampus circuit and the more lateral orbital frontal-temporal-amygdala circuit seem to exert modulating effects on mood and behavior. Bear (1983) has described two separate cortical circuits important for emotional responses, both of which feature frontal integration for final activation (Fig. 8-6). A number of investigators proposed that the major neocortical representation of the limbic system

FIG. 8-5. Two limbic circuits. The dense synaptic connections of the medial limbic circuit structures with the diencephalic-hypothalamic-tegmental reticular core are illustrated on top. The basal-lateral limbic circuit connections with the dorsal medial thalamus are shown in the bottom half of the figure. (From Livingston: In: *Neurosurgical Treatment in Psychiatry, Pain, and Epilepsy,* edited by Sweet et al. University Park Press, Baltimore, 1977, with permission.)

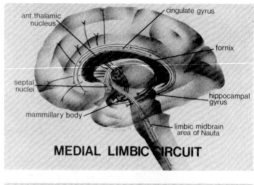

MEDIAL LIMBIC CIRCUIT

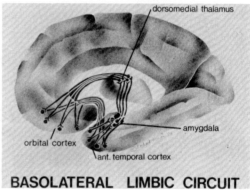

BASOLATERAL LIMBIC CIRCUIT

occurs in the prefrontal cortex (Fuster, 1980; Nauta, 1973): "The failure of affective and motivational responses of the frontal lobe patient to match environmental situations that he nonetheless can describe accurately could thus be tentatively interpreted as the consequence of a loss of modulatory influence normally exerted by the neocortex upon the limbic mechanisms by the frontal lobe" (Nauta, 1971, p. 182).

A second interpretation of frontal behavioral effects concerns the fact that information from the external environment, gathered through all modalities, converges only in the frontal lobe (Fuster, 1980). The ability to predict the consequence of a chosen behavior and to choose an alternative mode of action would thus be a frontal function. Damage to this "anticipatory selection process" may underlie some of the behavioral changes that follow frontal impairment. Such findings as flatness of affect, instability of intent, loss of ability to foresee the outcome of an action, socially inappropriate behavior, and so on may represent frontal loss (Nauta, 1971). Teuber (1964) hypothesized a corollary discharge mechanism for a number of complex mental functions, and Nauta (1971) postulated that such a mechanism would allow successive introceptive information to act as navigational markers and to provide "temporal stability of complex goal-directed forms of behavior."

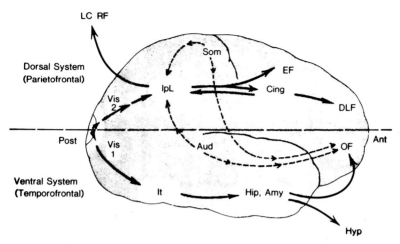

FIG. 8-6. Using the visual system as an example, two right hemispheric-dominant limbic pathways are depicted. The dorsal (parietal-frontal) system is important for surveillance of the internal and external milieu as well as appropriate arousal. The ventral (temporal-frontal) system has unimodal decoding and response responsibilities. LC, locus ceruleus; RF, reticular formation; Vis 1, ventral visual pathway; Vis 2, dorsal visual pathway; IpL, inferior parietal lobule; It, inferotemporal visual cortex; Som, somatesthetic pathway; Aud, auditory pathway; Cing, cingulate gyrus; EF, frontal eye fields; DLF, dorsolateral frontal cortex; OF, orbital frontal cortex; Hip, hippocampus; Amy, amygdala; Hyp, hypothalamus; Ant, anterior; Post, posterior. (From Bear: *Arch. Neurol.,* 40:195–202, 1983, with permission.)

Emotional changes resembling those seen following frontal pathology may follow damage to other areas of the brain. For example, Mesulam and Geschwind (1978) described emotional responses, similar to those that follow frontal damage, after right inferior parietal lobe pathology. Massive pathways connect the parietal lobes, the frontal lobes, and the cingulate gyri. Similar pathways connect the frontal and prefrontal cortices with most other portions of the CNS. "Frontal lobe" behavioral abnormalities could thus result from pathology at a distance based on separation of frontal structures from extroceptive sources. Behavioral differentiation of the effects of lesions at these different sites may be possible (Damasio and Van Hoesen, 1983).

In an attempt to correlate defined varieties of emotional behavior with neuroanatomically specific foci of damage, Benson (1984) outlined a complex matrix of interaction (Fig. 8-7). Mood, the underlying feeling tone, was linked with basal structures, including the upper brainstem, diencephalon, particularly the hypothalamus, and limbic structures. Affect was divided into four components—mood relevant affect, nonverbal affect, verbal affect, and pseudobulbar affect—each with a loose anatomical association. Thus mood relevant affect represented the outward demonstration of the basal activity. Right and left hemisphere activities were implicated with nonverbal and verbal affect, respectively, and of course pseudobulbar affect resulted from bihemispheric damage. Two additional factors in emotion—drive and cognitive control—were attributed to the frontal lobe, which served in a

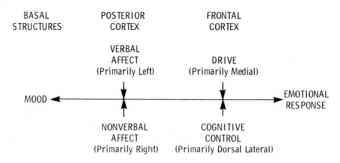

FIG. 8-7. Emotional responses as they are affected by various parts of the brain.

supervisory, executive role to the more posterior brain regions associated with emotion. The sum of these interacting factors produced an "emotional response." The number and variety of neuroanatomical regions involved in emotion is large, and most have direct connections to the frontal lobe. A wide variation in emotional behavior may occur on the basis of neuroanatomical damage in many brain areas, one of which is the frontal lobe.

SUMMARY

The complexity of the frontal lobes must be clearly recognized in any discussion of the position of their function in emotional behavior. The concept of a "frontal lobe personality" is woefully inadequate. Any study of emotion following frontal damage that is limited to a single factor (e.g., premorbid personality, response to specific testing, clinical syndromes, neuroanatomical locus of pathology) is not only inadequate but tends to be misleading. Any understanding of the effect of frontal lobe damage on emotional life demands integration of multiple studies over a broad spectrum of disciplines.

9

Sensory-Perception Functions

The frontal lobes are ignored by many in the analysis of sensation and perception (Luria, 1966/1980) for the obvious reason that they are generally known as motor areas, without primary sensory functions. Sensory-perception functions are viewed as complex but relatively passive processes. Many commonly used assessment techniques fail to discern deficits in sensation-perception in the face of prefrontal cortical pathology, particularly if simple tasks are used for evaluation. If perception is viewed as an active process, however, requiring coding and analysis of the perceived information, "there is every reason to suppose that a lesion of the frontal lobes, like a lesion of other parts of the cerebral hemispheres, is accompanied by changes in the various forms of perceptual activity" (Luria, 1966/1980, p. 328), although the changes are qualitatively different from impairment reported after damage in other brain areas.

This chapter reviews some deficits of sensory-perception functions that can be documented after frontal lobe damage. In theory, all sensory modalities are involved, but the focus is on the visual modality, where most research and observations have been performed. The material in this chapter is intimately connected with the chapters on visual-spatial abilities and awareness, the separation often being only arbitrary. Three major sections are covered: (1) unilateral inattention; (2) clinical disorders; and (3) visual search, followed by a brief summary of perception of melody after focal lesions.

UNILATERAL INATTENTION

The phenomenon of unilateral inattention has been experimentally demonstrated by both ablation (or lesion) and stimulation studies. The strongest and most consistent clinical observation is the production of unilateral neglect (hemi-inattention), an inability to attend, respond, or orient to stimuli presented to the side contralateral to the lesion. Although frequently a trimodal sensory deficit, unilateral inattention is most obvious in the visual modality and is emphasized here. Although the brain damage causing inattention is most commonly located posteriorly, particularly in the parietal-temporal-occipital junction (Hécaen 1962; Hécaen and Albert 1978; Heilman and Valenstein, 1972), frontal damage can produce unilateral inattention (see Crowne, 1983, for a detailed review). This may be secondary to dysfunction in connected subcortical regions (Deuel and Collins, 1983, 1984).

Frontal Eye Fields: Stimulation and Recording

The earliest experimental indication that the frontal lobes were actively involved in sensory-perception functions came with Ferrier's discovery that electrical stimulation in the frontal cortex caused conjugate eye deviation contralateral to the stimulation (1874; 1886). The finding was replicated and the technique used to delineate the so-called frontal eye fields (Barbas and Mesulam, 1981; Foerster, 1931; Rasmussen and Penfield, 1948; Robinson and Fuchs, 1969). The active zone lies just anterior to the face–hand junction of the premotor cortex, in the posterior part of the middle frontal gyrus. In monkeys the active area lies in the dysgranular periarcuate zone (Nauta, 1971). Denny-Brown (1951) noted that the deviation of both head and eyes follows stimulation in appropriate frontal, superior-temporal, or posterior parietal-occipital areas, but the lowest threshold for elicitation is in the medial two-thirds of Brodmann area 8.

Electrophysiological recordings from the frontal eye fields of normal rhesus monkeys, performed in the dark to minimize afferent sensory information from occipital regions, suggested that three types of cells discharged in the frontal eye field after eye movement has started (Bizzi, 1968; Bizzi and Schiller, 1970). The cells firing after initiation of eye movement were interpreted as the corollary discharge (Teuber, 1964) anticipating and preparing sensory areas for the future sensory input resulting from the movements of the eye, so that both elements can be incorporated into a perceptual behavioral unity (Fuster, 1980). In this manner some sections of the frontal cortex appear to subserve a combined sensory-motor function. There is suggestion of an additional specific voluntary command role. Certain visually triggered neurons in the frontal eye field show enhanced firing prior to the initiation of a saccade (Goldberg and Bushnell, 1981; Wurtz and Mohler 1976). Goldberg and Bruce (1981) have suggested that the essential signal activating the frontal eye field is the movement of the eye to the object to be perceived rather than the retinal location of the target. Stimulation and electrophysiological recording studies of the frontal eye field have gradually unfolded additional functions of this rather delineated frontal lobe area. The frontal eye field appears to play a role in the voluntary initiation of eye movements, as well as a combined sensory-motor activity after initiation.

Frontal Eye Fields: Ablation and Lesions

Animal research has long implicated the frontal lobes in visual inattention and more recently in a general sensory inattention syndrome. Munk (1881) reported temporary neglect in the contralateral visual field secondary to frontal eye field ablation, a finding that has been consistently replicated (Bianchi, 1895; Kennard, 1939; Kennard and Ectors, 1938; Welch and Stuteville, 1958). The full syndrome produced by this lesion includes the following: contralateral impaired head and eye movements; contralateral visual, auditory, and somesthetic neglect; ipsilateral conjugate eye deviation; ipsilateral deviated gaze fixation; relative disuse of the contralateral limbs; deficient tactile placing; and circling to the side of the lesion

(Crowne, Yeo, and Russell, 1981). Roux (1899) suggested that the causative lesion could directly involve the frontal eye field itself or connections with that area coursing through the internal capsule. Although visual signs have always been emphasized, trimodal sensory (auditory, visual, somesthetic) unilateral inattention has been reported secondary to frontal eye field lesions in animals (Crowne et al., 1981; Heilman, Pandya, and Geschwind, 1970; Welch and Stuteville, 1958). This inattention is commonly transient in nature. Whether a similar trimodal inattention occurs in man following frontal lobe damage is uncertain; clinical anecdotes support the possibility, but appropriate testing is rarely done.

A frontal source of unilateral inattention has been considered rare in man, perhaps reflecting the transient nature of the disturbance (Crowne et al., 1981; Doty, 1973). Reports of a "pseudohemianopsia," a lack of attention to visual stimulation from the contralateral side despite intact visual fields, are infrequent (Halstead, 1943; Jenkner and Kutschera, 1965; Thiebaut and Guillaumat, 1945). Even less common are descriptions of deficits similar to those described in the animal literature, such as forced circling (Silberpfennig, 1941). An incidence study covering all patients with frontal lobe pathology for 2 years in two hospitals uncovered only six patients with unilateral neglect (Heilman and Valenstein, 1972). Etiologies were varied, and the location of the lesion on the dorsal-lateral or medial aspect of the frontal lobe was mixed, three in each area. All had right hemisphere involvement, suggesting a preferential role of the right hemisphere for inattention, consistent with the reported predominance of right hemisphere pathology in patients with parietal lobe inattention (Heilman, 1979b; Heilman, Watson, Valenstein, et al., 1983b). The authors concluded that frontal lobe neglect was uncommon but not rare. Other reports have also indicated inattention after frontal pathology, certain cases having extension into other areas such as basal ganglia (Damasio et al., 1980; Stein and Volpe, 1983).

To date there is little documentation of differences between inattention caused by lesions in different areas. Heilman and Valenstein (1972) reported that, in man, few clinical signs (other than primary motor disability) differentiated frontal and parietal lobe neglect. In animal research, however, inattention secondary to frontal lobe lesions may be distinguished from those due to parietal pathology by signs such as head and eye deviation, forced circling, and a placing response deficit (Heilman et al., 1970).

In recent years two groups of experimenters have done a great deal of work to clarify the frontal lobe/inattention relationship. Heilman, Watson, and colleagues suggested that the basic deficit is an attention–intention impairment, controlled by a frontal-limbic-reticular loop. This theory is based on a series of experiments and observations that implicate, in addition to cortical areas, the cingulate gyrus, mesencephalic reticular formation, and intralaminar thalamic nuclei in inattention (Heilman, Schwartz, and Watson, 1978; Heilman et al., 1983b; Watson and Heilman, 1979; Watson et al., 1973, 1974). They proposed a right hemisphere dominant system involving cortical and subcortical areas mediating an attention–arousal–activation response as the basis for the frequently observed left-sided neglect.

Damasio and associates (1980) have replicated and embellished these findings. They suggested that the necessary lesion for unilateral inattention involves the supplementary motor area–anterior cingulate gyrus and their connecting pathways. Lesions in either the left or right frontal cortex, mesial or dorsal-lateral, can result in contralateral neglect (Damasio et al., 1980; Heilman and Valenstein, 1972). Damasio et al. (1980) suggested that mesial frontal pathology directly affects the supplementary motor area–anterior cingulate system and that dorsal-lateral frontal damage injures connections to this system. They included a striatal loop as well. In addition, although parietal area 7 is recognized as a command area for visually guided reaching and selective visual attention (Damasio and Benton, 1979; Mountcastle, Lynch, Georgopoulos, et al., 1975; Yin and Mountcastle, 1977), it also appears to be directed by the supplementary motor-cingulate zone, the "will" of visual attention (Damasio et al., 1980). Thus a frontal-parietal disconnection may underlie inattention, a concept postulated earlier by Mountcastle et al. (1975).

These theories successfully integrate much of the available information on inattention but lead to further questions. In particular, the role of the supplementary motor–cingulate gyrus connection must be clarified. Although Damasio et al. (1980) attributed an essential role to this area, Watson et al. (1973) could not induce neglect with ablation lesions in this region in monkeys. It remains uncertain if a correlation exists between components of the general inattention syndrome and specific lesion location. For example, Damasio et al. (1980) suggested that circling indicates involvement of the striatal portion of the loop, a postulate that deserves further evaluation. Stein and Volpe (1983) reported disordered sensory-motor activity with right frontal-basal ganglia lesions. Nevertheless, the entire relationship of unilateral inattention with the suggested anatomical substrates must still be considered theoretical and requires continuing investigation using techniques such as metabolic analysis (Deuel and Collins, 1984). While continuing this investigation, species differences in anatomy and function must be remembered (Markovitsch, 1984).

CLINICAL DISORDERS

Several sensory-perceptual disorders have been postulated as being secondary to frontal lobe pathology. Oneirism is a prolonged dream state even though the person is technically awake (Hinsie and Campbell, 1970). Many of the symptoms of delirium can be considered oneiristic. Oneirism is most often seen in conjunction with disorders that produce widespread symptomatology, e.g., toxic-metabolic disorders or subcortical lesions, but Hécaen and Albert (1978) suggested that oneirism may occur with frontal mass lesions. Although it can be conjectured that frontal tumors cause oneirism through pressure (cerebral edema) or disconnection of subcortical-frontal pathways, the symptom would still be related to frontal malfunction.

Paroxysmal hallucinations represent a second group of clinical disorders reported in patients with frontal tumors (Hécaen, 1964). These may be either unformed or complex visual hallucinations, auditory or olfactory hallucinations. Hécaen (1964) suggested that frontal pathology is not the direct cause; rather, invasion or compression of crucial brain areas is implicated. Others, however, have suggested that irritation of frontal-occipital or frontal-temporal pathways by frontal lesions may directly produce hallucinations (Shneider, Crosby, Bagchi, et al., 1961). In this view, the actual symptom is typical of distant cortical areas. From a clinical viewpoint, neither oneirism nor hallucination represents a primary sign of frontal disorder, but each can occur in patients with focal frontal lesions.

Anton's syndrome is a long-recognized clinical disorder in which the patient denies the presence of acquired blindness. The most frequent cause of the blindness in Anton's syndrome is bilateral posterior cerebrovascular occlusion infarcting the geniculocalcarine pathways bilaterally. The visual defect, however, may be entirely peripheral (Hécaen and Albert, 1978). In pure form Anton's syndrome manifests as an active, adamant denial of the blindness. The patient states that he can see, and no amount of contrary evidence alters this conviction, as illustrated in the case study in Chapter 7.

The degree of denial varies on a continuum. Some patients deny, some appear indifferent, and some admit to a visual problem but excuse the impairment as a secondary phenomenon due to poor lighting, old eyeglasses, and so on. A case study illustrates the latter phenomenon.

A 45-year-old man was involved in a head-on traffic accident that resulted in total blindness (due to bilateral optic neuropathy) and bilateral frontal lobe damage (Fig. 9-1). Upon recovery, he was alert and fully oriented, completely blind but without other obvious neurological deficit. He was referred because of denial of blindness, but his first complaint was of blindness. Although admitting blindness he explicitly stated that, with the proper light or in different circumstances (in his mother's kitchen), he would be able to see perfectly. He could accept that his statements were incongruous but would not or could not use such information to alter his conviction about the blindness. The blindness was due to a peripheral cause, but the inability to critically evaluate the deficit suggests an important malfunction due to the frontal lobe damage.

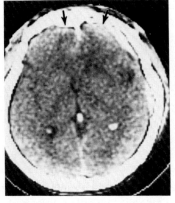

FIG. 9-1. X-ray CT scan of a patient with denial of blindness caused by bilateral optic neuropathy. The bilateral frontal lesions are indicated by the arrows. No pathology was noted in the occipital areas. (Courtesy of the Departments of Neurosurgery and Neuroradiology, Ottawa General Hospital.)

Some may prefer not to call this Anton's syndrome, reserving the eponym for cases with active denial. The difference appears to be one of degree only. Although denial was not active, the extreme indifference and unconcern, coupled with a failure to evaluate the opposing facts, produced a false conviction in the integrity of vision in other more familiar circumstances. This presentation is appropriately considered a defect of awareness (see Chapter 7); the similarity to Anton's syndrome and the implications concerning frontal disturbance cannot be ignored.

A number of theories have been postulated to explain Anton's syndrome. One implicates general intellectual deterioration (dementia) superimposed on the blindness, making it difficult to realize the blindness. Anton's syndrome has been reported, however, in a patient without any demonstrated intellectual, attentional, or memory deficit (Bychowski, 1920). Another theory postulated that the denial of blindness results from a simultaneous experience of visual hallucinations (Lagrange, Bertrand, and Garcin, 1929); many patients with Anton's syndrome report no visual hallucinations, however.

Another theoretical position notes the similarity of the Anton's syndrome mental defect with that of Korsakoff's disease, in terms of both the clinical characteristics and the vascular-anatomical distribution (Redlick and Dorsey, 1945). The denial can be compared to the confabulation frequently seen in Korsakoff's disease. The vascular distribution of the posterior cerebral artery includes the hippocampus and limbic circuit in addition to the posterior visual pathways, and pathology in this territory is known to result in a Korsakoff-like memory disorder (Benson and Blumer, 1982; Benson, Marsden, and Meadows, 1974). The blindness associated with the denial of Anton's syndrome does not have to be occipital, however, and this neuroanatomical-vascular explanation is appropriate only for this site of pathology.

Anton's syndrome has been explained as a disconnection syndrome, one that isolates the visual impairment from the cortical area necessary to evaluate and recognize the condition. Anton (1899) himself suggested that damage to the long association fibers would divorce the blindness from the rest of the brain, resulting in a deficit in recognition and awareness, outwardly portrayed as denial. Bychowski (1920) suggested that the essential problem was a deficit in the ability to criticize the erroneous statements concerning the derivation of stimulation. Although no new images are received, previous images are remembered, become elaborated, and are accepted as real. Thus Anton's syndrome would occur with impaired vision, dissociated from the frontal lobe evaluative and critical processes needed to recognize the defect. This description of impaired ability to monitor errors resembles other awareness deficits reported after frontal pathology (see Chapters 7 and 8).

In many respects, the last two propositions are similar. "Frontal" involvement has been suggested in Korsakoff's disease primarily because these patients are impaired on many psychological tests considered able to detect frontal pathology (Oscar-Berman, 1973). Confabulation itself has been postulated as a sign of frontal lobe disorder (see Chapter 7). The similarity of the behavioral characteristics of

Korsakoff's syndrome and of Anton's syndrome outlined above may be due to an underlying frontal system dysfunction common to both.

Another major clinical syndrome theoretically linked by some with frontal lobe disease is Balint's syndrome (Balint, 1909). Three signs characterize the syndrome: (1) a disturbance of gaze, called oculomotor apraxia by Cogan and Adams (1953), characterized by an inability to shift gaze voluntarily from a fixation point to a distant stimulus despite normal ocular movements (sticky fixation); (2) optic ataxia, a disorder of visually guided movements, demonstrated by the patient consistently missing when attempting to reach for a perceived object in space; (3) impaired visual attention, independent of any apparent general attentional deficit. Gaze is random until a salient stimulus enters the visual field and is seen and fixated.

Hécaen and Albert (1978) noted that all documented cases of Balint's syndrome had bilateral parietal-occipital lesions but that involvement of inferior-medial occipital zones was not mandatory. Many, but not all, cases of Balint's syndrome have frontal pathology, but the compulsory presence of frontal lesions is controversial. If it is conceptualized that both anterior and posterior lesions are required, the behavioral signs can be explained in the following manner (Hécaen and Albert, 1978). Bilateral parietal-occipital lesions would result in a sensory-perceptual deficit involving the peripheral fields. These areas are controlled, however, in an inhibitory manner by the frontal eye fields, Brodmann area 8. Unilateral posterior lesions cause no deficit of fixation, and bilateral posterior lesions would produce complete loss of inhibitory control and impairment of voluntary gaze control, allowing the eyes to wander in a disorganized fashion unless given a visual fixation. Similarly, when a stimulus crosses the central field, the frontal areas receive a proprioceptive impulse but no afferent impulse from visual responses, resulting in the psychic paralysis of gaze. Because of this, some have suggested that Balint's syndrome includes simultagnosia, although one defect is more pronounced (Milner and Teuber, 1968).

Even when posterior lesions alone are present, the frontal lobes may be involved through disconnection from the parietal-occipital area (Hécaen, DeAjuriaguerra, Rouques, et al., 1950); "it seems...that the full syndrome in its severe and complete form requires frontal lesions associated with those located posteriorly" (Hécaen and Albert, 1978, p. 234). The presence of frontal lesions is common (Milner and Teuber, 1968) and results in a syndrome that is "better defined and more persistent" (Hausser, Robert, and Giard, 1980). Variations in the syndrome and accompanying lesions, however, must be considered (Girotti, Milanese, Casazza, et al., 1982; Guard, Perenin, Vighetto, et al., 1984).

Thus evidence suggests that the clinical signs and syndromes of sensory-perceptual disorders associated with the frontal lobes appear to be either indirect manifestations based on proximity of frontal lobe pathology to other areas more directly involved or disconnection that separates a frontal controlling function from the associated brain areas. Frontal pathology can produce alterations in visual-sensory perception, but these are indirect.

VISUAL SEARCH

A disturbance in visual search is closely allied with visual inattention and is a prime illustration of impairment in the active aspect of sensory-perceptual functions. Luria (1973a, 1966/1980) divided the deficits of visual search into two categories: (1) disturbance of active searching; (2) inertia of gaze.

Disturbances of Visual Scanning and Searching

A visual search disorder is a deficit in the active component of perception. This active aspect selects, compares, analyzes, and integrates various optic stimuli. Clinically, it can be described as an inability to compensate for narrowed visual fields by scanning and/or by the perception of fewer details in a complex figure, and/or a defect in monitoring production, lack of motivation, impaired attention, and so on. The disorder is most strikingly demonstrated by simple but elegant experimental tasks. Analysis of the meaning of thematic pictures can demonstrate the basic deficit (Fogel, 1967; Luria, 1973a, 1966/1980; Luria, Karpov, and Yarbuss, 1966). For example, the patient may be presented with a picture of a man who has fallen through the ice. The picture contains a "danger" sign, e.g., people running toward the victim, as well as extraneous, irrelevant background information. Normal analysis of the picture would demand specific procedures. First, the theme or focus must be isolated from overall analysis of all details. A hypothesis concerning the meaning can then be formulated, compared to the picture content, accepted or rejected, and, if the latter, investigation continued.

Normal subjects have little difficulty performing the test. Patients with posterior lesions are adequate in their approach, although their perception may be distorted. Patients with frontal lesions tend to interpret the entire picture from a single detail, an isolate which may or may not be the central theme. The steps of purposeful searching, verification, hypothesis-making, and correction are limited. Verbal instructions from the examiner are not beneficial and do little to change the scanning strategy. Although the degree of disturbance may vary, the impairment in active analysis tends to be profound.

When the eye movements of a frontally damaged subject are monitored during the examination of thematic pictures, the disintegration of the active search process becomes visible (Luria et al., 1966) (Fig. 9-2). In free search conditions, the eye movements of normal subjects reveal an organized analytical searching pattern. When asked questions about the picture, their eye movements reflect a search for the relevant detail in order to answer the question. Frontally damaged patients, in contrast, show a disorganized, random search, a haphazard approach that is not altered by directing questions.

The Russian findings were replicated by Tyler (1969). Using a different technique for eye movement examination, he observed several deficits in two frontal lobe patients. Compared to normal subjects, there was little active scanning, longer gaze times at limited areas, but less gaze time on the informative areas. Frontal patients tended to analyze the picture in a "piecemeal" rather than an integrated, related

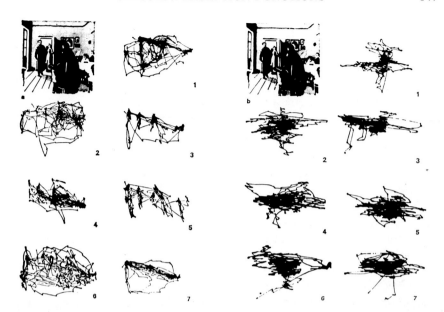

FIG. 9-2. Eye movements of two subjects while looking at a complex picture *(top left)*. Each number refers to a response to specific instructions (e.g., 4: How old are the people in the picture?). On the *left*, a normal subject has directed, organized eye movements. On the *right*, a subject with massive frontal lobe lesions has no direction in his analysis of the details of the picture. (From Luria: *Higher Cortical Functions in Man*, Consultants Bureau, New York, 1966/ 1980, with permission.)

manner; directed questions did not significantly change their visual exploratory behavior. There was a tendency to spend more time on the side of the picture ipsilateral to the pathology but no other apparent indices of unilateral inattention. Finally, the deficit was elicited only in the examination of complex pictures. The relationship to complexity was clearly described by Luria (1966/1980): "...the more complex the activity of perception, the more it necessitates a preliminary, planned approach to the material perceived, the more severely will the process of perception be disturbed in patients with frontal lobe lesions" (p. 331). Tyler (1969) concluded that the impairment is related to attention to and selection among different sensory inputs.

A more experimental psychological approach was used by Teuber and colleagues (Teuber, 1964; Teuber, Battersby, and Bender, 1949). Forty-eight patterns of various types (e.g., letters, numbers, shapes) were randomly distributed over the screen. The subject fixated a central window on the screen on which was projected one of the 48 stimuli. The subject's task, using necessary head and eye movements, was to search the entire screen to find the matching figure. Patients with frontal lesions, despite the absence of paresis of lateral gaze, had prolonged search times, particularly in the field contralateral to a unilateral lesion. This was interpreted as overactivity of posterior fixation functions, now acting independently of frontal eye field control. The deficit demonstrated by Teuber et al. resembles the disorders of impaired visual attention described for Balint's syndrome.

Guitton, Buchtel, and Douglas (1982) compared patients with unilateral lesions of frontal or temporal lobes in a voluntary saccadic eye movement task. In the standard saccade task, subjects had to look toward a target presented for 100 msec randomly flashed at a point 12 degrees to the right or left of fixation. Both groups of patients had normal latency and accuracy, regardless of visual field of presentation. In a second condition, termed the antisaccade task, stimuli were presented as in the first condition. However, the patient was now required to look away from the target stimulus to a corresponding position in the opposite visual field in order to detect the position of a gap in a square some 200 msec later. Although all subjects had difficulty inhibiting a response to the initial cue stimulus, the frontal patients were most impaired; there was no difference between normal control subjects and temporal lobe patients. Following this impulsive response to the initial cue, the normal and temporal lobe subjects executed a large corrective saccade to the appropriate visual field. Such corrective responses were almost impossible for the frontal eye field patients.

The Guitton et al. (1982) data appear to be consistent with reported frontal eye field electrophysiological recordings demonstrating firing before the onset of a saccade (Goldberg and Bushnell, 1981; Wurtz and Mohler, 1976). This anticipatory discharge suggests a directive, executive role as well as monitoring function for this frontal cortical area.

Inertia of Gaze

Inertia of gaze is closely allied to defective visual search and resembles the optic ataxia signs of Balint's syndrome. Clinically, it is observed as a difficulty in perceiving fast-moving objects and was considered a defect in shifting of attention by Luria (1973a, 1966/1980). If a severely damaged frontal lobe patient fixates on one object and the object is then moved, the patient may continue to fixate the original point in space. If two objects are presented, only one may be perceived (simultagnosia). In general, the inertia seems to reflect a deficit in attention that, in Luria's view, affects both sensory and motor processes.

This "pathological inertia of the nervous processes" is more than a disorder of scanning. When trying to disassociate pictures of figures that are superimposed on each other (e.g., Poppelreuter figures), frontal lobe patients cannot move from one pattern to another, tending to fix on one detail. Although most brain-damaged subjects fail on the detection of hidden figures, frontal lobe patients tend to bind to the strong, salient structure and cannot differentiate the pattern from the background, even after the pattern has been demonstrated (Luria, 1973a, 1966/1980; Teuber and Weinstein, 1956). A similar test requires the patient to isolate a structure (e.g., white cross) placed on a homogeneous background (e.g., checkerboard) (Luria, 1966/1980). The frontal lobe patient tends to be distracted by the irrelevant background. Yet another commonly noted example occurs if the patient is asked to draw one picture and then another; features from the first drawing tend to appear in the subsequent productions.

MELODIC PERCEPTION

Although the right temporal lobe has been primarily implicated in musical processing, a role of the right frontal lobe in melodic perception, particularly pitch alteration, has been suggested (Grossman, Shapiro, and Gardner, 1981; Shapiro, Grossman, and Gardner, 1981). Brown (1985) suggested that this was a spurious effect on the early processing stages of cognitive tasks. Zatorre (1985), dividing melodic processing into scale and contour components, and using signal-detection analysis, found no deficit in musical discrimination in patients with frontal lesions. Zatorre, however, did observe a response bias deficit in the right frontal patients, suggesting a frontal "control" problem.

SUMMARY

The above review indicates that the frontal lobes do play a role in sensory-perceptive functions. The role is specific but indirect. There is no involvement of simple, direct sensory functions. Frontal lobe damage does not result in loss of sensation; rather, it plays a role in the organization of perception (Luria, 1973a, 1966/1980). This includes the process of search, which implies anticipation, intention, attention, selection, and planning; it also acts to compare sensory data and create hypotheses based on the acquired information; finally, the frontal function includes verification of the hypotheses derived from the sensory data.

Differentiation of the sensory defect of frontal lobe damage from that due to pathology affecting other brain areas is usually apparent, but at times the sensory-perceptual organizational deficits secondary to frontal lobe damage can be difficult to disassociate from parietal-occipital damage. Luria (1966/1980) noted these similarities and suggested means of separating the mimicking effect: "The pseudoagnostic disturbances of perception accompanying lesions of the frontal lobes sometimes assume forms so outwardly similar to the manifestations of true optic agnosia that only by careful observation of the passive character of the perceptual activity and of the presence of the syndrome of generalized inertia and a lack of critical attitude towards performance will these defects be correctly diagnosed" (p. 461).

It appears that the frontal lobe, through its connections with other cortical areas, can produce effects that can resemble those caused by lesions directly affecting that area. Careful evaluation, however, usually demonstrates specific deficits characteristic of the frontal lobe function, allowing differentiation.

10

Visual-Spatial Functions

As noted in the previous chapter, the frontal lobes are not considered essential to visually oriented activities including visual-spatial discrimination. Hécaen (1972) specifically excluded the frontal lobe from involvement in "constructional apraxia," and Luria (1973a) noted that even with massive frontal lobe lesions there is little difficulty in the direct visual perceptions required to recognize or construct simple pictures or figures. A careful study of a patient with severe perinatal frontal lobe pathology showed no evidence of impoverished nonverbal abilities (Ackerly, 1964; Ackerly and Benton, 1947). Even when more complex measures such as the WAIS Performance scale tests were used, patients with frontal lobe damage from various etiologies and in various locations showed no significant deficit compared to normal subjects (Black and Strub, 1976; Stuss et al., 1981b).

These negative results differ from some findings of animal research where the spatial, positional cues appeared to be essential for frontal damaged animals in tasks such as the Delayed Alternation Test (Goldman and Rosvold, 1970; Konorski, 1967; Mishkin, Vest, Waxler, and Rosvold, 1969). There is little clinical literature on this subject. Many clinically oriented reports (Arrigoni and DeRenzi, 1964; Benson and Barton, 1970; Benton, 1968) that have utilized relatively demanding formal testing failed to suggest a frontal effect on visual-spatial functions. Others, however, did suggest frontal involvement in perceptual and constructive abilities (Black and Bernard, 1984; Kertesz and Dobrowolski, 1981; Kim, Morrow, Passafiume, and Boller, 1984). To reconcile these discrepancies and evaluate the role of the frontal lobes in visual-spatial functions, the themes initiated in the sensory/perception chapter are continued.

PSYCHOLOGICAL TEST RESULTS

Visual-Perceptual Ability

Visual-perceptual functions can be defined as those abilities in which organization and conceptualization of sensation occur but reconstruction of the percept is not required. Some tests, e.g., the WAIS Picture Completion, provide no evidence of deficit after frontal lesions (McFie, 1969; Stuss, Benson, Kaplan, et al., 1985). Teuber et al. (1951) demonstrated that frontal lobe patients performed poorly on a test of identification of hidden figures requiring perceptual closure in the face of distraction, but patients with parietal-occipital lesions were even more impaired, suggesting that the test was sensitive to general brain damage. It appears that frontal lobe patients make errors on figure-ground differentiation that are qualitatively specific, however, particularly distraction by irrelevant stimuli, and this disorder correlated with the complexity of the stimulus (Luria, 1966/1980).

Some pertinent findings may be noted in the area of orientation tasks. Topographical orientation, the localization of geographical places on maps, is not impaired after frontal lobe damage (Hécaen and Albert, 1978). Similarly, route-finding or maze-learning tasks (excluding the Porteus Maze), the use of visually or tactually guided orientation in space, are most disturbed by posterior lesions, particularly in the right hemisphere (Corkin, 1965; Hécaen, 1972; Hécaen and Albert, 1978; Milner, 1964, 1965). The frontal lobe patients, however, may be impaired for qualitatively different reasons. They make perseverative responses, fail to follow rules, and are less able to use feedback of erroneous responses to change their behavior (see also Walsh, 1977, 1978).

A comparison of two types of orientation demonstrated a double dissociation between function and hemispheric localization (Semmes, Weinstein, Ghent, and Teuber, 1963; Teuber, 1964). In an extrapersonal spatial orientation task, nine evenly spaced dots were placed in a 3×3 pattern on the floor. Maps, increasing in difficulty according to the number of turns required, provided routes to follow. The maps were presented visually or tactually and, in the latter, either ipsilateral or contralateral to the lesion. Subjects were required to pace out the map route following the dots on the floor. In the personal orientation task, subjects were presented with a front and back profile of a human figure (Fig. 10-1). Numbers were written on different parts of the body. The subject had to touch the indicated part on his or her own body in sequential order as indicated by the number. This task required body part finding and naming, right–left orientation, as well as rapid shifting of a principle.

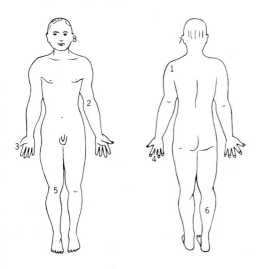

FIG. 10-1. Diagram used in the Personal Orientation Test (see text). (From Teuber: In: *The Frontal Granular Cortex and Behavior,* edited by Warren and Akert. McGraw-Hill, New York, 1964, with permission.)

Patients with parietal damage, right, left, or bilateral, were most impaired on the spatial orientation task; right posterior lobe patients were not impaired in the personal orientation task. Although the left frontal lobe patients had few problems on extrapersonal orientation, they were the most impaired on the personal orientation task. Patients with right anterior lesions were also impaired, but their performance was superior to those with left posterior lesions. An explanation for the frontal, particularly left frontal, deficit was not presented, but the demands of rapid sequencing, shifting, and reversals were suggested factors. Later research (described below) addressed this issue more directly.

Benson and Barton (1970) used a task demanding reversal of stick patterns in space: The subject, sitting across from the examiner, had to make a pattern that looked to him (the subject) the same as the examiner's model looked to the examiner. This task was the most difficult for patients with left posterior lesions, right anterior lesion patients being next worse, with the left anterior lesion patients performing at a level approximately equal to the control group. In a template matching orientation-rotation task, left frontal lobe damaged patients showed no impairment, but both right hemisphere groups performed poorly, the right anterior hemisphere group being the worse. In a basically similar task, requiring an abstract 180-degree rotation of an object, only parietal lobe patients showed impairment (Butters and Barton, 1970; Butters et al., 1970). Differences in lesion size, localization, and specificity of tasks make precise comparison of these two studies difficult, but the results suggest that, when frontal damage affects extrapersonal spatial orientation tasks, right hemisphere involvement is most prominent.

Butters, Soeldner, and Fedio (1972) readdressed the issue of personal and extrapersonal orientation by comparing results on the stick construction orientation test (Benson and Barton, 1970) to the Money Test of Directional Sense (Money, Alexander, and Walter, 1965). The latter test demands abstract personal spatial rotation as the subject travels back and forth on a circuitous path with many turns. At each turn the subect must consider how he is oriented to that corner and indicate if he should turn right or left. The patients compared were grouped by right parietal, left frontal, and right and left temporal lobe. The results suggested a qualitative dissociation between groups, with the left frontal lobe patients most impaired on the Personal Orientation Task and right parietal lobe subjects worst on stick reversal. The authors concluded that both frontal and parietal areas carried out spatial functions, but the actions were qualitatively different. This basic dissociation has been replicated in the animal literature, with the indication that frontal cortex has a superordinate role in spatial functions (Pohl, 1973; Ungerleider and Brody, 1977).

Additional experimental tasks appear sensitive to frontal pathology. In the perception of reversible figures (e.g., the Necker Cube), all brain-damaged patients perceived fewer reversals (Cohen, 1959; Teuber, 1964, 1966) and right hemisphere damaged patients fewer than those with left hemisphere lesions. Unilateral frontal lobe damaged patients had the fewest reversals of all, regardless of hemispheric localization of pathology. Surprisingly, subjects with bilateral frontal lesions perceived the most reversals. Lesion localization within the frontal lobes may have been relevant, however, as the bilaterally lesioned patients had less orbital involvement. Tests requiring perceptual figure rotation appeared especially sensitive to left anterior pathology, although pathology in any of the four quadrants produced deficits (Kim et al., 1984).

Finally, the Aubert task, the resetting of a tilted luminous rod to the apparent vertical with modifications allowing assessment of separate abilities, has proved sensitive to pathology in specific cortical areas (Teuber, 1964, 1966). Four conditions, two with the body upright and two with the body tilted, were administered. In the upright condition, the subject had to reset the rod to vertical in a simple manner (visual) or with a conflicting visual background created by oblique stripes (visual-visual) (Fig. 10-2). With the body tilted, the subject either returned the chair to apparent vertical (postural) or performed the same simple visual condition judgment under conditions of body tilt (postural–visual). Patients with chronic brain lesions showed an apparent double dissociation. Frontal lobe patients made

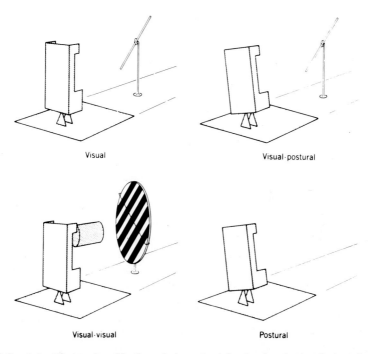

Visual

Visual-postural

Visual-visual

Postural

FIG. 10-2. Aubert Task and modifications. Judgments of visual and postural vertical are demanded under two conditions of body posture (upright or tilted). *Top left:* Pure visual control in which the subject, in an upright position, sets a luminous line to the vertical. *Bottom left:* Visual-visual control in which the subject, in an upright position, sets a black thread to the vertical against a conflicting visual background. *Top right:* Visual-postural control in which the subject tries to set a luminous line to the vertical, but with body tilted. *Bottom right:* Pure postural control in which the subject in a tilted position brings himself back to vertical. (From Teuber: In: *The Frontal Granular Cortex and Behavior,* edited by Warren and Akert, McGraw-Hill, New York, 1964, with permission.)

the most exaggerated compensatory errors in the postural-visual condition, but parietal lobe patients were most impaired in resetting the rod against a conflicting background.

In summary, visual-perceptual deficits can be found with frontal lobe lesions but appear to be qualitatively different from those following parietal lesions. Deficits occurred on complex tests that required sequencing, rapid switching of concepts, inhibition of interfering stimuli, or monitoring responses in an abnormal environment.

Visual-Constructive Functions

Visual-constructive functions include the abilities needed to perform a variety of tests that require a visual perception and then some type of manual response. Responses may include spontaneous production or copy of a two- or three-dimensional design, the reconstruction of block designs or cut-up objects, and so on.

Impairment in visual-constructive abilities is not obvious after frontal damage, and some deny frontal involvement in "constructional apraxia" (Hécaen, 1981). Negative findings, using many different constructional tasks, have been reported in patients with lesions of various etiologies and in various locations within the frontal lobes (Ackerly, 1964; Hamlin, 1970; McFie, 1969; Stuss et al., 1984a). Benson and Barton (1970), however, showed that a copy-draw test was a good general test of brain damage; abnormal copies occurred in subjects with damage in any of the four quadrants of the brain. Their task combined memory and copy scores, however, so any conclusions in relation to copying alone were tentative.

Impairment in patients with frontal lobe damage is less than that observed in patients with posterior pathology (Black and Strub, 1976; Hécaen, 1972). Several observations clarify this statement. Drawings of simple, independent figures almost never present a problem to a frontal lobe patient (Luria, 1973a, 1966/1980; Stuss et al., 1985), indicating that the basic visual-constructive ability is intact. The patient easily draws pictures of objects or copies simple designs. With complex figures such as the Rey-Osterreith, however, the frontal lobe patient often makes unnecessary intrusions and distortions (Taylor, 1979). Also, if asked to draw different pictures in a sequence, the process may break down, with repetition of one of the pictures or insertion of part of a previous image into subsequent drawings (Luria, 1973a, 1966/1980). The complexity of the design and the actual process required (individual or sequential) appear to be relevant.

A 53-year-old man with bilateral frontal infarcts was sufficiently well 1 month after admission to undergo neuropsychological testing. He performed within normal limits on Digit Span (eight forward), and could concentrate adequately to count by threes. Language functioning was not aphasic, although content was confabulatory. His performance on the Wechsler Adult Intelligence Scale (WAIS) revealed a verbal IQ in the low-normal range (92) but a significantly inferior performance IQ (74). His copy of the complex Rey-Osterreith figure included most details but was totally disorganized in its reproduction (Fig. 10-3A). On the WAIS Block Design subtest, he frequently broke the external configuration and focused on salient features such as the angle formed by the edges of the red blocks in order to reproduce the design (Fig. 10-3B). Neurological examination revealed mild left hemiparesis. Computed tomography (CT)

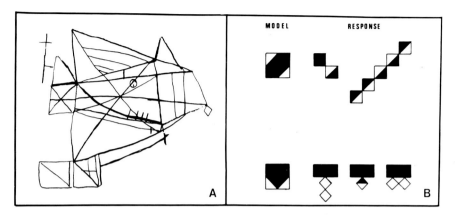

FIG. 10-3. Case study of a patient with a deep left frontal lobe lesion (see Fig. 6-1). Copy of the Rey-Osterreith complex figure **(A)** and attempts to do the Block Design subtest of the WAIS **(B)** show disorganization. (From Picton et al.: In: *The Brain, Cognition and Education*, edited by Friedman et al. Academic Press, New York, 1986, with permission.)

scan showed a deep left frontal infarct (Fig. 6-1A), and there was bilateral frontal slowing on the electroencephalogram (EEG).

The size and location of the lesion are relevant. Many of Luria's findings were derived from observations of patients with massive frontal lobe pathology. It is uncertain if similar findings are present with smaller, more focal lesions. The size variable does not account for all observed differences (Kertesz and Dobrowolski, 1981), and the relevance of the size of the lesion may also depend on location of pathology (Black and Bernard, 1984). In addition, there is considerable evidence indicating that, within the frontal lobes, damage in the right (particularly posterior) hemisphere is more likely to affect constructional abilities. This finding has been observed with reproduction of figures, the WAIS Object Assembly and Block Design, and other experimental tests, although the differences did not necessarily reach significance (Benson and Barton, 1970; Black and Bernard, 1984; Black and Strub, 1976; Kim et al., 1984; Taylor, 1979). Benton (1968) compared the ability of patients with right, left, or bilateral frontal lesions to copy the Benton Visual Retention test figures. Patients with bilateral pathology were most impaired; those with right frontal damage were nearly as bad, but there was little evidence of impairment for the left frontal patients. On a test of three-dimensional Block Construction, both the right and bilateral frontal lobe patients were significantly inferior to the left frontal lobe patients (Benton, 1968). Goodglass and Kaplan (1979) suggested that patients with large right hemisphere lesions involving the frontal lobe frequently show inertia on Block Design tests (the blocks are not turned over to examine other possibilities) and a disruption of external configuration focusing on one salient feature of the design. Kim et al. (1984) found that, within the right hemisphere, posterior lesion patients were more impaired on a number of perceptual and constructive tasks, but within the left hemisphere the anterior lesion patients were most impaired, having a greater deficit on specific tests than right posterior lesion patients. Kertesz and Dobrowolski (1981) suggested that constructional abilities may not be specifically localized within the right hemisphere, with possible qualitative differences in the types of error. Although these findings, taken together, suggest a predominance of right hemisphere activity in visual-constructive functions, the different results reported may indicate the importance of what type of test is used and how the impairment is measured.

Time of assessment in relation to onset of damage may be important, at least with certain tests and certain lesion locations. Digit Symbol and Object Assembly, for example, were effective indices of impairment in patients who had recently undergone topectomy for psychiatric treatment (Lewis et al., 1956). In a 14-year follow-up of the same subjects, Hamlin (1970) found no difference between control subjects and topectomy patients on either test.

To understand frontal lobe involvement in visual-constructive tasks, analysis of the process of performance as well as the end result is necessary. This is most clearly illustrated with block design tests (e.g., the WAIS Block Design, Koh's Blocks, or Link's Cube). When the design is simple and the visual patterns and block outline are compatible, frontal lobe patients perform normally, possibly because they do not have to break down what is perceived into its constituent parts for the purpose of reassembly (Luria and Tsvetkova, 1964). This results in the common observation of "normal" performance of frontal lobe patients on at least simple block design tests (Ackerly, 1964; Black and Strub, 1976; Hamlin, 1970; McFie, 1969; Stuss et al., 1984a). However, if the design or reproduction is indirect, requiring analysis and then reconstruction, errors may occur (Luria, 1973a, 1966/1980; Luria and Tsvetkova, 1964; Walsh, 1978). Frontal lobe patients may not divide the patterns into constituent parts, even having difficulty in determining the number of blocks needed. They often respond impulsively, are impaired in describing what they were doing, have no evident trial-and-error approach, and are satisfied with erroneous responses. Frontal lobe patients require detailed, exterior programming to help overcome the lack of internal, detailed programs. When these external programming cues are removed, failure occurs (Lhermitte, Derouesne, and Signoret, 1972; Walsh, 1977, 1978). These studies suggest that the disorder is not visual-spatial per se but a disorder of planning. Impairment in other "spatial tasks," such as Porteus Maze, that assess planning more directly are reviewed in Chapter 14.

Although constructional problems can occur with lesions in any of the four brain quadrants (Black and Bernard, 1984), deficits in visual-constructive tasks following frontal lobe damage appear to be qualitatively different from the dysfunction reported with posterior lesions, necessitating more complex tests to elicit the impairment.

INITIATION, INERTIA, SEQUENCING, AND ORDERING

Most hypotheses of the role of the frontal lobes in spatial functioning center on initiation of plans, performing sequences, pathological inertia, and the ability to correct performance.

Apathy, including decreased effort and initiation, is a frequent observation in patients with frontal pathology. Chapter 8 outlines the apathetic behavior noted with frontal lobe damage, and Chapter 11 reviews specific problems in the initiation of speech, particularly the generation of word lists, after focal left frontal damage.

Jones-Gotman and Milner (1977) probed the modality and hemisphere specificity of frontal disturbance with a test of the ability to generate visual, nonverbal forms. Two conditions were used, a 5-min "free" condition in which subjects produced as many drawings as they could invent that were neither namable nor mere scribbles and a second, 4-min fixed condition in which each figure had to consist of four lines. In the free condition, patients with right anterior lesions were the most impaired, with no impairment reported for those with right posterior lesions. In the fixed condition, all brain-damaged groups were impaired, including the right posterior lesion patients; only the left posterior lesion patients approximated the normal group. The right anterior lesion patients showed the greatest deficits, which were distinguished by perseverative responses. In the fixed condition, the left frontal lobe patients also showed a perseverative tendency, with the right posterior lesion patients exhibiting a lesser degree. The frontal lobes appear to be particularly important for the initiation and continuation of this behavior, with the greatest deficit in verbal or nonverbal material dependent on the side of lesion. This two-factor theory had been postulated earlier by Ramier and Hécaen (1970) in relation to verbal fluency.

Defective sequencing in drawing tasks was suggested by Luria (1973a). One commonly used psychological test, the WAIS Picture Arrangement Subtest, demands sequencing of perceived facts. Subjects are provided with a series of cards in a random order; if organized into the correct order, the pictures constitute a logical story. Frontal lobe patients often have difficulty understanding the meaning and frequently describe individual cards or focus on details (Luria, 1966/1980). It has been suggested that picture arrangement is not a sensitive localizing test, but McFie (McFie, 1969; McFie and Thompson, 1972) reported that right frontal lobe patients were notably impaired. They tended to leave the pictures in their original order, creating a story to fit the pictures as presented (Goodglass and Kaplan, 1979; McFie and Thompson, 1972). Even if their errors were pointed out, they were frequently unable to make the necessary corrections.

The WAIS Picture Arrangement appears sensitive to chronic frontal lobe pathology, at least as indicated in three long-term follow-up studies of the effects of psychosurgery (Hamlin, 1970; Medina, Pearson, and Buchstein, 1954; Stuss et al., 1984a). After 9 (Medina et al., 1954), 14 (Hamlin, 1970), and 25 (Stuss et al., 1984a) years, the Picture Arrangement subtest alone of all the WAIS Performance subtests significantly differentiated the psychosurgery patients from the control groups. Hamlin's (1970) results suggested that the deficit was location-specific, as orbital frontal topectomy patients were unimpaired. The negative results reported by Wehler and Hoffman (1978) raise questions about any interpretation of the long-term follow-up of other psychosurgery patients.

The perception of relative movement or of sequences of movement are at least generally related to the sequencing concepts of the WAIS Picture Arrangement. Albert and Hécaen (1971) devised a task in which two movable white discs were placed at a relative distance from the subject, one being closer. As the second disc approximated the first, the subject decided when the two discs were side by side. Although all brain-damaged patients performed worse than normals, the right hemisphere patients were worse than the left, and both frontal groups were most impaired. The authors postulated two factors in visual-spatial perception. The position is judged by the right hemisphere, more likely but not exclusively the right posterior. The kinetic factor is a bilateral frontal function, related to Teuber's corollary discharge. A high correlation between tasks of perception of relative movement and appreciation of visual coordinates occurred only in patients with right anterior lesions (Tzavaras, Albert, and Hécaen, 1972).

Deficits are also noted in tasks in which the subjects had to initiate and then organize and carry out a sequence of responses (subjective-ordered sequencing) (Milner, 1982; Petrides and Milner, 1982). Two verbal and two nonverbal tasks were administered. Patients with left frontal damage were impaired on all four tasks, whereas right frontal damaged patients were deficient only in the longest list of the nonverbal tests. In general, frontal lobe patients were less likely to group items in a meaningful way, a deficit apparently due to poor organization, poor monitoring of results, or both. *Post hoc* questioning revealed a deficient verbalization of strategy. The fact that left frontal damage caused impairment in all four tasks suggests a left hemisphere dominance for response programs, possibly because some verbal formulation is demanded. The temporal lobe patients were unimpaired unless there was significant hippocampal involvement.

Recency discrimination, although summarized among memory tasks, also reflects sequencing ability (temporal-ordered sequencing). Recency experiments indicate a material-specific frontal lobe effect and a more important role for the right frontal area in temporal judgment. Combining the two sets of experiments, there appears to be a hemispheric dissociation in response for temporal-ordered versus subject-ordered sequencing (Milner, 1982; Petrides and Milner, 1982). It was hypothesized that the right frontal predominance in temporal-ordered recency tasks reflects the right hemisphere dominance for visually guided attention. The left frontal lobe, on the other hand, appears dominant for programming and monitoring subjective-ordered voluntary actions.

SUMMARY

Whether the frontal lobes are involved in visual-spatial functions depends on the function. If the task demands merely knowledge of spatial relationships, especially the well-rehearsed, over-learned tasks used in familiar contexts, the frontal lobes do not appear to be significant. If the task directly or indirectly involves selection, initiation, direction, planning, flexibility, and/or monitoring, however, the frontal lobes may be significantly involved.

Many of the results described in this chapter have been interpreted in light of Teuber's (1964) corollary discharge theory (see Chapter 16) that visual-spatial tasks frequently demand sensory-motor coordination. The frontal lobes predict and anticipate, presetting sensory mechanisms with a corollary discharge so that the result of the motor output can be evaluated and changed if necessary. Damage to the frontal lobes inhibits the subject's ability to act as an active agent in behavior.

11

Speech and Language

A specific relationship of the frontal lobes to language functions was proposed by the phrenologist Franz Joseph Gall during the early nineteenth century (Lee, 1981). This relationship was restated by Bouillard (1825), Dax (1836), and Auburtin (1863), and was so powerfully demonstrated by Broca (1861a,b; 1865) that a left frontal localization for language became an accepted language/neuroanatomy correlation. The occurrence of "true" language deficits with frontal pathology was challenged by Marie (1906), who held that no part of the frontal convolutions was important to language; rather, damage here resulted in "anarthria," a defect in the mechanics of speech. The relative importance of the frontal lobes in language and speech function has been controversial since then, but most investigators now accept that portions of the frontal lobe do play an important role in both functions.

Frontal involvement in speech and language functions are reviewed in the four sections of this chapter. The first section reviews frontal aphasic syndromes using the comparatively accepted divisions of classic aphasiology. Within this classification, Broca aphasia, aphemia, transcortical motor aphasia, supplementary motor area language disturbance, and the subcortical language disturbances are relevant to the discussion of frontal communication disorders. Against this background two striking frontal language disabilities, agrammatism and the limited ability to handle sequences of words, can be presented; this comprises the second section. A third section addresses the frontal speech disorders: mutism and hypophonia, dysarthria, apraxia of speech, and aprosodia. The fourth section presents disorders based on frontal lobe malfunction that affect language including verbal adynamia and the regulatory power of language.

FRONTAL APHASIC DISORDERS

Broca Aphasia

A number of terms have been used to describe Broca aphasia, including expressive aphasia, Broca aphasia, motor aphasia, efferent motor aphasia, anterior aphasia, and verbal aphasia. Broca aphasia is the most widely accepted term, and the syndrome ranks among the most widely accepted signs of frontal lobe pathology. Traditionally, pathology found with this syndrome involves the dominant posterior-inferior frontal lobe, particularly the pars triangularis and pars orbitalis of the third (inferior) frontal gyrus, also labeled F3 or Brodmann area 44. A number of localizing methods link this area to Broca aphasia: clinical/postmortem correlation (Broca, 1861a; Mohr et al. 1978); war-related brain damage (Luria, 1970b; Russell and Espir, 1961; Schiller, 1947); radioisotope brain scan (Kertesz, 1979; Kertesz, Lesk, and McCabe, 1977); and computed tomography (CT) scan (Kertesz, 1979; Naeser and Hayward, 1978).

Although still controversial, it is now generally accepted that infarction of the Broca area alone or its immediate surroundings (a lesion that could be called "little Broca") is insufficient to produce the full syndrome of Broca aphasia, at least not permanently (Foix, 1928; Kleist, 1934b; Mohr, 1973; Mohr et al., 1978) (Fig. 11-1A). The full, permanent syndrome (big Broca) invariably indicates larger dominant hemisphere destruction affecting much of the operculum, including the area of Broca but extending deep into the insula and adjacent white matter and possibly including basal ganglia (Brunner, Kornhuber, Seemuller, et al., 1982; Naeser, Hayward, Laughlin, and Zatz, 1981) (Fig. 11-1B). The severity, persistence, and evolution of the language deficit appears to be dependent on the size of the original infarct, whereas the symptom picture apparently depends on the specific neuroanatomical areas involved (Alexander, 1984).

Accompanying neurological signs with Broca aphasia include a right-sided motor weakness in 80% of patients (Howes and Geschwind, 1964), most often full hemiplegia or hemiparesis with the upper extremity maximally involved. In addi-

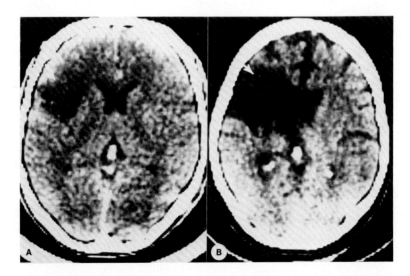

FIG. 11-1. A: X-ray CT scan of a 29-year-old man with acute mutism and Broca aphasia which resolved into a fully grammatical but hesitant speech with word-finding problems. The lesion is in the distribution of the upper left middle cerebral artery and primarily undercuts Broca's area, although there appears to be some cortical involvement (*arrow*). The lesion is relatively circumscribed. **B:** X-ray CT scan of a 69-year-old woman with clinically diagnosed persistent Broca aphasia. The large size and deep extension of the lesion is apparent with involvement of frontal operculum, insula, and subjacent white matter (*arrow*).

tion, left (nondominant) ideomotor limb apraxia is usually present (see Chapter 5). Right limb apraxia cannot be demonstrated because of paralysis, but theoretically the right limb should also be apractic. Sensory findings are variable, dependent on lesion extent; visual field defect is uncommon (Benson, 1977).

The language signs have been well documented (Benson and Geschwind, 1971; Kertesz, 1979; Lecours, Lhermitte, and Bryans, 1983; Lichtheim, 1885). The most visible feature is the nonfluent verbal output, which is sparse, dysarthric, hesitant, and effortful, has short phrase length (one word or telegraphic), and has agrammatical verbal content (relative infrequency of syntactically significant functor words). Persistent nonfluency appears to require involvement of the left hemispheric rolandic cerebral cortex and underlying frontal-parietal white matter (Knopman, Selnes, Niccum, et al., 1983). In some instances speech is limited to a verbal stereotype, a repetition of single words or phrases. Comprehension of spoken language, although variable and usually imperfect, is always better than conversational speech. The comprehension disturbance appears to center on the meaning of syntactical structures, the parts of speech omitted from conversational speech (Samuels and Benson, 1979; Zurif, Caramazza, and Myerson, 1972). Repetition is always impaired, although not to the extent of spontaneous speech in many cases. Maximum repetition deficit is observed with grammatically rich phrases, such as: "When he comes, I will go away." For instance, when asked to repeat "the big boy is eating an apple," the Broca aphasic characteristically omits functors, repeating "boy—eat—apple." Relatively automatic speech output such as recitation of numbers or the days of the week often improves the quality of spoken output.

The ability to name presented objects or pictures of objects is always impaired, although it may appear better than spontaneous output. A characteristic feature of the naming disorder in Broca aphasia is the ability to benefit from cues, both phonetic (presentation of initial phoneme) and contextual (presentation of an openended statement) (Barton, Maruszewski, and Urrea, 1969; Goodglass, Kaplan, Weintraub, and Ackerman, 1976; Goodglass and Stuss, 1979; Pease and Goodglass, 1978). Reading aloud is at least as impaired as spontaneous speech, but the ability to understand written material may be better. Most Broca aphasics have difficulty understanding written material, however, particularly the words important for syntactical relationships (Samuels and Benson, 1979). The frontal lesion thus produces a specific type of alexia (Benson, 1977; Benson, Brown, and Tomlinson, 1971; Krischner and Webb, 1982). Comprehension of spoken language and comprehension of written material are defective in a similar manner. Thus most Broca aphasics comprehend some written material, usually nouns and action verbs (e.g., they may interpret a headline correctly but cannot understand the more detailed article). Frontal alexia is characteristically a literal alexia [an inability to name individual letters even though some full words are recognized (Benson et al., 1971)].

Frontal lobe pathology has been implicated in the production of acquired writing disability (agraphia). Even allowing for clumsiness due to use of the nonpreferred left hand, patients with Broca aphasia produce abnormal written output that is clearly deficient in both language and mechanical aspects. Individual letters are characteristically oversized and poorly formed; misspellings and letter omissions are common; and grammatically significant words are routinely omitted, even when the patient writes to dictation. A lesion involving the lower end of the middle frontal convolution (just superior to Broca's area) has been said to result in pure agraphia, independent of any other language disability (Aimard, Devic, Lebel, et al., 1975; Exner, 1881; Hécaen and Albert, 1978; Mahoudeau, David, and Lecoeur, 1951), interpreted by some as a frontal lobe kinesthetic disorder (Aimard et al., 1975). Such reports have been infrequent and the specificity of lesion location questionable; some degree of verbal expressive difficulty is described in most reports (Botez, Lecours, and Bérube, 1983; Hécaen and Angelerques, 1966). Pure frontal agraphia remains a questionable entity.

Other causes of "pure" agraphia further cloud the picture. Chédru and Geschwind (1972) considered confusional states to be the most common cause of pure agraphia. Agraphia presenting as the sole aphasic disturbance has been described after focal left temporal pathology (Rosati and DeBastiani, 1979). Pure agraphia has also been described after dominant angular gyrus lesions (Gerstmann, 1930). Some consider writing as too complex a function to have localizing value (Leischner, 1969). To date, few studies have convincingly correlated qualitative differences in defective written output with discrete anatomical foci of pathology. If such studies are forthcoming, the possibility that a "frontal" writing defect could be discovered that is clearly distinguishable from other writing defects appears plausible.

A 69-year-old woman was examined 9 years after a cerebrovascular accident (CVA). She lived at home with her husband and assisted in daily chores. She had persistent right hemiparesis and could walk only with assistance of a cane. Speech was effortful, hesitant, agrammatical, and had many paraphasias. Repetition was moderately impaired; writing was effortful and clumsy. Comprehension was excellent, with impairment only in understanding complex relational sentences. X-ray CT scan revealed a large left anterior lesion (Fig. 11-1B). The diagnosis was of a persistent Broca aphasia, a "big Broca."

A right-handed university graduate computer analyst suffered an embolic left anterior CVA, demonstrated in Fig. 11-1A. Originally the patient was mute, with severe buccofacial apraxia, limb apraxia, and agraphia, but there was only mild right-sided motor weakness. Comprehension was relatively preserved, although deficits were elicited with questions requiring the comprehension of passive tense or possessives. Recovery was rapid. In the early stages speech was effortful with a tendency to be agrammatical, although complete phrases were uttered. Examination 4 months after the CVA revealed recovery from the hemiparesis. Speech was fully grammatical, with long, complete sentences, but hesitations were noted and fluent transition from phoneme to phoneme and word to word was impaired. The patient complained of problems in correct use of syntactical structures, such as tense agreement. Evidence of apraxia, comprehension, or repetition disturbance could be elicited only with complex, rapid demands. A mild to moderate problem in naming on visual confrontation remained, and generation of word lists was severely impaired. The patient originally presented with the symptom complex of Broca aphasia, but the rapid amelioration and subsequent pattern of speech warrants a "little Broca" description.

Aphemia

Aphemia, the term originally used by Broca to identify the aphasic disturbance that now bears his name, was later used to refer to a purely vocal output problem with no true language abnormality (Bastian, 1898). Other terms identifying the same syndrome include pure word dumbness, pure motor aphasia, cortical anarthria, and subcortical motor aphasia. The necessary lesion appears to be a direct but limited involvement of Broca's area or a subcortical undercutting of area 44 (Bastian, 1898; Dejerine, 1914/1977; Lichtheim, 1885; Souques, 1928). The lesion is similar in location, but not size, to the little Broca lesion described above. Schiff, Alexander, Naeser, et al. (1983) reported small lesions in pars opercularis, inferior prerolandic gyrus, or white matter deep to these areas. The clinical characteristics of aphemia and little Broca have been considered similar (Albert, Goodglass, Helm, et al., 1981; Benson, 1979), but differentiation can be suggested (Mohr et al., 1978). It now appears that both the clinical signs and the anatomical location of aphemia, little Broca, and apraxia of speech can be differentiated (see below).

Basic neurological signs reported in cases of aphemia include an initial but usually transient right-sided hemiplegia or paralysis, recovering without evident neurological deficit. A residual clumsiness and sensory disturbance of the right hand may persist, especially involving the thumb and index finger. There may be an apraxia; in some cases this is limited to buccofacial activities with no limb or whole body apraxia. Dysphagia may be present early. Although suggested as most commonly representing a residual of Broca aphasia (Albert et al., 1981; Mohr, 1973; Ruff and Arbit, 1981), the following description emphasizes the uniqueness of the syndrome.

> A 32-year-old left-handed man presented at the hospital alert and mobile but mute, with the ability only to phonate (utter) gutteral sounds. Although the history later revealed very transient right arm weakness, physical and neurological examinations at the time of admission were essentially normal. There was no evidence of primary laryngeal pathology. There was a striking buccofacial apraxia. Comprehension was normal, except for minimal errors when fatigued. He expressed himself correctly in grammatically complete writing. Within days, he was asymptomatic except for oral apraxia and breathy speech with diminished voice volume. He gradually recovered to a normal voice volume. The limited frontal lesion resulting in this aphemia is demonstrated in Fig. 11-2.

One striking clinical sign of aphemia is initial acute mutism without primary laryngeal pathology. Verbal output recovers, evolving into a poorly articulated, hypophonic, slow, breathy speech. Even from the beginning of recovery, however, no deficit in syntax is present, a striking difference from the output in Broca aphasia. On recovery, a change in speech pattern in some produces a "foreign accent" output, described as dysprosody by Monrad-Krohn (1947). This may persist. Comprehension (spoken or written) and production of language through writing are normal. The apparent deficits in naming and repetition reflect the mutism, not a language deficit. In a very real sense, then, aphemia is not an aphasic disorder, but it is a good indicator of focal frontal pathology. It is better considered

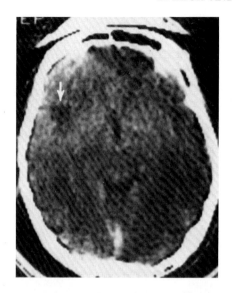

FIG. 11-2. X-ray CT scan of the small frontal lesion undercutting the frontal operculum *(arrow)*, resulting in aphemia.

a severe articulatory problem secondary to disruption of the cortical motor system for articulation (Schiff et al., 1983). Although aphemia may occur coincidentally with either Broca or little Broca aphasia, it is seen as a separate entity in some instances.

Transcortical Motor Aphasia

Transcortical motor (TCM) aphasia, also known as dynamic aphasia (Luria, 1966), adynamia of speech (Kleist, 1934b), and the anterior isolation syndrome (Benson and Geschwind, 1971), was originally described by Lichtheim (1885) who ascribed it to a separation of general conceptual brain processes from the Broca motor output area. Luria (1966, 1970b) viewed it as a loss of the predicative function of inner speech, necessary for transformation of thought into verbal output. The causative lesion has long been considered to involve the middle or anterior portion of the third (inferior), second (middle), and even possibly the first (superior) frontal gyri of the dominant lobe, i.e., frontal tissues anterior or superior to Broca's area (Goldstein, 1917, 1948; Luria, 1970b) (Fig. 11-3, top). Rothman (1906) described the syndrome in a case with a small white matter lesion under the motor speech region. Kertesz (1979), based on radioisotope scan studies, proposed two lesion areas: (1) the prerolandic speech area in the anterior cerebral artery distribution, the "supplementary speech area"; (2) smaller lesions in or immediately under Broca's area. Botez et al. (1983) proposed cingulate and supplementary motor area (SMA) pathology as sources of the syndrome. The most common causes include frontal intracerebral hematoma, frontal glioma, and internal carotid artery occlusion with infarction of the border zone (watershed) area between the middle and the anterior cerebral territories. A right hemiparesis is common but not constant. Left-sided limb apraxia and oral apraxia are often present. Sensory loss or visual field defect is uncommon, although transient conjugate deviation to the side

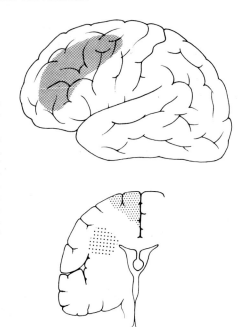

FIG. 11-3. The lesions necessary to cause transcortical motor aphasia and the supplementary motor area language disturbance. TCM aphasia has been ascribed primarily to pathology anterior or superior to Broca's area in the dominant frontal lobe **(top)**, but it may be predominantly subcortical, with convergence of pathology in the white matter anterolateral to the left frontal horn of the lateral ventricle (*light stippling*, **bottom**). SMA language disturbance involves the anterior cerebral artery distribution in the medial superior frontal lobe (*heavy stippling*, **bottom**).

ipsilateral to the lesion, with or without unilateral right visual field inattention, may be seen, apparently indicating involvement of the frontal eye field (see Chapter 9).

The clinical syndrome of TCM aphasia superficially resembles Broca aphasia (Benson and Geschwind, 1971; Goodglass and Kaplan, 1972). The nonfluent, agrammatical conversational speech is often characterized by striking difficulty in articulatory initiation, most prominent when the patient attempts to generate detailed narrative discourse (Albert et al., 1981). A transcortical motor aphasic may prompt verbal output by movements such as waving the hands, tapping the feet, walking, etc. Once started, serial speech is produced much better than spontaneous speech, although perseverations may occur. Both Broca aphasia and TCM aphasia patients show dysarthria, but the latter is characterized by greater repetition of phonemes and words, stumbling, and stuttering. Comprehension is relatively intact but with some deficit in understanding sequences and relational words. These similarities may be due to lesion overlap, and more precise clarification appears possible (see later discussion of SMA).

The key difference between Broca and TCM aphasias is the good to excellent ability to repeat spoken language in the latter, theoretically linked to sparing of the arcuate fasciculus and the speech reflex arc (Geschwind, 1970). Although frequently repeating what has been said by the examiner, the repetition is not mandatory; grammatically incorrect phrases are corrected, wrong tenses changed, and nonsense words rejected in the repetition (Benson, 1979). A strong completion tendency is common (Stengel, 1947). The normal repetition in contrast to the severely abnormal spontaneous verbal output is dramatic, offering absolute evidence that TCM aphasia is fundamentally different from Broca aphasia.

Naming is impaired in TCM aphasia, as in all true aphasic disorders. It is difficult to determine, however, whether the naming deficits represent true word-finding problems or merely a disturbed ability to initiate verbalization (Benson, 1979). Contextual and phonemic cues are often beneficial. Reading aloud tends to be poorly articulated, but reading comprehension has been described as normal to perhaps mildly impaired. Written output is usually large and clumsy, and the output is frequently agrammatical and shows spelling errors.

SMA Language Disturbance

The effect of SMA pathology on verbal output has been recognized for years (Foerster, 1936b; Penfield and Roberts, 1959). It appears to be the only cortical area outside the perisylvian language area in which electrical stimulation reliably results in speech arrest (Penfield and Roberts, 1959). Focal seizures from the left SMA produce speech arrest (Peled, Harnes, Borovich, and Sharf, 1984). The lesion necessary for production of SMA language disturbance lies in the medial frontal area, in the distribution of the anterior cerebral artery, just anterior to the medial extension of the motor homunculus. Etiology may vary, including interhemispheric subdural hematoma (Tijssen, Tavy, Hekster, et al, 1984). The classic neurological findings following involvement of this area include weakness, hyperreflexia, extensor plantar reflex, and sensory loss of the contralateral lower limb, with mild weakness of the shoulder (Fisher, 1975). Arm, hand, and face strength, in contrast, are normally strong although some involuntary motor activity of the right arm may be seen (Alexander and Schmitt, 1980; Goldberg et al., 1981; see also Frontal or Magnetic Apraxia, Chapter 5, this volume).

An evolving clinical description of SMA language disturbance has appeared in recent years (Alexander and Schmitt, 1980; Goldberg et al., 1981; Masdeu, 1980; Masdeu, Schoene, and Funkenstein, 1978; Rubens, 1975). An initial period of muteness is followed by a stage of sharply decreased verbal output, in both spontaneous production and response to questions, although some capacity for brief response is present. A striking feature is the lack of spontaneous initiation of speech, an adynamia that may extend to facial expression, gesture, and language production through writing. Speech, when produced, lacks paraphasias [although Masdeu et al. (1978) state otherwise] and is well articulated. Sentences are usually short and lack full lexicon but are grammatically correct. Confrontation naming may be relatively well preserved, but lengthy hesitations are common. The relatively preserved ability to name real objects contrasts with severe impairment in the generation of word lists belonging to a specific category. Repetition is absent during the mute stage but then becomes relatively effortless and well articulated. Rubens (1975) described perseveration, echolalia, and a strong completion phenomenon, but this has not been observed by all (Masdeu et al., 1978). Comprehension appears intact, but some problems with relational, syntactic, linguistic structures have been noted. Agraphia and left-hand limb apraxia have been reported.

The lack of dynamism in spontaneous activities that disappears during automatic responses closely resembles that seen in TCM aphasia. As noted, Kertesz (1979) localized two forms of TCM aphasia, listing SMA aphasia as one type. Although the basic language disturbances of TCM and SMA aphasias are similar, several differentiating factors have been proposed (Albert et al., 1981; Alexander and Schmitt, 1980). Lesions in the SMA (frontal parasagittal zone) start with total muteness or severe dysphonia. A grasp reflex (see magnetic apraxia) is usually present. The electroencephalogram (EEG) offers a unique differentiating finding, a medial frontal slow-wave focus. TCM aphasia lesions, on the other hand, by involving lateral cortical and subcortical areas, usually produce some dysarthria, phonemic paraphasia, and agrammatism. The difference between repetition and spontaneous speech may be less striking in TCM aphasia than SMA language disturbance.

Although language output is affected, the SMA disturbance may not be true aphasia. Damasio and Van Hoesen (1980) described the deficit as an impairment in the energizer necessary for the initiation of willed movement. Botez and Barbeau (1971) similarly interpreted the deficit as a fault in the "starting mechanism" for speech, adding the function of maintenance of fluency. A position of the SMA as an extension of the limbic system and the role of limbic input to speech has been noted (Sanides, 1970). Volitional control was also indicated from animal research on the anterior cingulate cortex (von Cramon and Jurgens, 1983). Alexander and Schmitt (1980) noted the role of the SMA in the primitive system of speech organization. Thus the SMA may be a component of the entire motor system including speech, playing a supervisory rather than a specific language role. The similarity of SMA language disturbance and TCM aphasia is explained by pathology involving the language initiation system in both (Freedman et al., 1984). A lesion in the SMA apparently affects an energizer, resulting in either muteness or a difficulty in initiation of speech. TCM aphasia produces a similar disturbance by separation of the SMA from Broca's area (Fig. 11-3), a suggestion originally proposed by Goldstein (1917, 1948). In addition, however, the lesion of TCM often involves frontal dorsal convexity areas important for language (e.g., Broca's area) and is contaminated by true aphasia findings.

Arseni and Botez (1961) proposed three clinical varieties of SMA: (1) a parox-ysmal disturbance with speech arrest lasting 1 to 2 min; (2) a transient disturbance lasting 2 to 7 days; (3) a permanent type. The paroxysmal type usually indicates a seizure phenomenon, to be distinguished from speech arrest due to seizure focus elsewhere in the brain. The transient disturbance most often follows parasagittal tumor resection or acute occlusion of an anterior cerebral artery. The third variety is rare and most often indicates infarction or removal of the dominant SMA.

Subcortical Language Disturbances

In recent years a syndrome or syndromes of language impairment following subcortical pathology have been reported, usually under the term subcortical aphasia.

At least three distinct subcortical aphasias have been suggested, but only one features extension into subcortical frontal areas (Alexander, 1984; Alexander and LoVerme, 1980; Damasio, Damasio, Rizzo, et al., 1982; Naeser, 1983; Naeser, Alexander, Helm-Estabrooks, et al., 1982). Lesions have been reported in the putamen, caudate, and anterior limb of the internal capsule. The pathology often extends anteriorly to implicate periventricular white matter deep to Broca's area, as well as superiorly into periventricular white matter and corona radiata deep to the precentral gyrus facial area. Clinically, patients with such lesions resemble Broca aphasics in that they have good comprehension, impaired articulation, and right hemiparesis. Verbal output, however, retains complex syntactic structures and longer phrase length, similar to that seen in Wernicke aphasics. Whether language impairment with such frontal lobe lesions requires extension into pertinent cortical regions remains controversial; there is no doubt that left frontal subcortical lesions do affect motor speech.

AGRAMMATISM AND THE SEQUENCING OF LANGUAGE

One of the more striking findings in the evaluation of aphasia is the telegraphic style of language abbreviation that characterizes nonfluent verbal output. As Zurif et al. (1972) noted, the term agrammatism aptly characterizes the form of speech typified by omission of articles, prepositions, and inflectional forms, even after the patient recovers a considerable speaking vocabulary. Major writings on the grammatical disturbances of aphasia appeared in the German literature from 1902 to 1922 and again in the American literature from 1960 to the present. Careful study divides abnormal grammatical output of aphasia into two types: agrammatism, the reduction of language to the use of substantives (Jakobson, 1964), or paragrammatism, the improper use of grammatical structures. It has been suggested that the omission of syntactical structures merely represented an economy measure in effortful language output (Lenneberg, 1967), but numerous evaluations (Goodglass, 1968; Jakobson, 1964; Luria, 1970b) have clearly demonstrated a more specific disturbance. Agrammatism has been described as the result of disturbance to mechanisms that subserve the ability to structure a string of words syntactically (Zurif and Caramazza, 1976), a feature of some, but not all, aphasias.

Agrammatism has been defined simply as the telegraphic verbal output caused by brain injury in which grammatical modifiers are missing, but there is relative preservation of nouns, verbs, and substantive words (Kertesz, 1979); however, psycholinguistic investigations into the ability of aphasics to handle the syntactical structures of language suggest a more complex problem (Caramazza and Berndt, 1978; Goodglass and Berko, 1960; Von Stockert and Bader, 1976; Zurif et al., 1972). Many studies now demonstrate that the patient with agrammatism comprehends and produces the salient features of linguistic output best, whereas nonlexical syntactic structures tend to be omitted, misused, or simplified in relation to their meaningfulness in the sentence. Although it is the most obvious, the problem is not limited to verbal output; the patient with agrammatism has the same difficulty, apparently to the same degree, in comprehending these same syntactical structures. Agrammatism is a significant language disorder for some aphasics.

All studies of agrammatism describe the language of patients with Broca aphasia, and it is widely accepted that a frontal lesion is necessary for the condition. Nonetheless, proof that agrammatism represents a frontal abnormality is tenuous. Although the studies feature Broca aphasia and therefore assume a frontal lesion (Zurif et al., 1972), there are almost no correlations of locus of pathology within the frontal lobe with agrammatism. Agrammatism is not a feature of either TCM aphasia or aphemia. Tonkonogy and Goodglass (1981) suggested that agrammatism occurs with damage to tissue in or near Broca's area or a subcortical extension. Levine and Mohr (1979), however, demonstrated in a single, well-studied case that bilateral damage to the third frontal gyrus did not produce Broca aphasia. Many more correlation studies are needed if agrammatism is to be localized in a more exact manner. It appears clear, however, that the damage underlying agrammatism involves either frontal cortex or direct connections to frontal language areas. The implication that this aspect of syntax, the use of grammatical structures, is a frontal lobe function is strong.

A related but even less well studied problem concerns another significant aspect of syntax, the ability to handle sequences of material. Patients with anterior aphasias routinely recognize single lexical items (e.g., point to a named object) but fail to handle sequences of items (e.g., point to three or more objects in sequence) (Albert, 1972; Benson, 1979; Luria, 1966). In a similar manner, individuals with anterior lesions often fail to carry out multistep commands, cannot reproduce sequences in drawing or motor activities, cannot replicate a tapped-out rhythm, etc. Chapter 5 outlines a number of such disturbances. Very few formal studies have investigated sequencing as it applies to language forms (Albert, 1972; Samuels and Benson, 1979). These few studies suggest that frontal lesions can produce sequencing disturbances, even in the absence of other major language problems.

The specific location within the frontal lobe responsible for problems in handling sequences remains unknown except for the anticipated left greater than right involvement when language is tested (Albert, 1972). Investigations of disturbed sequencing in language are greatly hampered by similar failures in patients with posterior aphasia. Although apparently based on totally different abnormalities (e.g., defective lexical comprehension), many posterior aphasics fail to handle sequences of language material. Although this complicates localization studies, good evidence indicates that frontal lobe pathology alone can lead to an inability to handle sequences of language material despite intact comprehension of lexical items. Thus another facet of syntax, sequential relationship, appears to be related to frontal lobe function.

FRONTAL SPEECH SYNDROMES

Mutism and Hypophonia

Abnormalities of voice volume may occur for a number of reasons (Adams and Victor, 1977/1981; Benson, 1979). Hypophonia (lowered voice volume) and aphonia (total lack of voice) are the most common disorders of voice volume secondary to noncortical disease. The most common cause of hypophonia and/or total aphonia is laryngitis due to disease of the larynx or its innervation. In such cases, language and articulation remain intact, and the patient can either whisper or mouth full language output.

Abnormal voice volume can be secondary to brain disease and may coexist with aphasia, at least temporarily, but it may be caused by cerebral pathology without any language disorder. Cerebral areas in which pathology can produce abnormality of vocalization include the following:

1. *Supplementary motor area:* Damage to the SMA can result in mutism (Foerster, 1936b; Penfield and Roberts, 1959; Schwab, 1926), and speech arrest may be produced by electrical stimulation of this zone (Penfield and Roberts, 1959). Dominant hemisphere SMA pathology is most common, but at least two documented cases with mutism or speech arrest have been reported following right SMA lesions (Botez and Carp, 1968; Caplan and Zervas, 1978). Current hypotheses emphasize the executive function of the SMA, which energizes willed movement including initiation of speech. Mutism after SMA pathology appears secondary to damage at the source of all motor activation including speech production.

2. *Broca's area:* Acute pathology in the dominant hemisphere opercular area can produce transient mutism; language disturbance may not be present if the lesion is limited to Broca's area (aphemia). Electrical stimulation of this area consistently results in speech arrest (Lesser, Lueders, Dinner, et al., 1984; Ojemann and Whitaker, 1978). The mutism apparently reflects damage to the brain area essential for organization of motor speech.

3. *Frontal border zone area:* Mutism is a common but not consistent finding in TCM, apparently dependent on lesion proximity to either Broca's area or the SMA. Whether the lack of output in these patients is true aphonia may be debated. Albert et al. (1981) expressed it in this manner: "The deficit in spontaneous speech may approach muteness in severe cases" (p. 94).

4. *Putamen and internal capsule:* Lesions in the putamen and internal capsule have been demonstrated in cases of mutism (see section on subcortical aphasia). Transient mutism secondary to subcortical basal ganglia damage has also been reported after severe closed head injury (Levin, Madison, Bailey, et al., 1983).

5. *Mesencephalic reticular area:* Pathology in the reticular area of the mesencephalon (reticular activating system; RAS) may produce akinetic mutism. Most commonly, however, it results in some degree of hypophonia (Botez and Barbeau, 1971; Segarra, 1970).

6. *Frontal septal area:* Lesions at the other end of the median forebrain bundle from the RAS, the posterior, inferior, medial portion of the frontal lobe known generally as the septal area, can also cause akinetic mutism (in this instance a form of coma vigil). As could be anticipated, mutism or hypophonia can also result from bilateral pathology involving the median forebrain bundle as it courses through the hypothalamus from the mesencephalon to the septal area.

7. *Thalamus:* Altered vocalization, to the level of total mutism, was a feared complication of left thalamotomy performed as treatment for parkinsonism (Riklan and Levita, 1970). With experience, surgeons came to consider hypophonia in parkinsonian patients as a strong contraindication to stereotactic thalamotomy because mutism so often occurred. The greatest danger for the vocal changes appeared in the face of thalamic pathology (Bell, 1968). Stimulation in the pulvinar and ventral-lateral thalamus, however, produced total speech arrest in only 1 of 13 nonparkinsonian patients (Ojemann, Fedio, and Van Buren, 1968; Ojemann and Ward, 1971) and dorsal-lateral thalamic lesions, even if bilateral, do not appear to cause mutism (Guberman and Stuss, 1983; Winocur, Oxbury, Roberts, et al., 1984), although lowered voice volume may occur. Thalamic tumor, especially if left-sided, has also been reported to diminish voice volume (Smythe and Stern, 1938).

8. *Bilateral motor system:* Finally, bilateral cerebral pathology involving the motor system can cause mutism or hypophonia by producing the pseudobulbar or the locked-in syndrome. The finding is inconsistent, however, and may well represent pathological involvement of one of the areas mentioned above.

Mutism and alterations in voice volume have many causes that reflect different neuroanatomical sites. Many of these sites are in or near the frontal lobes, and additional findings of frontal dysfunction should be sought in the evaluation of a mute patient. Conversely, these findings demonstrate that frontal structures play important roles in voice volume.

Dysarthria

The act of speaking depends on the integrated activity of a number of functions in which the frontal cortex, as the motor brain, plays an important role. The motor cortices act through the corticobulbar tracts on the vagal, hypoglossal, facial, and glossopharyngeal cranial nerves and the phrenic nerve to control the musculature of the larynx, pharynx, palate, tongue, and lips as well as respiration. Dysarthria is the term used for motor speech disorders based on impaired control of this complex speech musculature system and, by tradition, refers to those motor speech abnormalities caused by neurological dysfunction (Darly et al., 1975). Some aphasiologists suggest that dysarthria does not result from pathology in brain areas that also serve language. Others, however, insist on cortical sources of dysarthria, usually when part of anterior aphasic syndromes (Trost and Canter, 1974). A number of concepts of "cortical dysarthria" are presented later in the discussion of apraxia of speech. Pathology anywhere in the motor pathways for the act of speaking apparently affects speech, regardless of language involvement. Nevertheless, in "pure" form dysarthria traditionally refers to speech disorders based on peripheral motor dysfunction.

Distinct variations of dysarthria have been described (Adams and Victor, 1977/ 1981; Darley et al., 1975).

1. *Flaccid paretic dysarthria:* Paralysis of lower motor neurons results in paretic or flaccid paralysis characterized by hypernasality, breathy phonation, and audible inspiration (stridor). Dysphagia and drooling are present. Pathology involves the motor nuclei of the medulla and lower pons or their cranial nerve extensions. Recognized causes include bulbar paralysis: amyotrophic lateral sclerosis, poliomyelitis, tumor, cerebrovascular accident (CVA), and myasthenia gravis.

2. *Spastic paretic dysarthria:* A second paralytic type is due to upper motor neuron disorder producing a spastic verbal output. Speech characteristics include a slow rate, low pitch, harsh quality, imprecise articulation, and difficult phonation. Pathology involves the cortical-bulbar tracts. Because the cranial nuclei innervating the bulbar muscles receive connections from both hemispheres, spastic dysarthria usually indicates bilateral lesions. Hemiplegia or pseudobulbar palsy is frequently present.

3. *Ataxic or cerebellar dysarthria:* A distinct speech disturbance occurs with cerebellar dysfunction and is characterized by slowness, irregularly broken articulation, harsh, irregular tonal quality, equalization of stress on words and syllables, and prolongation of phonemes. Dramatic, uncontrolled variations in the force of speaking produce the so-called explosive speech. Disease processes such as multiple sclerosis, Friedreich's ataxia, cerebellar atrophy, cerebellar injury or infarction, or heat stroke may be present.

4. *Hypokinetic dysarthria:* This distinctive speech disturbance is characteristic of parkinsonism. Features include decreased variability of pitch and loudness (monotonous output), hypophonia, inappropriate silences, imprecise articulation, and reduced stress.

5. *Hyperkinetic dysarthria:* A rapid verbal output with episodic hypernasality, breathiness and loudness in speech, harshness of voice, variable articulation, and slow rate of speaking with prolonged pauses and equalized stress or a second disorder with slow output, irregular articulation, prolongation of both phonemes and intervals, and variable harshness and breathiness have been reported with certain disorders (Tourette's syndrome, athetosis) (Hanson, 1983).

When analyzing dysarthria, each variety of motor speech disorder must be considered before accepting that the output represents cortical pathology. Nonetheless, there is strong suggestion and some evidence suggesting an important cortical influence on motor speech output.

Cortical Dysarthria—Apraxia of Speech

Dysarthria is present in many cases of anterior aphasia but rarely occurs in aphasia with focal postrolandic pathology. A number of labels have been proposed for the speech disorder(s) that accompany anterior aphasic syndromes including cortical dysarthria, spastic dysarthria, verbal apraxia, cortical anarthria, and efferent motor aphasia. One early, extreme position suggested that anterior cerebral lesions produced only dysarthria (anarthria): Any accompanying aphasic disturbances were secondary to involvement of the language (Wernicke's) area (Marie,

1906). Another extreme position, popularly held at present, is that dysarthria always indicates subcortical involvement.

The terms (implied mechanisms) suggested for speech difficulty with frontal lobe lesions have made specific categorization difficult, but some clarification can be made by correlation with known frontal aphasia syndromes. Clinical experience indicates that lesions in the SMA do not usually result in articulation problems with exceptions based on lesion extension (Schiff et al., 1983). Broca aphasia, on the other hand, characteristically features serious articulation problems. Categorizing Broca's area lesion syndromes into little and big Broca aphasia provides a framework for differentiation. Little Broca is defined by a lesion limited to the anterior operculum involving Broca's area and/or immediate surroundings. Clinical signs include some impairment of speech, the most severe being mutism. Improvement is rapid (hours to days) but varies with initial severity. Some degree of language impairment is present in spoken and written language, and the degree is a good indicator of recovery. These patients may have facial, oropharyngeal, lingual, and respiratory (i.e., nonverbal) apraxia, deficits that extend and complicate any language problem. Little Broca resembles aphemia, but the two are separable, as aphemia never includes "dyspraxia or language deficit in writing or in auditory or visual testing" (Mohr et al., 1978). Little Broca lesions appear to result in "dyspraxia of speaking aloud," a "speech apraxia," but may include other evidence of language disorder.

Levine and Mohr (1979) suggested that the third frontal gyrus is not essential for well-articulated speech, even if destroyed bilaterally. Rather, a more central region, the inferior two-thirds of the prerolandic cortex and the rolandic operculum, represent cortical control of articulation, a localization tentatively confirmed by Tonkonogy and Goodglass (1981) (Fig. 11-4). The latter reported that a limited lesion in the foot of the left third frontal gyrus (F3), including parts of the pars triangularis, opercularis (Broca's area), and orbitalis, produced a transient, mild language disorder with word-finding, comprehension, reading, and writing problems, but no articulation disorder. There was, however, a slowness in speech and difficulty in transition from one articulation to another. If pathology involves the lower motor strip including the rolandic operculum, a deficit in articulation occurs (Kleist, 1907; Lecours and Lhermitte, 1983; Luria, 1966/1980; Marie, 1906). It can be suggested that a lesion limited to Broca's area (F3) can cause "apraxia of speech," making the transition from one articulation to another difficult. This area may also be important for integrating other complex motor acts including writing (Lesser et al., 1984).

Based on these tentative observations, it may be preferable to use the term cortical dysarthria for output abnormality secondary to prerolandic pathology and adopt a term such as "apraxia of speech" or "melodic speech disturbance" for the area 44 disturbance. Luria (1969, p. 733) discussed the problem as follows:

> If the lesion is situated in the inferior portions of the premotor area of the dominant (left) hemisphere, phenomena similar to the disturbances of kinetic melodies described above [for motor functions] may also appear in speech and verbal thinking. The patients

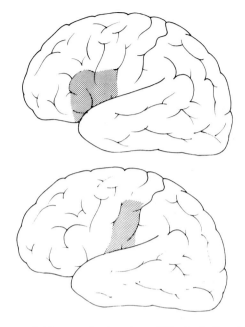

FIG. 11-4. Frontal cortical areas producing a mild, transient language disturbance but no significant articulation problem **(upper)** or causing a deficit in articulation **(lower)**. (Based on Tonkonogy and Goodglass: *Arch. Neurol.*, 38:486–490, 1981, with permission.)

of this group begin to have difficulty in fluent speech, their speech becomes interrupted, and difficulties arise in the transition from one element of articulation to another. Similar phenomena of the loss of smoothness (and sometimes of perseveration) may also appear in writing.

Right Hemisphere Involvement in Speech and Language

It has become increasingly apparent that the right hemisphere also plays a role in speech and language. As early as 1878 Hughlings Jackson suggested that the right hemisphere of the brain might control emotional aspects of speech. Affective components of communication, including emotional prosody and gesturing, have been linked to right hemisphere activity by many researchers (Heilman, Scholes, and Watson, 1975; Larsen, Skinhoj, and Lassen, 1978; Ross and Mesulam, 1979; Tucker, Watson, and Heilman, 1977). Ross (1981) studied separate functions (affective quality of spontaneous verbalization and gestures, repetition, and comprehension; affective verbalizations and gestures) and classified variations following right hemisphere pathology in a manner similar to the language disturbances of aphasic patients with left hemisphere pathology. Two right hemisphere disturbances of speech and language appeared to be specifically frontal. Patients with lesions in the right posterior inferior frontal gyrus, analogous to Broca's area (Fig. 11-5), understood emotional gestures and recognized emotionality in verbal output but had difficulty repeating the affective quality of sentences and showed limited affective quality in spontaneous gesture. The second right frontal variation resembles transcortical motor aphasia in that the only deficit was a lack of spontaneous output of emotional melodic verbalizations. Spontaneous speech was presented in

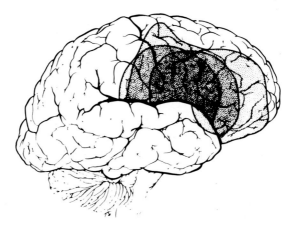

FIG. 11-5. Right frontal area involved in disturbance labeled motor aprosodia. (From Ross: *Arch. Neurol.* 38:561–569, 1981, with permission.)

a flat, nonemotional manner, but emotional verbalizations were repeated accurately. No cases with the lesions in the SMA of the right hemisphere were reported.

The work of Ross and others thus suggests that the right frontal lobe plays a role in communication, particularly that dealing with emotion. The right frontal language function appears limited to gestural and melodic expression, and it can be postulated that the left frontal lobe could carry out similar communication roles with syntactic and semantic language. Both the right and the left frontal lobes appear to have important communication roles in emotion (see Chapter 8).

RELATED CONSIDERATIONS

Verbal Adynamia

One of the more characteristic frontal language features, present to some degree in all frontal language disturbances, is the altered dynamic qualities of TCM aphasia and SMA language disturbance. Diminished speech spontaneity (*"adynamie der sprache"*) was originally reported after damage to the left frontal area by Kleist (1934b). The deficit has been characterized as difficulty in speech initiation or disinclination for sustained verbal output (Luria, 1969; Zangwill, 1966). In most instances adynamic verbal output accompanies general apathy, an overall decrease in spontaneous motor activities. The verbal and general motor adynamic qualities may not be equivalent, however. Reports of dissociation or uneven recovery with greater verbal than general motor disturbance are not uncommon (Damasio and Van Hoesen, 1980; Rubens, 1975), particularly in TCM aphasia and SMA language disturbance.

One clinical test that illustrates this function is the word fluency test, more aptly described as a word generation task. The patient is asked to produce a series of words derived from a category presented by the examiner (i.e., animals, professions, words beginning with a specific letter). Using an accepted procedure (Thurstone and Thurstone, 1943), Milner (1964) demonstrated a verbal generation deficit in frontal lobe damaged patients. Patients were required to write, within a 5-min time period, as many words as they could beginning with a specific letter. Frontal lobectomy patients, with no demonstrable language disorder, were significantly worse on this task than patients with excisions localized elsewhere. Milner's results have been widely replicated, most frequently using an oral version of the test, i.e., F-A-S (Spreen and Benton, 1969), requiring verbal production of a word list (Borkowski, Benton, and Spreen, 1967; Benton, 1968; Hécaen and Ruel, 1981; Perret, 1974; Ramier and Hécaen, 1970).

Caution is required when interpreting word generation tests as the specificity of the finding must be questioned. Impaired word list generation occurs with all types of aphasia and with cortical and subcortical types of dementia. Depressed word list generation cannot be considered pathognomonic of frontal adynamia.

It was first thought that significant word fluency problems did not occur after right frontal dysfunction (Feuchtwanger, 1923; Kleist, 1934b; Milner, 1964; Zangwill, 1966). Benton (1968), however, demonstrated disordered verbal fluency in patients with right frontal damage, although the frequency (38%) was not as great as it was following left frontal damage (70%). These findings of relative asymmetry of deficit for the two frontal lobes have been replicated (Hécaen and Ruel, 1981; Perret, 1974; Ramier and Hécaen, 1970) although not consistently (Bruyer and Tuyumbu, 1980). Ramier and Hécaen (1970) proposed a two-component deficit: (1) a nonverbal deficit in spontaneity or initiation; (2) a left hemisphere verbal problem. A similar effect has been found in a test of nonverbal design generation. Patients were requested to draw as many nonsense designs as they could within a time limit (Jones-Gotman and Milner, 1977); both left and right frontal lobe damaged patients performed worse than patients with lesions in posterior areas or normal subjects, and right frontal lobe damaged patients were significantly more impaired than those with left frontal lobe damage.

Lesions in the orbital frontal cortex do not impair performance on verbal fluency tests (Luria, 1966, 1970b; Milner, 1964; Stuss and Benson, 1983b). The inferior lateral cortex immediately anterior to Broca's area has been suggested as most important for word generation, (Luria, 1966/1980, 1970b), but this appears to be the case only if patients are aphasic (Hécaen and Ruel, 1981).

Perret (1974) hypothesized that a list of words beginning with a specific letter stresses symbolic factors, whereas category list generation emphasizes semantic factors. Semantic fluency tasks would draw on well-established associations and are more readily performed by frontal lobe patients. Newcombe (1969) did not demonstrate a significant deficit in left frontal lobe patients asked to generate a list of specific semantic categories (e.g., flowers). Symbolic tasks, on the other hand, not only demonstrated a deficit in language initiation but demanded inhibition of strong but incorrect associations.

Another explanation may be proposed for decreased word list generation with frontal pathology, a verbal adynamia based on SMA damage or separation of the energizer (SMA) and motor control (Broca) areas.

Regulatory Power of Language

Based on the theoretical writings of Vygotsky (1962), Luria (1960, 1967, 1973b) suggested that inner speech has an important programming and regulating role in behavior. Inner speech was thought to be responsible for the most complex forms of voluntary behavior by selecting the most salient features, creating an internal plan, and then monitoring the performance by comparison with the original intention. Damage to the frontal lobe can disturb this regulatory power of language. Frontal lobe patients may verbalize a task correctly but fail to use this information to direct their behavior. Ackerly and Benton's (1947) patient "had an excellent sense of right and wrong when talking about it in an abstract manner, but showed no such sense in his actions" (p. 490). Patients may state that they want to return to work, but they cannot mobilize the resources to actually do anything.

Luria provided several examples to illustrate this deficit. A patient with a left frontal tumor, when asked to lift his hand, can easily do so if his hand is above the blanket but fails if the hand is under the blanket, even though he correctly repeats the command (Luria, 1973a; Luria and Homskaya, 1964). In another task, Luria requested both frontally and parietally damaged patients to squeeze hard or soft to a specific signal (red/hard, green/soft). The groups could be differentiated by their ability to use verbal cues as an aid. Parietally damaged patients improved dramatically whereas patients with frontal damage could not use the programming influence of the verbal instructions (Luria, 1973a).

The loss of the regulatory power of language may also involve involuntary behavior (Luria and Homskaya, 1964). A novel stimulus normally elicits an orienting response, measured physiologically by the galvanic skin resistance. With repetition, the orienting response habituates unless a unique meaning such as requesting the subject to count the stimuli is appended. Patients with massive frontal lobe lesions produce few or no orienting responses, and verbal instruction has little effect. With less massive damage, verbal instruction helps stabilize the orienting response, but only temporarily. With parietal lesions, on the other hand, the orienting response may be stabilized by verbal instructions.

Further research is required before Luria's concept of the loss of verbal control of behavior can be fully accepted. First, lesion specificity within the frontal lobes must be sought. The most characteristic deficits apparently occur in patients with left dorsal-lateral frontal convexity pathology, and some negative evidence comes from an absence of the deficit in patients with large bilateral orbital frontal lesions (Benson and Stuss, 1982). Kaczmarek (1984) suggested lesion specificity of verbal utterances within the frontal lobes. In general, the left dorsal-lateral frontal lobe appears to be involved in the sequential organization of linguistic information. The orbital region monitors and compares the actual utterance with the intentions, leading to directed development of a narrative. The right frontal lobe is also involved in organization but of nonlinguistic information. Second, the overall deficit may not be as general as initially suggested. Drewe (1975b) found verbal/action dissociation on only a few tests given to frontal patients. Petrides (1985) and Milner (1982), based on deficits shown in frontal lobe patients on both spatial and nonspatial conditional learning tasks, argued for a more general deficit in the utilization of external cues to guide responses rather than a selective verbal regulation of behavior impairment. Nevertheless, verbal/action disassociation, a decrease in the control of actions by verbalized thought, deserves consideration as another example of frontal language disturbance.

SUMMARY

The following summary of the role of the frontal lobes in speech and language can be proposed for deliberation and future research.

1. Initiation of speech is a predominantly frontal lobe function that is based on a frontal volitional system, from the SMA to Broca's area. The press of speech described in certain posterior aphasias might be interpreted as a release of frontal speech activation from the normal control of posterior cortical zones.

2. Almost all language disturbances secondary to frontal lobe pathology have extension into underlying white matter and subcortical areas. These may be essential for the requisite aphasia syndrome.

3. There appear to be two frontal speech organization zones. The lower motor strip (area 4) seems to control the actual motor articulatory programs. The area anterior to this (Broca's area and immediate surround) appears to be important for the organization, speed, and smooth transition from articulation to articulation, comparable to the limb-kinetic apraxia of smooth motor movements secondary to premotor disturbance, described in Chapter 5.

4. Both left and right frontal areas are active in speech and language in accordance with their respective roles in cerebral activity.

5. Frontal pathology disturbs sequencing and relational organization for both verbal output and comprehension when multistep tasks are presented.

6. Frontal lobe damage results in impaired verbal control of behavior.

Whether any or all of the above postulates are proved true, there can be little doubt that the frontal lobes play an important role in speech and language functions, both directly and through interaction in a controlling manner with functions subserved in other brain areas.

12 ————————————

Memory

The function of memory occupies a prominent position in many theories concerning the role of the frontal lobes in human behavior. Nonetheless, several obvious difficulties preclude acceptance of an underlying deficit in memory as a fundamental defect of frontal lobe damage. Although memory function may be affected by frontal damage, present evidence for a frontal input to memory function is weak: (1) it is extremely difficult, almost impossible, to construct a memory task that is not affected by other known dysfunctions of frontal damage; (2) control of various factors such as age, education, size, and extent of lesion has been virtually impossible; (3) results have been inconsistent, especially when comparing animal and human research. This chapter probes the role of the frontal lobes in memory.

A brief summary of salient animal research introduces the human clinical observations and research studies. The controversy generated by conflicting results leads to related behavioral research which helps clarify the part the frontal lobes play in memory.

ANIMAL STUDIES

"Loss of recent memory" was one of the earliest theories used to explain the behavioral deficit noted in animals with frontal lesions (Jacobsen, 1935, 1936). This interpretation, which influenced thinking about frontal lobe functions for many years, was based on the poor performance of frontally lesioned animals in delayed response and delayed alternation tasks. The Wisconsin General Testing Apparatus (Fig. 12-1) was frequently used for these tests. The animal sits in a transport cage in a sound-shielded room facing two identical covered food wells situated at a specified distance from each other. The dishes may be shielded from the animal by an opaque screen that can be raised or lowered by the examiner. Behavior is shaped by first leaving food in open food wells, then in enclosed food wells. In the delayed response task, a reinforcer (food) is placed in one of the containers in full view of the animal. The wells are covered, and the opaque screen is lowered. Following a defined interval, the screen is raised and the animal must select the container with the food. In the delayed alternation task, the screen is lowered immediately after the animal selects one of the food wells, whether the response was correct or incorrect. If correct, food is placed in the alternate food well, both wells are covered, and the screen is raised after the defined delay

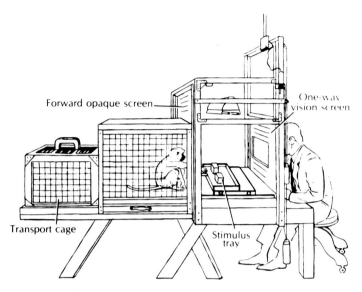

FIG. 12-1. Wisconsin General Testing Apparatus, used in testing discrimination, delayed response, and delayed alternation tasks in primates. (From Hinde: *Animal Behavior*. McGraw-Hill, New York, 1966/1970, with permission. Originally published by Harlow: *Psychol. Rev.*, 56:51–65, 1949.)

interval. If incorrect, food remains in the original well, and the trials are repeated until correct.

Bilateral frontal lobe damage in monkeys caused impaired performance on both the delayed response and delayed alternation tasks. Because the animals performed normally under conditions of no delay, a logical interpretation of the deficit appeared to be "a loss of recent memory."

Explanation of this frontal lobe dysfunction as a memory defect has been subject to modifications and criticisms. An alternate theory suggested that the deficit indicated disturbance in handling positional and orientational cues based on the inherent spatial quality of the tasks (Goldman and Rosvold, 1970; Mishkin and Pribram, 1956). Negative evidence was used to attack the memory theory. No deficit was demonstrated in frontal lobectomized monkeys given a delayed paired comparison task (Weiskrantz, 1978). This criticism itself came under attack, however, in that the task was difficult; the animals needed much training, obliterating the significance of differences after lobectomy. Another series of experiments demonstrated that, after bilateral frontal lobectomy, animals had no difficulty on delayed response tasks if distractions were minimized and their attention was fully captured. For example, if lights were turned off during the delay period or if reward was obtained before as well as after the delay period, no deficits occurred (Finan, 1942; Malmo, 1942). Similar negative results were observed if animals were trained under the influence of sedatives or if the relevance of the discrimination was emphasized by prolonged training (Campbell and Harlow, 1945; Wade, 1947). Results from these and related experiments gradually replaced the concept of a memory deficit per se, and other explanations were offered: distractibility (Finan, 1942; Malmo, 1942); decreased drive (Pribram, 1950); hyperactivity (Orbach and Fischer, 1959; Richter and Hines, 1938); hyperreactivity (Buffery, 1967; Ruch and Shenkin, 1943); deficit in habituation (Grueninger and Pribram, 1969; Kimble, Bagshaw, and Pribram, 1965); and stimulus and task specific disturbances (Jacobsen and Nissen, 1937; Pribram, 1961).

Two types of animal experiment exemplify the increasing understanding of the quality of the deficit in delayed tasks. Pribram and Tubbs (1967) modified the classic delayed alternation task by placing a 15-sec interval between each pair of responses (RL–RL–RL). Animals with prefrontal lesions, who fail on the classic delayed alternation task, performed normally in this modified version. Because performance was adequate over a 15-sec delay, the deficit after frontal lobe damage was not well explained as an impairment in maintenance of a memory trace for a short period. Rather, the frontal lobes were interpreted as important for programming, that is, parceling information into workable "chunks" to provide an organized division of the information, an important feature in short-term memory. Tubbs (1969) extended these experiments by inserting a light or a sound on every other trial during the intertrial period of delayed alternation tasks. The "syntactical prosthesis" superimposed by the light or sound failed, indicating that temporal structuring of information input was the most efficient means of compensating the original frontal lobe deficit.

Fuster and Bauer (1974) investigated the hypothesis that the lateral prefrontal cortex, specifically the sulcus principalis, was important for spatial information-processing and for short-term memory. They trained four monkeys on a delayed matching-to-sample task. The control condition was simultaneous matching-to-sample. Cooling probes were inserted in the prefrontal and parietal areas bilaterally. Monkeys were investigated under three experimental manipulations: localized cooling of frontal areas, localized cooling of parietal areas, and inoperative coolers, i.e., normal brain temperature. The results indicated no difference in reaction time across conditions, eliminating the concept of motivation as an explanatory factor. Most errors occurred under the condition of frontal (unilateral but particularly bilateral) cooling, increasing with the length of delay. If a distracting stimulus was inserted, performance deteriorated for all conditions but was significantly more impaired with prefrontal cooling. The authors proposed that the basic function of the prefrontal cortex was to provide "consistent and purposive attention during and beyond the time of exposure to relevant stimuli."

Frontal lobe lesions in animals also impair performance on specific conditional-learning tasks (Gross and Weiskrantz, 1962; Milner, Foreman, and Goodale, 1978; Stamm, 1979). Lesion localization for at least certain tasks is specific. For example, periarcuate pathology severely impairs motor conditional-associations, whereas principalis region lesions result in mild impairment (Petrides, 1982). These results are useful in providing a framework to interpret similar deficits in humans with frontal lobe damage (Milner, 1982).

Mishkin (1982), based on monkey ablation studies, has proposed two parallel circuits as the neuroanatomical bases of memory: (1) amygdala and thalamic dorsal/medial (DM) nucleus; (2) hippocampus and anterior thalamic nuclei. Based on the known projections of the DM nucleus to the frontal cortex, Mishkin and Bachevalier (1983) tested object recognition memory in monkeys with either dorsal-lateral or ventral-medial frontal lesions. Ventral-medial prefrontal cortex, connected to the magnocellular division of DM, was more important in general memory processes than the dorsal-lateral prefrontal cortex. Whether this represents memory function in the accepted manner or is another example of frontal control is undetermined. Monkeys with inferior prefrontal convexity lesions had a deficit in relearning due not to a memory loss but to perseverative interference (Kowalska, Bachevalier, and Mishkin, 1984).

In summary, research with animals originally led to the memory hypothesis of frontal lobe functioning, but additional research with more specific designs gradually led to the interpretation of the deficit in terms of attention. It is still possible that the appropriate localization or combination of lesions, or extent of pathology, might result in a true memory disorder after frontal lesions.

HUMAN CLINICAL DESCRIPTION

Despite the relatively consistent and generally negative results in the animal literature, controversy over the role of the frontal lobes in human memory functions has continued. Gardner (1975), in his textbook on neurology, stated that "it is interesting that extensive bilateral lesions of the prefrontal cortex interfere with short-term memory" (p. 426). Disturbances of memory are frequently observed in patients with frontal lobe tumors (Hécaen, 1964), and some even state that disturbances of memory and orientation are the most striking feature of frontal lobe tumor (Stookey et al., 1941). Kolodny (1929) reported that 43% of patients with frontal lobe tumors had subjective or objective evidence of memory problems (compared to 50% of cases with temporal lobe tumors), and memory disturbance could be considered an early symptom of frontal lobe tumor.

The memory disturbance described with frontal abnormality primarily involves recent events. Hécaen and Albert (1978) described a "forgetting to remember" in which an intended act or memory is forgotten, although it may be retrieved later. An example from the information subscale of the Wechsler Adult Intelligence Scale illustrates this deficit. A patient who had undergone bilateral frontal leukotomy many years earlier was asked what the Vatican was and replied that he did not know. Later in the examination, while discussing religion, the patient stated that he was a Catholic, that the Pope was the head of the Church, and that he was situated in the Vatican in Rome. Although he "knew" the answer when originally asked, he could not "remember" without the cue of religion.

A 55-year-old patient who had sustained bilateral frontal polar injury in a traffic accident was evaluated for diabetes insipidus through a water limitation program. He was instructed by his doctor: "Don't drink any water, don't go near the water fountain." Within 10 min the patient was seen getting a drink at the fountain. When confronted he was asked what he had been told and immediately replied: "Don't drink any water, don't go near the water fountain."

Such divorce of the verbal thought from the action characterizes many reported frontal lobe memory losses; this important problem has been discussed elsewhere (see Chapter 11).

The most common source of reports of memory impairment following frontal pathology concerns rupture and/or surgical correction of anterior communicating artery aneurysms. Neurosurgeons have long been aware of impaired memory function as a common and serious residual of this disorder. It has been interpreted that frontal lobe damage underlies the memory loss, suggesting that the medial, posterior orbital frontal area be included among neuroanatomical loci of memory function. Subarachnoid hemorrhage is common in these situations, however, and tends to have widespread consequences. Pathological studies consistently fail to correlate focal frontal pathology with amnesia. There is one exception, a well-studied case of post-cerebrovascular accident (CVA) amnesia which at autopsy had evidence of anterior cerebral artery occlusion. The infarction subsequent to the occlusion did not involve only the frontal lobes, however; bilateral destruction of the columns of the fornix was also demonstrated. The amnesia may not have been a product of frontal lobe involvement (Brion, Pragier, Guerin, et al., 1969).

A 40-year-old taxi driver suffered two episodes of subarachnoid hemorrhage based on anterior communicating artery rupture. The course following the second bleed was stormy, but he was eventually stabilized and the aneurysm successfully treated by surgery. Postoperatively both physical and mental conditions were abnormal. He showed a serious motor problem, mild generalized spasticity complicated by pronounced ataxia. Mentally he was demented, showing among other problems a total inability to learn new information and long retrograde amnesia. He was incontinent. A diagnosis of normal-pressure hydrocephalus was eventually made, proved by appropriate laboratory studies, and treated by ventriculoatrial shunt. Twelve hours after the surgery all of the physical and mental problems had disappeared; he had a full return of memory function with the exception of a hiatus of about 2 months' duration (the time from the second bleed to the shunting) for which he had no memory.

This case illustrates another explanation for the amnesia secondary to anterior communicating artery hemorrhage, a complicating normal-pressure hydrocephalus (Hakim, 1964). Both the loss of memory function and the rapid total return of memory following therapy are dramatic. Not all patients with normal-pressure hydrocephalus show memory disturbance, and not all improve with therapy. It appears that when memory loss follows anterior cerebral artery occlusion it cannot be confidently ascribed to frontal lobe pathology.

A 54-year-old business analyst without previous medical history suffered bilateral paramedian thalamic infarcts. Early in the course the most striking impairment was diminished arousal. He gradually improved but remained somewhat hypersomnolent, apathetic, unconcerned, with little initiative or spontaneity. General abilities appeared to be inferior to estimated premorbid levels, although verbal IQ and most language skills had returned to normal limits. Memory, attention, and visual-spatial abilities remained severely impaired.

This case was interpreted as a subcortical dementia, with a severe memory disorder secondary to the bilateral dorsal medial nucleus lesions (Guberman and Stuss, 1983). A second interpretation is possible (Stuss, Guberman, Nelson, et al., 1984/b). The monitoring and attentional disorder may be secondary to the dorsal-medial lesions, known to have important connections with prefrontal cortex (see Chapter 2). The memory disorder, on the other hand, is hypothesized as being due to two factors: (1) an attentional-frontal memory problem secondary to the thalamic lesions; (2) a true amnesia, due to involvement of the mammillothalamic tract coursing proximal to the dorsal medial nuclei. Even with focal circumscribed lesions, the possibility of involvement of proximal pathways must be considered. Care must be taken to dissociate a true amnesia from secondary problems.

Although observations of memory impairment in humans with frontal pathology are numerous, correlation of the clinical picture with the pathological findings is tenuous at best. No consistent demonstration of frontal structural abnormality associated with memory disturbance in the classic amnesia pattern has been presented in the human.

HUMAN PSYCHOLOGICAL TEST RESULTS

Positive Evidence of Frontal Memory

In addition to the clinical reports, several formal psychological studies have suggested memory deficits following frontal lobe damage in human patients. In a 14-year follow-up, Hamlin (1970) noted that decreased digit span differentiated patients with superior frontal lobe topectomy from normal controls. Digit span backward, a task that requires immediate memory plus manipulation of this information " in abstracto," was also said to be impaired postleukotomy (Vidor, 1951).

Memory problems following rupture of anterior communicating artery aneurysms were formally assessed (Lindqvist and Norlen, 1966; Talland, Sweet, and Ballantine, 1967). Both studies suggested that a Korsakoff type of amnesia can occur in which the ability to learn is most affected (Benson, 1978). It was suggested that the memory problems following rupture of an anterior cerebral artery aneurysm reflect the proximity of the pathology to the base of the third ventricle, "a site where lesions may affect new learning whilst leaving other aspects of intelligence unimpaired" (Logue, Durward, Pratt, et al., 1968). The full amnesia syndrome is not observed in all patients with this disorder, however, and whether the extent or the location of the lesion is the crucial factor remains unknown. In fact, it is entirely possible that the brain abnormality underlying this memory disorder may not affect the frontal lobes at all. Damage of anterior communicating artery perforators that feed the anterior hypothalamus or septum may be necessary for the syndrome (Alexander and Freedman, 1984).

A frontal memory deficit was suggested by Lewinsohn, Zieler, Libet, et al. (1972), who compared left and right, frontal and nonfrontal brain-damaged patients. Aphasia was controlled by a six-point language scale, but differences in etiology were not considered. Four memory tasks involving visual, auditory, perceptual, and kinesthetic patterns were administered. All stimuli were presented for 1 sec, with memory tested after delays of 0 sec (registration) or 10 sec (retention) by having the subject point to the target stimulus embedded among all possible stimuli. For the 10 sec delay, the subjects counted out loud forward to prevent rehearsal over time. For the visual and auditory short-term memory task, each stimulus contained more than one bit of information. For example, on the visual short-term memory task, each slide contained a picture of an object, a background color, and a background pattern. For each trial, the subject had to respond either immediately or after the 10-sec delay by naming or pointing first to the object, then the color, and then the pattern of each slide in the order in which they were presented. All brain-damaged patients performed worse than normal subjects, but no difference was found between those with left and right hemisphere lesions. The frontal lobe damaged patients performed the worst, with the greatest decrement for the auditory conditions followed by visual, somewhat less for the perceptual, and least for the kinesthetic modality. The authors (Lewinsohn et al., 1972) noted that their results were consistent with those reported following anterior cerebral artery aneurysm rupture and concluded that the frontal lobe was significantly involved in memory. Other possible reasons for the apparent memory deficits were not well controlled. All patients had large, acute cerebrovascular or neurosurgical lesions, and the characteristics of aphasia were poorly defined. In addition, the experimental design introduced a number of possible confounding manipulations; the interference (counting out loud), the temporal ordering (recall of information in sequential order), and the visual search (recall by pointing to a stimulus embedded among other stimuli) demand a variety of mental skills in addition to memory. Each of these manipulations has been demonstrated to be sensitive to frontal lobe damage in nonmemory tasks.

Pribram, Ahumada, Hartog, et al. (1964) reported a deficit in delayed alternation in lobotomized psychiatric patients when compared to unoperated control patients, and Freedman and Oscar-Berman (1986) found that bilateral frontal lobe patients were impaired on both delayed response and delayed alternation tasks. These results cannot be accepted as evidence of a primary memory disorder based on frontal lobe damage, however. Although of considerable interest, the results of these studies more likely suggest a sensitivity to interference.

Negative Evidence Against Frontal Memory

In contrast to the limited number of investigations reporting positive results, many studies have failed to demonstrate a clear-cut effect of frontal lobe damage on memory functions. Comparison of patients with frontal lobe damage from a variety of etiologies with normal control subjects revealed little or no difference in immediate memory as measured by auditory and/or visual-motor span tests (digit span, Knox Cube) (Ghent, Mishkin, and Teuber, 1962; Mettler, 1949; Partridge, 1950; Stuss et al., 1978, 1982b; Teuber, 1964). Similarly, in contrast to the findings of Pribram et al. (1964) and of Freedman and Oscar-Berman (1985), humans with frontal lobe pathology did not show unique or outstanding impairment when tested on a delayed response task, the test most sensitive to frontal lesioning in the animal literature (Chorover and Cole, 1966). Negative results on single and double alternation and delayed response tasks, as well as on Goldstein's stick test, were reported in a patient with partial bilateral frontal lobectomy (Hebb, 1945). Assessment of a patient with congenital bilateral frontal lobe disorder disclosed no discernible memory deficit (Ackerley and Benton, 1947). Testing at varying durations of follow-up after bilateral frontal leukotomy has revealed no significant memory deficit in comparison to normal control subjects on almost all measures of memory (Baker, Young, Gauld, et al., 1970; Malmo, 1948; Medina et al., 1954; Struckett, 1953; Stuss et al., 1982b; Vidor, 1951). This lack of specific effect of relatively gross frontal lobe abnormality on memory test performance has been observed with a variety of etiologies (epilepsy, tumor, trauma, lobectomy including cingulotomy) and a variety of memory tests (Wechsler Memory Scale, paired associate learning, Benton Visual Retention Test, recall of narrative prose) (Black, 1976; Butters, Samuels, Goodglass, et al., 1970; Delaney, Rosen, Mattson, et al., 1980; Medina et al., 1954; Milner and Teuber, 1968; Mirsky and Orzack, 1977; Struckett, 1953; Stuss et al., 1982b; Teuber, Corkin, and Twitchell, 1977; Vidor, 1951). Thus a preponderance of reported studies suggest that the frontal lobes have little, if any, role in the memory process.

Related Studies

Delayed Response Tests

The role of the frontal lobes in memory functioning can perhaps be better understood by reviewing individual areas of research and focusing on specific theoretical issues. One major point concerns the validity of the delayed response effect in humans. Milner and Teuber (1968) suggested that the negative results with the procedure reported by Chorover and Cole (1966) may be attributed to the fact that humans can verbally encode and thus mediate a longer delay. Ghent. et al. (1962) devised a more difficult delayed response task that could not easily be verbalized and tested the hypothesis that the delayed response deficit was not specific for either positional or orientational cues. All subjects had frontal or nonfrontal brain damage from penetrating gunshot wounds and were compared to a normal control group. Four spatial tests were devised, with recall after 0 or 15 sec delay. In the first test a 36-inch illuminated rod 10 feet distant from the subject was tilted. The rod was then returned to the vertical and the subject asked to return the rod to the angle of the tilt. A second test required memory for tactile point localization on the palm, and a third localized a lighted point in space. A fourth test, comparable to the rod tilt test but without a delayed recall, was designed for personal body tilt. No overall impairment could be demonstrated on any task in the frontal lobe damaged subjects. The authors concluded that damage to the frontal lobes does not necessarily produce a specific recent memory deficit, regardless of positional or orientational cues. Possible reasons suggested for the failure to demonstrate a frontal memory deficit included size or etiology of the lesion, length of interval for delayed recall, and the absence of a control for possible rehearsal effects as there was no interpolated task. Nevertheless, these results stand as negative evidence for the involvement of frontal lobes in memory functions.

Prisko (1963; Milner and Teuber, 1968) extended the investigation of the effect of delayed response in humans by adapting a delayed paired comparison procedure using the compound stimuli originally developed for animal research by Konorski (1959). Two stimuli from the same sensory modality were separated by a delay, and the subject had to judge if the second stimulus was identical to the first. Chance probability of correct identity was 50%. The task was designed to demand memory of the first stimulus for comparison with the second stimulus rather than for discrimination. The procedure demanded inhibition of the memory of the previous trials. Five stimuli were used: clicks, flashes, tones, colors, and irregular nonsense patterns. Five stimulus values were used in each task, making verbal rehearsal difficult. Experimental conditions included stimulus modality, duration of delay before recall (up to 60 sec), and the presence or absence of interpolated distraction. Subjects assessed were normal controls, those with unilateral left or right temporal lobectomy, and those with unilateral left or right frontal lobectomy. The normal subjects found all tasks easy. The unilateral temporal subjects performed all tests within the normal range, with the exception of the right temporal lobe patients who had difficulty with the visual pattern recognition test. On the other hand, unilateral frontal lobe patients were significantly impaired on the tests of clicks, flashes, and colors, but their performance on the irregular nonsense patterns was equivalent to normal control subjects.

The following conclusions and interpretations were offered: (1) the delayed comparison test in the human was considered equivalent to the delayed response test in the monkey because both had intertrial delays; (2) the results implied a similar memory impairment following frontal lobe damage; (3) a susceptibility to interference and not a deficit in memory in the narrow sense was offered as the reason for the disturbance; (4) the frontal lobe subjects did well on the nonsense figure recall task because these figures were unique; (5) frontal damage may affect time marking and temporal distinction, producing problems in discriminating recent from prior stimuli. This inability to keep separate trials distinct appears to be similar to the deficit reported by Pribram and Tubbs (1967) in monkeys.

Continuous Recognition Tests—Recency

Continuous recognition or recurring stimuli techniques have been considered sensitive indicators of the effect of frontal lobe damage on memory functioning. A number of recurring figures tests exist. Single stimulus items are presented one at a time, and the subject must decide whether each item has been seen before (Milner and Teuber, 1968). Most tests are designed with high similarity among items, tending to maximize interference effects. In a recurring nonsense figures test (Kimura, 1963), patients with frontal lobe damage were as severely impaired as those with right temporal pathology, even though the former had normal visual pattern recognition. The frontal lobe patients responded perseveratively or randomly, changed responses, showed little concern about their judgment, yet could verbalize the test instructions perfectly. The deficit in the frontal lobe patients was interpreted as a "heightened susceptibility to interference." Corkin (1964; Milner and Teuber, 1968) administered a test of recurring tactile pattern recognition to patients with frontal damage, temporal pathology, and posterior parietal pathology, all having normal sensation. Forty irregular abstract patterns were presented. Patients with posterior lesions had no impairment on this task with either hand. If the lesion involved the frontal lobe, however, a deficit was found in the hand contralateral to the lesion. This was interpreted as suggesting a close link between central and frontal cortex functions within the same hemisphere.

Others have reported results that are not consistent with the reported deficits. Delaney et al. (1980) compared nonverbal recurring figures in patients with frontal and temporal lobe epileptic foci. Milner's suggestion that unilateral frontal lobe damage produced heightened susceptibility to proactive interference was not substantiated. Similar negative results with recurring figures tests of various content and modality were reported following bilateral frontal leukotomy (Stuss et al., 1982b). In this study, to maximize interference, an independent introductory set of figures containing the recurring figures was not identified. Not only was there no difference from normal control subjects, a first-half/second-half difference was not demonstrated, negating a gradual buildup of interference as a memory defect in frontal lobe damaged patients. Finally, recognition of recurring bird songs was performed normally by frontally damaged patients (Milner and Teuber, 1968). It was postulated that the bird songs were more interesting, thereby compensating for the boredom and interference normally present in the continuous recognition procedure.

In summary, results from a variety of continuous recognition tasks administered to a variety of frontal lobe damaged subjects have yielded interesting but inconsistent results. The possibility that a heightened susceptibility to interference underlies much of the apparent memory disturbance in frontally damaged patients is raised, a possibility proposed by Malmo (Malmo, 1948; Malmo and Amsel, 1948). If interference accounts for the apparent memory deficit, the continuous recognition tests does not provide a reliable measure of the impairment.

A related line of inquiry suggests that the ability to discriminate items in memory temporally may be impaired by frontal lobe damage. Corsi (1972) and Milner (1971, 1974, 1982) directly addressed the concept of temporal recency using both verbal and nonverbal modalities in patients who had sustained left and right frontal or temporal lobectomy. For each modality, 184 cards were prepared, two items on each card. For the verbal modality, two "spondaeic words" were presented (e.g., cowboy, railroad). For the nonverbal task, reproductions of abstract art or representational drawings were used. Two task conditions were administered. In the recency condition, cards were presented one at a time, certain cards having a question mark between the two words or works of art. Both items on the card had been presented on previous cards, and the subject was asked which of the two items had been seen most recently. In the recognition condition, a question mark again occurred between the two items presented on one card, but only one item had been presented previously and the subject was asked to identify the item seen before.

The results demonstrated both modality and lesion specificity. In the recognition condition, the temporal lobe damaged patients were impaired for either verbal or nonverbal material, dependent on the left or right hemispheric site of the lesion, respectively. In the verbal recency condition, both temporal groups performed more accurately than the left frontal and left frontal-temporal patients. The right frontal and right frontal-temporal groups were inconsistent but better than the two left frontal groups. Patients with left frontal damage were unimpaired for nonverbal recency judgments. It appeared that judgment of verbal recency was sensitive to frontal, particularly left frontal, damage. Right frontal patients, in contrast, were impaired for nonverbal recency judgments (more severe for abstract), as well as the verbal recency task, suggesting a right hemisphere dominance for recency discrimination. This involvement of the frontal lobes in the temporal structuring of behavior appears similar to the concepts proposed by other authors (Fuster, 1980; Pribram and Tubbs, 1967; Tubbs, 1969).

Maze Tests

Milner (1965) tested whether memory defects were the reason that frontal lobe damaged patients perform poorly on visually guided maze learning. The subjects were required to discover and remember one correct path on a 10×10 grid of boltheads. Trials continued until three successive errorless performances were achieved. Patients with damage in either parietal lobe or in the left temporal areas were equivalent to normal subjects in performance, whereas patients with right temporal, right temporal-parietal, and either left or right frontal lobe damage were markedly impaired. Both quantitative and qualitative differences in performance were locus-dependent (Milner, 1965). Frontal lobe patients had problems obeying test instructions; they frequently broke the rules and had higher intitial time scores because disobeying of rules occurred most often in the early stages (Milner, 1965; Walsh, 1978). It appeared that the deficit in the frontal patients was best explained as an inability to follow instructions, not as a memory disorder. Corkin (1965) observed similar results in a tactually guided maze learning test.

Conditional Associative Learning Tasks

Animal research suggests that frontal lesions impair conditional associative learning tasks (Petrides, 1982). The presence of the deficit for spatial and nonspatial tasks suggested that the deficit was generally a problem in response selection. Petrides (1985) and Milner (1982) tested this hypothesis by comparing lobectomized patients on spatial and nonspatial associative learning tasks. Left and right frontal lobe patients were impaired on both tasks, whereas hippocampal lesion patients had a modality-specific effect (spatial–right; nonspatial–left). General impairment in the utilization of external cues as a means of response guidance was suggested, not the selective verbal regulation impairment suggested by Luria (1973a).

Frontal Amnesia—A Disorder of Organization

The accumulated evidence implies that lesions of the frontal lobe in humans do not cause a primary disturbance of memory, but that they do interfere with mnestic activity (Goldstein, 1936a). Luria (1973a) suggested that frontal lobe damage leaves the operative function of memory intact, but "the ability to create *stable motives* of recall and to maintain the *active effort* required for voluntary recall, on the one hand, and the ability to *switch from one group of traces to another* [*are deficient*], with the result that it is the process of recall and reproduction of material which is significantly impaired" (p. 211). In other words, the frontal lobes are involved in the process of organizing methods of memorization and retrieval, and in comparing the results with the original intention. Frontal lobe damage does not interfere with putting material into storage (memorizing) but does impair essential associated mnestic activities including attention, motivation, programming, regulation, and verification.

Luria demonstrated the influence of the frontal lobe on memory by a series of tests. When a frontal lobe patient is required to memorize a long series of spoken or written words, those items that make a direct impression and require little effort to memorize are best remembered. The total number of items remembered does not significantly increase with repetitions of the list as it does with normal subjects, but different words may be recalled on subsequent trials. It is suggested that the passive imprinting of material is intact but that a deficit exists in the control of retrieval. If given one series of words to remember, followed by a second series to remember and then a request to remember the first list, frontal lobe patients perform less well than normal subjects. The second list may be presented, or, more often, words from both lists are offered. Luria (1973a) noted that although any patient with brain damage is susceptible to the effects of interference, patients with focal frontal lobe pathology have a greater tendency to repeat the more recent memory trace.

These concepts were assessed by administration of a battery of memory tests to patients with orbital-medial prefrontal leukotomy lesions (Stuss et al., 1982b). The results suggest that orbital frontal pathology does not affect memory functioning per se. Leukotomized subjects performed as well as normal subjects on standard memory tests (e.g., the Wechsler Memory Scale). No significant differences were noted on tests of continuous recognition or recall of a series of words. These patients were sensitive, however, to the effects of interference as defined by the Brown-Peterson technique in the consonant trigrams test (Brown, 1958; Cermak and Butters, 1972; Peterson and Peterson, 1959) (Fig. 12-2).

Material from the literature plus our own work strongly support susceptibility to interference as an important source of underlying impaired performance on

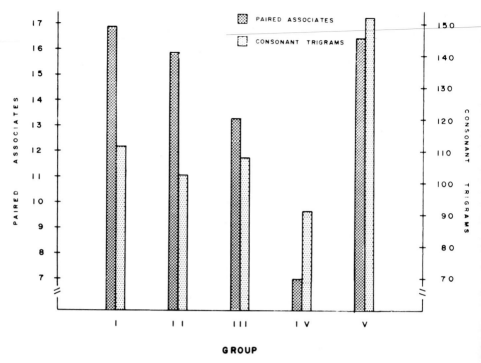

FIG. 12-2. Comparison of the Wechsler Memory Scale easy paired associates with the consonant trigrams total score depicts the comparable performance on both tests for the normal control group (V) and the nonleukotomized schizophrenic control group (IV). The leukotomized psychiatric patients with orbital frontal lesions, particularly those in group I, the good recovery patients, had a dissociation in performance, with deficits on the interference test. Maximum score for the paired associates is 18, for consonant trigrams 180. (From Stuss et al.: *J. Comp. Physiol. Psychol.*, 96:913–925, 1982, with permission.)

memory tests in animals and humans with frontal lobe damage. If it is only the reason is not yet determined. This susceptibility to interference appears to be nonspecific as it is reported following both orbital and dorsal-lateral cortical frontal pathology. It can be further suggested that this deficit reflects a frontally damaged patient's inability to maintain consistent, directed attention over time based on an inability to control interfering stimuli (Fuster and Bauer, 1974). Although not directly affecting operative memory, the prefrontal cortex does play a directive, organizational role in the processes of memory.

SUMMARY

Memory, as suggested by lesion research, is subserved by a variety of complex neuroanatomical circuits. Pathology at different points in the circuit might result in qualitatively different disorders of memory functioning (Butters and Cermak, 1975). The frontal lobes are closely interconnected with the limbic-diencephalic system of memory. Most current research demonstrates that damage to the frontal lobes does not produce classic amnesia but, rather, results in frontal cognitive impairments that influence the successful functioning of memory (Barbizet, 1971). Knowledge of this qualitatively different memory disorder may be helpful in identifying the neural basis of deficits in other populations such as the elderly (Moscovitch and Winocur, 1983).

13

Cognition

No greater confusion concerning the function of the frontal lobes has occurred than the turmoil surrounding the question of their role in cognition. Reflecting ongoing disagreement as to the meaning of cognition, the problem has been intensified by fanciful notions of the functions of the frontal lobes. Many early authors attributed the highest possible functions to the frontal lobes; these included will, recent memory, abstract behavior, foresight, ethical behavior, and so on. It was as if the frontal lobes were *"sedes sapientiae totae,"* the seat of all wisdom. The neurosurgeon Percival Bailey (1933) related how this background affected his judgment when faced with amputating a frontal lobe: "This procedure is always followed by more or less alteration in character and defects in judgment.... [*In a*] professional business man, who must make decisions affecting many people, these results may be disastrous" (p. 433).

On the other hand, others could not identify specific functions associated with the prefrontal lobes. Most unexpected, intellectual functions appeared to be unaffected by frontal amputation. In contrast to the hesitations described by Bailey, examples of improved functioning after bilateral frontal lobectomy were documented (Hebb, 1945; Hebb and Penfield, 1940). It was concluded that the frontal lobes had no specific role or, rather, research to date had not identified specific functions dependent on the frontal zones (Hebb, 1945; Meyer, 1960).

The "riddle" of the frontal lobe in cognition (Teuber, 1964) is largely relegated to neurohistory at present, but paradoxes and questions remain. Advances have been made on several fronts: greater care in selection and identification of subjects; less reliance on case studies; innovative experimental designs; and development of clearer operational definitions.

This chapter and the next one, although divided logically, should be viewed as representing a gradual evolution of concepts becoming clarified over time. Chapter 14 presents the executive functions, those abilities that appear to depend more directly on the integrity of the frontal lobes. The present chapter, titled "Cognition" to represent the historical development of frontal lobe investigation, actually provides an overall description of this group of functions. The absence of an operational definition of cognition is accepted, and throughout the chapter the term is used only in a general descriptive manner. The chapter has four sections. The first briefly reviews reports of cognitive functions from case studies of frontal lobe pathology. The second section examines the effects of frontal lobe damage on intellectual functioning as defined by scores on tests of intelligence. The third explores the function of abstraction in frontal lobe patients, and the final part presents Halstead's concept of biological intelligence in relation to the frontal lobe.

CASE STUDIES

Clinical observations and case studies have been remarkably consistent in their descriptions of the cognitive changes that follow extensive frontal lobe damage. The famous description of Phineas Gage (Harlow, 1868) included many behavioral changes, including astute observations on intellectual ability. Gage's "mental operations were perfect in kind, but not in degree or quantity"; that is, although impaired or diminished, his cognitive functions were not lost. Phineas Gage was by no means "demented." Similarly Welt (1888), describing a furrier who severely injured his right frontal lobe in a 100-foot fall, noted that although his personality changed radically the patient's intellect appeared intact and he was able to return to work, slower but still capable. Another patient who had extensive portions of both frontal lobes removed (Brickner, 1936) had IQ scores within the normal range.

In one extensively investigated case study of an individual with extensive bilateral frontal lobe defect, probably on a congenital basis (Ackerly, 1935; Ackerly and Benton, 1947), the right frontal lobe was totally absent and the left had extensive cystic degeneration. The patient was always considered to have good intelligence, although he failed grades 4 and 5. He was noted to learn quickly, and IQ tests administered at several points during his life provided scores that indicated no gross intellectual impairment (e.g., Stanford-Binet measures showed an IQ of 90 at age 11, 92 at age 13, and 97 at age 20, and he obtained an IQ of 100 on the Army Alpha test).

Case studies of this type are open to criticism. Even though IQ scores were obtained, no comparison measure was available; an IQ score within the normal range may reflect impaired functioning in comparison to a noninjured state. IQ tests do not adequately reflect cognition. Regardless of deficiencies, however, these presentations are important as they clearly demonstrate that despite the presence of gross frontal damage objective measurement of cognitive deficit was not easy.

IQ SCORES

A well-educated professional suffered a severe head injury in a nine-story fall down an elevator shaft, resulting in coma of 48 hr. Six months after injury, CT scan (Fig. 13-1) showed mild bilateral frontal atrophy. His behavior was generally appropriate even though punctuated with emotional lability. Neuropsychological testing performed after stabilization of the physical condition indicated a Wechsler Adult Intelligence Scale (WAIS) Verbal IQ in the superior range (120). The Wechsler Memory Quotient was 112, suggesting an ongoing mild amnesia. He could perform his previous occupation at a high level, and his advice was sought by colleagues, even while he was still in hospital. Despite the apparent cognitive recovery, he showed a tendency to confabulate and remained mildly slow at new learning.

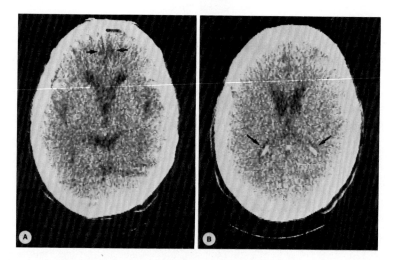

FIG. 13-1. A: Slight focal cortical atrophy is seen in the interhemispheric fissure *(arrows)*, and the anterior horns of the lateral ventricles are prominent. **B:** At the next CT scan level, the anterior horns are seen to be enlarged relative to the small trigonal portions *(arrows)* of the lateral ventricles. The findings are indicative of generalized bilateral frontal lobe atrophy.

This case study illustrates the frequently negative findings on IQ tests observed in patients with frontal lobe pathology (see below). Some of the results using objective measures of intellectual functioning in patients with frontal lobe pathology are presented here. Most were standardized tests of intelligence, expressed as IQ scores. These reports are also open to criticism, mainly the shortcomings of this type of brain damage/psychological battery research. Nevertheless, the sheer weight of evidence derived from these studies overshadows the shortcomings.

Positive Findings

Many reports discuss intellectual changes following frontal lobe damage. Goldstein (1944) reported a change in abstract attitude; Rylander (1939, 1948) suggested a defect in reasoning; Brickner (1936) suggested a loss of the power of synthesis; Robinson (1946) implied that the intellectual changes were due to impairment in attention; Pippard (1955) noted that 58 of 114 patients who had had rostral leukotomies showed evidence of impaired intellectual functioning, primarily affecting memory and conceptual thinking. The definitions of intellectual ability were so varied that it was virtually impossible to decide what had happened from these reports (Meyer, 1960).

Many reports of positive findings after frontal lobe damage are limited to IQ scores as determined by one of the commonly used tests: Stanford-Binet, Wechsler-Bellevue (W-B), or WAIS. Yacorzynski, Boshes, and Davis (1947) reported a total W-B IQ loss of 22 points in one patient. Malmo (1948) suggested that frontal lobe operations, either gyrectomy or lobotomy, produced a general IQ loss unrelated to the amount of tissue removed. Drewe (1974) reported that frontal brain-damaged patients were worse than nonfrontally damaged patients on performance IQ but not verbal IQ. Nonsignificant decreases in IQ scores postsurgery were reported by DeMille (1962), Rylander (1948), Strom-Olsen, Last, Brody, et al., (1943), and Vidor (1951).

One demonstration that frontal lobe damage does affect IQ was provided in a study of five military veterans who developed paranoid schizophrenia and, as part of their treatment, underwent the standard Freeman-Watts lobotomy (Malmo, 1948). Results of follow-up tests using the Wechsler Intelligence Test and the Army "M" test administered 1 to 3 months postsurgery were compared to two preoperative scores, an enlistment Army "M" test and a prelobotomy Wechsler test. The Wechsler comparisons did not achieve significance, but a definite deterioration of IQ from premorbid abilities was demonstrated with the Army "M" test comparisons. This study is unusual in having a premorbid comparison and suggests that lobotomy can cause intellectual deterioration. The effect of the schizophrenia demands clarification, however, and if the decreased IQ reflected the frontal damage remains in question.

Reported findings of IQ deterioration after frontal damage are rare, whereas the number of studies reporting negative results is overwhelming. Even studies that do report IQ deterioration admit that other factors may be important. Struckett (1953) suggested that the decrease may be temporary with a return to preoperative levels after about 1 year. Petrie (1952a,b) indicated that differences in IQ scores in his subjects were dependent on the location of the leukotomy, the more anterior lesions not demonstrating the IQ changes seen with more posterior lesions. In addition, analysis of subscales suggested to some that the "intellectual loss" actually reflected a personality alteration and/or social comprehension deficit. Malmo (1948) interpreted the IQ deterioration not as a loss of facts or abilities but as a problem in adapting and maintaining a set or attitude in the face of interference until a specific goal was obtained or abandoned. The inconsistencies in findings and the multiple interpretations produced demonstrate that the positive findings are not sufficient to provide a definitive correlation.

Negative Findings

The absence of deterioration on intellectual testing in frontal lobe patients can also be interpreted in several ways. Test results may have been inconsistent, observed changes may not have been interpreted as intellectual changes, or the deterioration noted was not sufficient to reach significance. In this section the reported negative results are briefly, and in a general way, summarized. Interpretation is difficult as the comparisons vary. In various studies the results from frontal lobe damaged patients are compared to normal test score ranges as well as to the results from normal control subjects, patients with brain damage in other areas, or in cases of psychosurgery nonoperated patients with similar psychiatric problems.

Excluding the studies following topectomy, the evidence is overwhelming that "the average intelligence test scores after psychosurgery do not differ significantly from those of the population at large" (Valenstein, 1973, p. 321). The reliability of this finding can be observed by comparison across different types of frontal brain damage (including different kinds of psychosurgery), as well as across different researchers. Negative results were reported subsequent to both unilateral and bilateral lobectomy (Hebb, 1939, 1945; Hebb and Penfield, 1940; Milner, 1964; Stookey et al., 1941), open or closed lobotomy or leukotomy, including orbital undercutting (Baker et al., 1970; Freeman, 1971; Halstead, 1947a,b; Halstead, Carmichael, and Bucy, 1946; Hunt, 1942; Medina et al., 1954; Mirsky and Orzack, 1977; Porteus and Peters, 1947a,b; Robinson and Freeman, 1954; Rylander, 1973; Smith et al., 1977; Strecker, Palmer, and Grant, 1942; Strom-Olsen and Northfield, 1955; Struckett, 1953; Stuss, Benson, Kaplan, et al., 1983; Stuss, Kaplan, and Benson, 1982a; Walsh, 1977; Wehler and Hoffman, 1978), cingulumotomy and other types of limbic leukotomy (LeBeau and Petrie, 1953; Long, Pueschel, and Hunter, 1978; Meyer, McElhaney, Martin, and McGraw, 1973; Mitchell-Heggs, Kelly, and Richardson, 1976, 1977; Teuber et al., 1977), other types of frontal system psychosurgery including stereotactic capsulotomy (Bingley, Leksell, Meyerson, et al., 1977), and prefrontal sonic and multitarget bilateral stereotactic lesions (Mirsky and Orzack, 1977), as well as various nonsurgical causes of frontal damage (Black, 1976; Drewe, 1974; Jarvie, 1954; Logue et al., 1968; Reitan, 1964; Teuber, 1964, 1966; Weinstein and Teuber, 1957).

Although decreased IQ performance was present in some early postoperative state tests (Struckett, 1953), later follow-up assessments revealed negative results: 1 to 3 months (Mitchell-Heggs et al., 1976, 1977); 1 to 2 years (Mitchell-Heggs et al., 1976, 1977; Struckett, 1953); 2 to 5 years (Smith et al., 1977); 5 to 10 years (Hebb, 1945; Medina et al., 1954); greater than 20 years (Stuss et al., 1983; Wehler and Hoffman, 1978). The negative results appear to be consistent across types of surgery and time of postoperative assessment.

Topectomy Studies

The effects of frontal topectomy are presented separately because they alone, of all major studies, followed a preconceived research plan that included pre- and postsurgical studies using specific measurements. Topectomy results came from two large investigations: the Columbia-Greystone project (Mettler, 1949, 1952) and the New York State Brain Project (Lewis et al., 1956). The psychosurgery employed in these projects was a measured ablation of frontal cortical surface area in one of two locations: lower forebrain (orbital topectomy) or upper forebrain (superior topectomy). Postsurgical results may be divided into three epochs: early follow-up, approximately 8-year follow-up, and approximately 14-year follow-up.

The early assessment failed to show any significant decrease in intellectual functioning for either location of surgery (Heath and Pool, 1948a,b; Landis, 1949; Sheer, 1956). An early loss in "psychological test efficiency" was noted, but there was no loss or gain on the W-B IQ score. The frontal lobes did not appear to play an active role in intelligence as indicated by psychometric testing. Although no differences were noted between the superior and the orbital ablations, patients appeared to make a slower recovery after the former (Sheer, 1956).

The 8-year follow-up did indicate impaired function (Smith and Kinder, 1959). When compared to nonoperated schizophrenic controls, both groups of topectomy patients were significantly inferior on WAIS tests of Digit Span, Mental Arithmetic, and Digit Symbol, and the superior topectomy patients showed a significant FSIQ and VIQ decline ($p < 0.05$) from the preoperative baseline. Among the orbital topectomy patients, some impairment was noted in the older subjects but not in the younger patients. These general findings were confirmed by a 14-year follow-up (Hamlin, 1970). Although little change was noted for the nonoperated controls, the superior topectomy patients (removal of Brodmann areas 8, 9, sometimes 10, and 32) showed an approximate 10 point lower IQ. All verbal subtests except information were lower, with Digit Span the most affected. Among the performance subtests, only Picture Arrangement demonstrated a deficit. There was little difference at the 14-year follow-up between the orbital topectomy patients and nonoperated schizophrenics.

Hamlin (1970) concluded that ablation of the upper frontal lobe did affect problem-solving (comprehension and manipulation), sustained attention and concentration, and other intellectual functions. These basic problems persisted over the years, even though their manifestation varied, different tests being significant at different times.

ABSTRACTION

One of the more prevalent concepts used to explain the change in cognitive behavior after frontal lobe damage was the "incapacity for abstract behavior" proposed by Goldstein (1936a,b, 1939, 1944; Goldstein and Scheerer, 1941). Goldstein (1936a) illustrated this difficulty with an example. A frontal lobe patient had little difficulty constructing a design using wooden sticks when the design was based on a concrete image such as the roof of a house. He could not, however, complete a seemingly similar construction task when the design had no concrete meaning. Similarly, although frontal lobe patients easily performed the physical act of throwing balls into boxes situated at various distances, they could not judge the distances or estimate the relative proximity of each box unless the distance was physically measured. Although simple pictures could be understood, complex pictures remained a mystery. Petrie (1952a,b) studied 70 standard leukotomy patients pre- and postoperatively with Stanford-Binet proverbs and concluded that there was a significant loss in the ability to generalize. Identification of differences between pairs of words was impaired in patients with frontal lobe damage (Rylander, 1939; Tow, 1955). Benton (1968), using Gorham proverbs, suggested that frontal lobe patients had a tendency for concrete thinking; others have also concluded that the basic deficit following frontal damage involves abstraction (Ackerly and Benton, 1947; Nicholls and Hunt, 1940; Willett, 1960).

Other studies, however, contradicted the hypothesis of a basic disorder of abstraction. Luria (1969) stated that there was no evidence of a general disturbance of abstract intellect. Well-consolidated information, for example, is not impaired after frontal damage. Maslow (1955) indicated that lobotomized schizophrenics had neither a specifically disturbed abstract behavior nor a deficiency in concept formation. Topectomy patients, regardless of the area of lesion, did not demonstrate a specific disturbance in abstract behavior on seven tests of abstraction (W. R. King, 1949; Landis, 1949).

The apparent incongruity is partially resolved by examination of the operational definitions of abstraction. Goldstein (1944) specifically defined the loss of abstract attitude. *"Their mental capacity may be sufficient for executing routine work*, but they *lack initiative, foresight, activity, and ability to handle new tasks.* They are *impaired in voluntarily shifting and choice.* That corresponds to the personality changes due to impairment of abstract attitude" (p. 192). The deficits associated with impairment of abstract attitude were outlined (Goldstein and Scheerer, 1941). Many of the listed functions are now associated with the concept of the executive system (described in Chapter 14) and are not necessarily defined by tests such as WAIS similarities or the interpretation of proverbs. Thus when Valenstein (1977) concluded that problems in "abstract thinking" do occur after frontal surgery, he cited tests such as the Wisconsin Card Sorting Test and admitted that readily available tests of abstract or divergent thinking are rare.

Stuss et al. (1982a, 1983) addressed the problem of abstract thinking in an operational manner by administering four tests of cognitive functions to three groups of leukotomized schizophrenics and two control groups. The WAIS, administered as a standard test of intelligence, confirmed earlier results showing little or no deficit in overall IQ after frontal lobe pathology. On the Visual Metaphor test (Winner and Gardner, 1977), a test probing for dissociation of the ability to understand a metaphor from the ability to verbalize the meaning of the metaphor, frontal lobe patients had little difficulty in identifying the correct metaphor but had trouble explaining why it was chosen. Goldstein (1944) had earlier noted this distinction between the ability to "think" abstractly and the ability to use abstract (metaphoric) words.

The third test, the Visual-Verbal test (Feldman and Drasgow, 1960), also demanded a type of abstraction. The subject was required to tell how three of four figures on a card were alike in some way. Patients with frontal lobe lesions did not show significant impairment. When requested to perform a conceptual shift, however, by telling how three of the same four figures were alike in some other way, they had considerable difficulty in shifting, apparently independent of abstraction competence, as demonstrated by the first abstraction (Fig. 13-2). The fourth test, the Wisconsin Card Sorting Test, revealed impaired performance by the frontal lobe subjects based on perseveration of incorrect responses and difficulty in maintaining sequences of correct responses (Stuss et al., 1982a, 1983).

Terms can be misleading and interpreted to match the investigator's perceptions and theoretical predispositions. The abstraction problems of patients with frontal lobe pathology is not a simple inability to interpret proverbs. Several specific deficits appear to underlie the failed performances, including: (1) an inability to

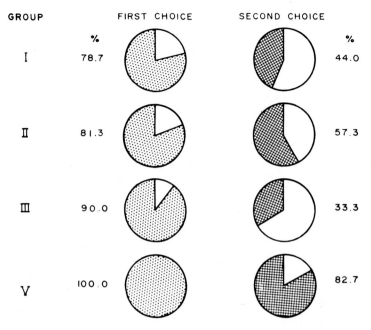

FIG. 13-2. Results from visual-verbal tests of three leukotomy groups (I = good recovery, III = no recovery) and matched normal subjects (V). Percentage of correct responses to initial and second concept formation demands are shown. (From Stuss and Benson: In: *Localization in Neuropsychology*, edited by A. Kertesz. Academic Press, New York, 1983, with permission.)

translate knowledge of specific facts into appropriate action; (2) a problem in shifting from one concept to another or changing a behavior once started; (3) a tendency to respond to a fragment with failure to grasp the totality or the key feature of a complex situation; (4) a deficit in relating or integrating isolated details; and (5) a deficiency in handling simultaneous sources of information. Each problem has been described as a deficit in abstraction but seems better explained under the concept of executive ability, described in Chapter 14.

BIOLOGICAL INTELLIGENCE

Halstead's concept of biological intelligence (Halstead, 1947a,b; Halstead et al., 1946) represents an important attempt to assess "usable intelligence" rather than measure specific knowledge as shown by standardized psychometric tests. Halstead believed that Freud's concept of a controlling ego or intelligence, adaptive behavior dependent on the normal functioning of a healthy nervous system, could be objectively defined and measured. His efforts provided a direct attack on the paradox of someone with a high psychometric IQ who was obviously impaired in adapting to daily life.

With a battery of 27 tests, Halstead studied 237 brain-damaged patients of varied etiology and lesion location. Factor analyses of these data suggested a four-factor theory of biological intelligence (Halstead, 1947a,b). The C (central integrative) factor represented the ego or organized experience where the new and familiar became incorporated. Psychometric tests loaded highest on this factor, suggesting that at least some of its parameters are reflected in standardized IQ tests. The A (abstraction) factor was the "fundamental growth principle of the ego," representing the ability to group according to criteria and to understand how things are the same or different. The Category and Tactual Performance (memory) tests were represented in this factor. The P (power) factor serves to counterbalance or regulate the affective forces, thereby freeing the growth principle of the ego for further ego differentiation. The fourth factor, the D (directional) principle, was defined by the motor speed on the Tactual Performance Test and by a peripheral vision test, with the suggestion that it represents the way the process factors became exteriorized. Later formulation interpreted factor A as related to abstraction, factor C to verbal intelligence, and factor P to vigilance (Shure and Halstead, 1958).

Based on his research comparing patients with frontal lobectomy and lobotomies to other brain-damaged subjects, Halstead concluded that although biological intelligence was represented throughout the cortex it was maximally represented in the frontal lobes. This interpretation came under criticism. Petrie (1952b), for example, observed that the index differentiated lobectomy but not leukotomy patients, and therefore a generalization could not be made to the frontal lobes per se. Other criticisms included insufficient documentation of or concern about several factors, including anatomical and pathological information, group age differences, and variation between groups (Crown, 1951; Meyer, 1960; Zangwill, 1949).

Revisions have been made to Halstead's neuropsychological approach, now commonly referred to as the Halstead-Reitan test battery. Current usage does not emphasize the localization of the battery results to the frontal lobes. Reitan's (1964) extensive research suggested that such a localization is not tenable or, at the very least, demands extreme care with control of the many variables and that large subject samples must be used before reaching such a conclusion.

SUMMARY

In summarizing the "cognitive abilities" associated with the frontal lobes, this chapter mirrors the problems of research on frontal lobe functioning. One serious difficulty concerns inadequate definitions of the functions under discussion, particularly intelligence, cognition, and abstraction. Contradictory claims are gradually being reconciled as operational definitions become more precise and conclusions are limited to the test used (Meyer, 1960). It is now recognized that intellectual processes deal with both old and new information (Luria, 1969). Old information and well-established processes appear to be unaffected by frontal lobe damage. However, ". . . when intellectual operations demand the creation of a program of action and a choice between several equally probable alternatives, the intellectual activity of patients with a marked 'frontal syndrome' is profoundly disturbed" (Luria, 1969, p. 749). "Higher cognition," defined more as a deficit in motivation and failure in real life situations, can be impaired after orbital/lower mesial frontal damage despite adequate to excellent performance on general psychological and even "frontal lobe" tests (Eslinger and Damasio, 1985). The frontal lobes do participate in cognitive functioning, the mode of participation dependent on the operational definition of "cognition." Reciprocal cortical-cortical connections between the frontal lobes and the major association areas provide a neuroanatomical map for this role (Nauta, 1971).

In one sense, the intellectual operations of the frontal lobes underlie all brain activities demanding a certain level of complexity or requiring new procedures. This chapter was opened with a concept of the frontal lobes as *sedes sapentiae totae* and can conclude with the observation: *"Le lobe frontal . . . n'est pas le siège de l'intelligence, mais il intervient au cours de toutes les activités intellectuelles"* ["the frontal lobe . . . is not the seat of intelligence, but it intervenes in all intellectual activities"] (Lhermitte et al., 1972, p. 416). The following chapter, on executive functions, reviews research on the specific nature of the intervention by the frontal lobes.

14

Executive System

Frontal lobe patients are said to suffer impaired intellectual functioning yet have normal IQ levels on psychological tests, as outlined in Chapter 13. A major source of confusion stems from the definition of terms such as intelligence, cognition, mental function and others; concepts beyond simple IQ test results are demanded. As Hunt (1942, p. 154) stated: "Whether this frontal lobe deficit is purely a matter of intelligence, however, is debatable unless the term 'intelligence' is broadened to include planning capacity and enterprise, the setting of a goal, and planning the course to attain it and adaptability to the occupation." One must find how to gauge this diverse yet specific group of attributes. Additional problems were noted by Hebb and Penfield (1940, p. 437): "It may be that no laboratory study will be adequate to reveal whatever defects follow frontal lobe injury in man because of insufficient control of environmental factors and the difficulty of obtaining a good premorbid rating of ability."

A 30-year-old man was referred for neurobehavioral evaluation because of school failure. At age 23, while in his third year of college, he had attempted suicide by shooting himself in the right frontal-temporal area with a .44 caliber revolver. Following a long convalescence (including about 8 months of amnesia) his general behavior appeared intact, and after psychological evaluation and counseling he reentered college. Despite limited class loads, he failed and had to drop out on two occasions. The neurobehavioral evaluation showed no neurological residua, no significant depression or memory problem, and an IQ of 123. The patient was adamant that he could understand and remember the material in his college courses but stated he could generate no interest in it (or in anything else). X-ray computed tomography (CT) (Fig. 14-1) revealed marked right frontal and lesser left frontal areas of lucency; the electroencephalogram (EEG) showed bifrontal slowing. There was no evidence, from neurological or psychological examinations or from the physical laboratory studies, of any except frontal brain damage.

This chapter reviews clincal observations and selected research on human deficits in planning and control based on frontal lobe damage. Research is reported in two sections. The first presents innovative uses and/or analyses of commonly used psychological tests to enable assessment of frontal impairment, and the second presents experimental procedures designed to measure planning disorders.

Terms such as anticipation, goal establishment, planning, response trials, monitoring of results, and use of feedback, although more explicit than "intelligence," are still vague and again reflect our lack of knowledge of the specific roles played

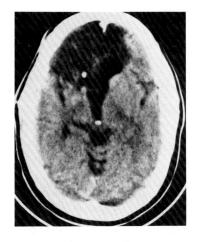

FIG. 14-1. X-ray CT showing massive right frontal and lesser left frontal damage caused by a gunshot wound. Right and left are reversed in the figure.

by the frontal lobes. For the time being we consider each of these important functions (and probably others) as an integrated portion of an overall function to be called executive function. A growing refinement can be anticipated as the experimental paradigms become more sophisticated and better directed. The executive functions remain among the most significant of human frontal lobe accomplishments.

CLINICAL OBSERVATIONS

Early observations provided good descriptions of the basic deficits that follow frontal lobe pathology. Bianchi (1895), on the basis of crude animal experiments, hypothesized that the frontal lobes were essential for gathering and analyzing sensory data originally perceived in the other hemispheres and then acting on this information. The frontal lobes could be considered the origin of the final common pathway, a motor, executive function, but even then their function was considered considerably more complex. Selective observations in human frontal lobe cases help analyze some of the complex functions that are apparently dependent on the frontal lobes.

Penfield and Evans (1935) described a housewife (later known to be the senior author's sister) who, after removal of much of the right frontal lobe to treat a tumor, could prepare individual dishes yet was unable to plan and prepare an entire meal for her family. Brickner (1936) detailed the performance of a 39-year-old New York stockbroker who had extensive, bilateral frontal resection for removal of a frontal meningioma. Although seemingly intact intellectually, he was unable to focus his attention, show initiative, plan meaningful activity, or complete his verbalized intentions. Autopsy revealed several additional meningiomas, but it is unlikely that they influenced the behavior at the time of the original observation (Damasio, 1979).

Studies of brain damage from war wounds include many individuals with frontal injury. Reports of behavioral alterations are common, including many descriptions of impaired ability to direct appropriate actions. Thus Kleist (1934b) described loss of initiative, aspontaneity of motor activity, and mutism; and a general decrease in motor activity, apathy, has been reported by many (Faust, 1955; Feuchtwanger, 1923; Forster, 1919; Lishman, 1966, 1968; Walch, 1956). Ruesch (1943) noted that the major mental effects of head injury include impairment of speed and sustained effort. Many others, however, have emphasized amnesia, psychiatric disability (both psychosis and neurosis), and "the posttraumatic syndrome." Some exclude, or fail to note, motor defects. The diversity of symptomatology, the lack of precise descriptive terminology, and the inconsistency of the frontal area involved in different patients make observations of brain injury cases inexact and difficult to interpret.

> After partial resection of both frontal lobes, an executive secretary still obtained an IQ score of approximately 120 and had little problem completing the Kohs blocks test (Nichols and Hunt, 1940). Nevertheless, he showed great difficulty in alternating attention between two aspects of a topic, in shifting hypotheses once started, in generating novel solutions to problems, and in envisaging the totality of a situation.

A number of observational studies have reported on patients following frontal lesioning and one or more of the following faults reported: lack of insight and foresight; diminished capacity for planning; decreased initiative (Freeman and Watts, 1942, 1944; Hutton, 1943; Schrader and Robinson, 1945). Ackerly and Benton (1947) studied an individual who suffered bilateral frontal lobe damage during the perinatal period or at birth. Although memory, IQ, perceptual speed, and visual-motor coordination were within normal limits on standard testing, he was mentally disabled and showed two striking disorders. The first was a deficit in goal establishment and planning. His interest involved only the immediate present, with little concern for the past, and almost no planning for the future. The second was an inability to maintain or shift a mental set. Thus on a puzzle test he could not keep a directing goal in mind, particularly if there were competing stimuli and interests. If doing one action, he could not be requested to do a second. He worked successfully as a gas station attendant for a time but lost the job when he became extremely angry at a customer who requested that he wash the windshield when he was pumping gas. Slomka, Tarter, and Hegedus (1984) reported a patient with apparent agenesis of the frontal lobes who was extremely distractible and hyperactive, and showed many emotional and motivational disorders. This patient was considered moderately retarded, and the agenesis probably involved both cortical and subcortical areas.

An apparently conflicting case study was reported by Hebb and Penfield (1940; Hebb, 1945). At age 28, a patient had bilateral frontal lobe ablation to remove scar tissue caused by a compound frontal fracture sustained at age 16. After surgery, no gross defects in behavior were noted. Indeed, the patient appeared to improve in many aspects. Although he had no concern about the future, Hebb denied that this showed lack of foresight as he could verbalize plans for days or weeks in the future. Although apparently contradicting previous reports, Hebb (1945) stated, "it is still possible that long-term planning and initiative (Penfield and Evans, 1935), creative work and capacity for radical readjustment may be notably impaired by lesions of the frontal lobe" (p. 23).

Executive functioning after frontal lobe damage in the human may be quite disabling but has proved difficult to characterize; interpretations beyond the actual data are necessarily suspect.

INNOVATIVE USE OF COMMON PSYCHOLOGICAL TESTS

There are many examples of tests designed for another purpose that have been used to assess the executive functions of the frontal lobe. In many respects, this epitomizes Luria's insight into the functions of the frontal lobes (Christensen, 1975; Luria, 1973a, 1966/1980) and characterizes the qualitative approach to neuro-psychological assessment that advocates study of how the final solution to a problem is achieved in addition to or even instead of concern about the actual result (Kaplan, 1983). Most of the diverse malfunctions attributed to the frontal lobe described elsewhere in this book—memory, language, visual-spatial skills, and so on—reflect disorder of the executive system. A few specific examples are highlighted.

"Abstraction" (as discussed in Chapter 13) is not lost with frontal damage, provided that it represents the identification or awareness of well-established concepts. The frontal lobe patient has no difficulty completing analogy problems such as "father–son; mother. . . ." (Luria, 1969). If a well-established response is not known, however, if alternatives are not clearly differentiated, or if a previous response must be overcome, the frontal lobe patient will fail, reverting to familiar associations. Frontal lobe patients are not attracted to the literal interpretation of simple metaphors and readily perceive similarities of items in tests such as basic grouping tests, Wechsler Adult Intelligence Scale (WAIS) similarities, or the visual-verbal test (Hebb, 1945; Stuss et al., 1983). They show impairment, however, when asked to shift concepts or to complete complex concept formation tasks (Cicerone, Lazar, and Shapiro, 1983; Milner, 1964; Stuss et al., 1983). Only by analyzing the process of the response can such deficits be observed.

Even simple functions such as arithmetic may help to assess frontal lobe deficit (Lhermitte et al., 1972; Luria, 1969, 1973a; Walsh, 1978). Intact performance with the basic written operations of addition, subtraction, and so on verify the absence of outright acalculia, and even phrasing an arithmetical operation into a simple algorithm provides no problem for the frontal lobe patient. (For example: Jack has four apples, Jill has three apples. How many apples have they in total?) If an intermediate step is introduced, however, defective performance may be demonstrated. Thus if the patient is requested to give the total number of apples when Jill has two more than Jack, who has four, the frontal lobe patient cannot divide the task into component parts and often guesses or responds with a simple mathematical operation.

Luria (1973) outlined at least two additional levels of complexity. One demands a recoding of the question, e.g., "There are 18 books on two shelves; there are twice as many books on one shelf as on the other. How many books are on each shelf?" This question necessitates the understanding that there are two shelves and that the number of books must be divided into three parts. Although frontal patients have no difficulty doing the fraction ⅔ of 18, they fail the task when phrased in the manner above. They may focus on the two shelves and answer "18 times 2 equals 36" or "half of 18 is 9." A second, more difficult, situation sets up a conflicting condition that requires inhibition of an impulsive response. For example: "A candle is 6 inches long, and the shadow from the candle is 18 inches longer. How many times is the shadow longer than the candle?" The impulsive response, common in frontally damaged patients, is to divide 18 by 6 and respond 3.

Analysis of the processes required to solve these tasks helps to understand the impairment (Lhermitte et al., 1972; Luria, 1969, 1973a). First, the information is analyzed, next identification and selection of the mathematical operations are necessary, then a logical, step-wise solution is selected, and finally the answer is verified. Frontal patients tend to give impulsive responses lacking one or more of the necessary steps, or they may fail to create the needed strategies or insert (perseverate) other activities into the problem-solving task. If the examiner assists by breaking the problem into appropriate stages, demanding a response at each step, a correct answer may be achieved.

A similar frontal disturbance may be demonstrated by block design tests (e.g., WAIS block design, Kohs blocks). Patients with frontal damage show no basic visual-spatial or constructional disturbance (see Chapter 10) and may perform block design tests normally (Ackerly and Benton, 1947; Bailey, Dowling, and Davies, 1977; Hunt, 1942; Stuss et al., 1984a). Nevertheless, several researchers have demonstrated consistent deficits in frontal lobe patients on block design tests (Goodglass and Kaplan, 1979; Lhermitte et al., 1972; Luria, 1969, 1973a, 1966/1980; Walsh, 1978). Frontal lobe patients, particularly those with right frontal damage, tend to be pulled by the salient features of the design and break the external configuration although maintaining the general features (e.g., angle) of the inner design (Goodglass and Kaplan, 1979). Difficulty in figure-ground differentiation may be present. Also, frontal lobe patients are impulsive and often fail to assess whether their output differs from the original example (self-monitoring). Lhermitte and colleagues (1972) outlined specific steps in the solution of a block design, similar to the steps proposed for solving an arithmetic problem, and found that frontal lobe patients could fail at any stage. Again, if given partial assistance in the planning of the response (e.g., presenting the block design model divided with superimposed lines), performance improves (Lhermitte et al., 1972; Luria, 1969; Walsh, 1977, 1978). If the assistance or partial detail is removed, however, performance deteriorates (Luria, 1973a).

The Picture Arrangement subtest of the Wechsler Intelligence Scale demands that a subject analyze the individual cards, identify and differentiate relevant from irrelevant details, perceive the logical relationship among the cards, and rearrange them in logical order. The patient's strategy can be analyzed by asking that the story of the arranged cards be told. Many reports show that this test is selectively impaired among WAIS performance subtests administered to patients with frontal lobe pathology even though the general IQ score remains within normal limits. Impaired performance has been reported following ruptured anterior cerebral aneurysms (Logue et al., 1968), bilateral anterior cingulotomies (Bailey et al., 1977), and frontal lobotomy and topectomy in chronic schizophrenics (Hamlin, 1970; Medina et al., 1954; Stuss et al., 1984a). McFie (McFie, 1969; McFie and Thompson, 1972) reported that right temporal and right frontal lobe patients moved the cards little or not at all, attempting to provide a story to fit the original arrangement of the cards. Among the visual-spatial and/or visual-constructive tests administered to bilaterally leukotomized schizophrenics, only the picture arrangement test was impaired in all groups, even the good recovery patients (Stuss et al., 1984a). These subjects did attempt to rearrange the cards, but they failed to make even simple logical relationships.

SPECIFIC TESTS OF THE EXECUTIVE SYSTEM

Certain standardized tests—sorting and category tests and maze tests—appear to be particularly sensitive to defects in the planning functions of the frontal lobes. In addition, a number of experimental procedures have been designed specifically to assess this aspect of the executive function.

Sorting and Category Tests

There are several types of sorting and category tests. Although superficially similar, the mode of administration makes them remarkably different. One common procedure is to present the patient with a series of objects randomly arrayed on a table, either real objects (e.g., Tow, 1955) or figures of varying shapes, sizes, and colors (W. R. King, 1949; Weigl, 1941), with the request that items be grouped or sorted according to specific principles. Alternative procedures demand category identification or discovery of a sorting principle. The most widely used category identification test is the Halstead Category Test (Halstead, 1947a) which consists of seven subtests, the first six measuring nonverbal abstraction-concept formation and the last testing memory (Boll, 1981; Trites, 1977). For the first six subtests, a series of slides are presented, each with different figures and patterns. The subject is instructed that something will suggest a number between 1 and 4; he then presses one of the four buttons and receives a feedback tone or buzzer telling him if the answer is correct. At the completion of each group, the examiner states that another group of items will be presented and that the main idea may be the same or different. The seventh and final group demands memory of previous stimuli.

A variation on this theme demands a shift of the discovered principle. The Wisconsin Card Sorting Test (WCST) (Grant and Berg, 1948) is the most widely recognized example. The patient is presented with four stimulus or target cards, each different in number, color, and form: one red triangle, two green stars, three yellow crosses, four blue circles. The subject is given a deck of cards with similar stimuli to be sorted by placing each card in front of one of the four target cards based on one of the three categories. The subject is told only whether he is correct or incorrect for each response. Using this feedback, the subject gets as many correct as possible. Unknown to the subject, the examiner selects one criterion as the correct one and bases the feedback on the relationship of the response to this criterion. After 10 consecutive correct responses, the examiner alters the sorting criterion without telling the subject. The subject must shift until a new principle is discovered, and this is again changed after 10 correct responses. The score reflects the number of sets of 10 correct responses attained by the subject, as well as the number of various types of error.

Results

The Halstead Category Test is considered a good measure of bilateral and left prefrontal pathology because of its conceptual nature and the necessity for organization and "purposive behavior" (Golden et al., 1981). Although frontal lobe patients are frequently impaired on this test (Golden et al., 1981; Shure and Halstead, 1958), other studies suggest that it is actually a sensitive test for brain damage without a localizing function (Chapman and Wolff, 1959; Doehring and Reitan, 1962; Golden, 1978). This is certainly true if impaired functioning is observed on other tests (Golden et al., 1981). Swiercinsky (1978), in a factor analytical study, found that the Halstead Category Test did not correlate highly with any single factor.

Grouping, sorting, and the identification of simple categories may or may not be impaired in patients with frontal lobe pathology. Halstead (1940) found that frontal lobe patients produced smaller numbers of spontaneous groupings than patients with lesions in other areas. Tow (1955) also reported that leukotomized patients showed decreased ability to sort real objects according to four principles. Difficulty at the level of concept formation may be a factor (Cicerone et al., 1983). Milner (1963, 1964), on the other hand, reported that frontal lobe patients had no difficulty identifying the three correct sorting criteria in the WCST, and Stuss et al. (1983) noted that concept identification per se was not impaired in frontal lobe patients. W. R. King (1949) reported relatively intact ability in isolated sorting tasks by frontal lobe patients. The relevant issue did not appear to be the ability to perceive the relevant category, but performance of the task could be impaired for one of several specific reasons. One appeared to be a deficit in "shifting," i.e., to move to a new task or criterion from an established position (Ackerly and Benton, 1947; Goldstein, 1944; W. R. King, 1949; Nichols and Hunt, 1940; Poppen, Pribram, and Robinson, 1965; Rylander, 1939; Smith, 1960; Stuss et al., 1983; Weigl, 1941; Yacorzynski and Davis, 1945). Although patients with frontal lobe pathology usually verbalized task requirements correctly, they still had problems completing the task (Milner, 1963, 1964; Rosvold and Mishkin, 1950; Walsh, 1977). Overt verbalization may actually impede performance (Benson et al., 1981; Stuss et al., 1983).In addition, frontal lobe patients, performing category tasks that required shifting, showed disinterest, made random responses, were unable to maintain correct responses, and, most frequently, perseverated erroneous responses

(Drewe, 1974; Milner, 1964; Mirsky and Orzack, 1977; Robinson, Heaton, Lehman, et al., 1980; Rosvold and Mishkin, 1950; Smith, 1960; Stuss et al., 1983); these deficits can even be elicited with less complex and unambiguous material (Nelson, 1976).

Teuber and his colleagues (Teuber, 1964; Teuber, Battersby, and Bender, 1951) administered the WCST to patients with penetrating missile wounds and showed that patients with posterior lesions performed worse than patients with anterior lesions (both groups were impaired in comparison to normal subjects). This investigation, however, eliminated the problem of shifting by informing the subjects of each criterion change, making the task one of simple category identification. In contrast, Milner (1963, 1964) administered the task without instruction. Despite normal IQ, her dorsal-lateral frontal lesion patients performed significantly worse than those with more posterior lesions. Not one of the 25 dorsal-lateral lesion patients achieved more than three of the possible six categories (maximum in Milner's administration), whereas 51 of 69 patients with inferior frontal or posterior lesions achieved this level. The dorsal-lateral lesion patients showed a strong perseverative tendency despite being repeatedly informed that their response was incorrect.

A middle-aged man with suspected bilateral frontal lobe pathology secondary to a severe closed head injury suffered 20 years earlier was referred for neuropsychological evaluation when he was unsuccessful even at a simple task of sorting mail. He had worked in a clerical position but over a period of 15 years had never been promoted. His own explanation of failure to sort mail was lack of interest due to being overlooked for promotions. On two basic tests he achieved an IQ of 138 on the WAIS-R and was at the 99th percentile on Raven's Progressive Matrices; thus he belonged to a select group of individuals with extremely high IQs. The WCST, on the other hand, clearly demonstrated the source of his work difficulty. He obtained only four sorting criteria over the 128 cards and made innumerable perseverative errors. A control subject of the same age and educational background, in contrast, achieved 10 sorting criteria with few perseverative errors. Despite excellent performance on IQ tests, the patient was severely impaired in performing executive tasks, reflecting the bilateral frontal lobe pathology of the closed head injury.

This case study illustrates that the dissociation of the deficit on sorting tasks from the intellectual performance as measured by standard psychological tests can be striking.

Sorting tasks, particularly when used to assess the ability to change, appear to be particularly sensitive to frontal lobe damage. They are not, however, differentially sensitive to frontal lobe dysfunction, as generalized or diffuse brain damage can produce similar deficits (Golden et al., 1981; Robinson et al., 1980). The sorting tasks are not diagnostic unless normal functioning is observed on a majority of "nonfrontal" tests. Moreover, no clear deficits in sorting tests were reported following small frontal system lesions such as cingulotomy (Teuber et al., 1977). Finally, the absence of impairment on sorting tasks does not exclude frontal pathology, at least in certain locations (Eslinger and Damasio, 1985).

Maze Tests

The maze tests may be classified into two general types: the Porteus Maze test and all other maze tests. The non-Porteus mazes more directly measure spatial learning and are included here as a comparison to the Porteus Maze test. Subjects are presented with a series of points on a board and asked to find the correct route from a starting point to an end point using a trial and error method. The subject continues until he makes an incorrect guess, then returns to the starting point and repeats the same process until he learns the route or exceeds a maximum number of trials. The Porteus Maze, on the other hand, assesses visual-motor planning (Porteus, 1950; Porteus and Kepner, 1944; Porteus and Peters, 1947a,b). The test consists of a number of labyrinths, each increasing in difficulty. The subject must find the most direct route from beginning to end without entering blind alleys or crossing through lines. The subject must not lift the pencil while tracing the route and must keep within the side boundaries. As soon as an error is made, the same labyrinth is presented for a second trial, with a limit of two to four trials depending on the degree of difficulty of the test. Two types of scores are obtained. A test age compares the particular achievement based on the number of repeated trials with a maximum score of 17, and a qualitative score assesses the type of production errors (e.g., cutting corners, touching the side).

Results

Although the spatial maze learning tasks do not directly assess planning, they do allow demonstration of frontal deficits in a manner similar to that described for sorting and category tests. Benton, Elithorn, Fogel, and Kerr (1963) found the Elithorn (1964) maze test sensitive to brain damage, but not specifically frontal brain damage. Some researchers suggest that qualitatively specific errors are made by frontal lobe patients (Corkin, 1965; Milner, 1964, 1965; Walsh, 1977, 1978). These patients understand the rules but do not follow them; they make the same erroneous response on repeated trials, break the rules, and fail to use their own knowledge to change their behavior. On these measures, frontal lobe patients were more impaired than patients with localized lesions in other cortical areas. The tendency to break rules on maze performance declines over time but remains a characteristic of frontal lobe patients (Canavan, 1983).

The Porteus Maze has been suggested as the most sensitive indicator of early and long-term changes after frontal lobe psychosurgery (Smith, 1960), but there are negative reports. Fabbri (1956) reported improvement in performance after transorbital lobotomy. Teuber et al. (1977) could find no pre/postoperative difference with anterior cingulotomy (Brodmann area 24, defined as part of the frontal cortex by some). Little if any deficit was observed after orbital topectomy, particularly if the patient was young (Smith, 1960; Smith and Kinder, 1959). Nevertheless, a majority of studies have reported deficits on Porteus Maze performance after psychosurgery, including cingulectomy (Bailey et al., 1977—tested with Wechsler Mazes), and leukotomy or lobotomy (Malmo, 1948; Medina et al., 1954; Petrie

1952a,b; Porteus, 1950; Porteus and Kepner, 1944; Porteus and Peters, 1947b; Walsh, 1977).

A more controversial aspect of the effects of frontal surgery on the Porteus Maze has been whether the deficit is permanent or transient. Some authors contend that the deficit is permanent, as indicated in follow-up studies ranging from 3 to 8 years (Medina et al., 1954; Walsh, 1977). Smith (Smith, 1960; Smith and Kinder, 1959) suggested that patients with superior topectomy showed a continual deterioration (a "drop and drop"). Other authors report only a temporary deficit. Porteus and Peters (1947a,b), in an early study on the effects of prefrontal lobotomy, reported a sharp drop in performance during the first month, but repeated assessments over 2 years showed a gradual improvement until the prelobotomy level was regained. The improvement correlated with social improvement. Also, the recovery level was low, suggesting that the preoperative performance may have been impaired. A similar drop and rise were reported in early topectomy studies; although the deficit in maze ability appeared to last for about 3 months, a gradual recovery correlated with good social recovery (H. E. King, 1949; Landis, 1949; Sheer, 1956). These early reports also hinted that superior topectomy patients recovered somewhat slower. An 8-year follow-up study (Smith, 1960; Smith and Kinder, 1959) showed that the superior topectomy patients had not improved over the long term. Conclusions must be interpreted in light of the baseline used, the effects of test practice (Porteus and Diamond, 1962; Riddle and Roberts, 1978), and the surgical procedure employed, leaving considerable room for uncertainty.

The Porteus Maze appears to be a sensitive measure of frontal lobe dysfunction, nonetheless, at least after psychosurgery. Although a primary purpose was a measure of social adaptation among delinquents (Porteus and Peters, 1947a), and the test has been interpreted at times as a measure of introversion-extraversion (Willet, 1960), it is best considered an index of the ability to perceive a complex situation as a unity, plan the correct action while anticipating errors, and execute the response (Medina et al., 1954; Porteus, 1950; Walsh, 1977). The Porteus Maze, against the background of normal functioning in other areas, appears to isolate and test the executive functions hypothesized for the frontal lobes.

Experimental Procedures

A number of experimental procedures have been designed to test one or more aspects of the executive system in humans. Lezak (1976/1983) proposed the "Tinkertoy" test as a means of assessing independent initiation, planning, and implementation of a potentially complex activity. Shallice and Evans (1978) reported that frontal lobe patients had difficulty making a "cognitive estimation." For example, they had difficulty judging the size of common objects or distance from one place to another. Based on his theoretical concept of the "supervisory attentional system" (see Chapter 16), Shallice (1982) used a "look-ahead" puzzle, the Tower of London, borrowed from the artificial intelligence literature (Fig 14-2). This task does not allow the use of well-rehearsed, overlearned programs of behavior; instead, it demands planning the appropriate order of subgoals to reach the final goal.

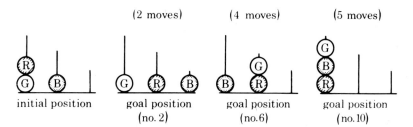

FIG. 14-2. Three subproblems (Nos. 2, 6, 10) from the Tower of London test. Each subtest requires a different number of moves for solution. The starting position *(far left)* is the same for all subtests. (From Shallice: In: *The Neuropsychology of Cognitive Function,* edited by Broadbent and Weiskrantz. The Royal Society, London, 1982, with permission.)

The Tower of London Puzzle consists of three differently colored beads or rings and three sticks (pegs) of different length. A starting order of the beads on the pegs is constructed by the examiner. The subject must then build a new order, as defined by the examiner, in a minimum of moves. The level of difficulty is manipulated by the number of required moves.

Sixty-one patients with brain lesions of various etiology localized to one of four brain quadrants were compared to 20 control subjects (Shallice, 1982). Although all four groups of brain-damaged patients were impaired in comparison to the control subjects, the left anterior lobe damaged patients were most impaired, particularly as the items became more complex. The errors could not be considered impulsive errors, as defined by the time to the first move, because left anterior lobe patients were the slowest. The differences could not be attributed to short-term memory, as use of digit span as a covariate did not change results. Moreover, the deficits in planning could be ascertained during the very first move. The possibility that the deficit represented a verbal disturbance (the impairment was maximal in left anterior lobe patients) was raised, but verbal interference created by partial alphabet recitation did not alter the performance. The author concluded that a specific deficit in planning was present (Shallice, 1982). In many respects the Tower of London test resembles block design tests in that both are visual-motor and utilize verbal mediation. A double dissociation has been found between the two tests in some patients, suggesting a relative difference. Although the block design requires planning and may reflect frontal lobe damage, its primary component is visual-spatial; the Tower of London offers a more direct assessment of planning competence.

Petrides (1985) and Milner (1982) have assessed the role of the frontal lobes in the use of external stimuli to regulate behavior. They compared left and right unilateral frontal lobe damaged patients with left and right temporal lobe damaged patients, the latter divided into those with and those without hippocampal involvement. Spatial and nonspatial conditional associative learning tasks were administered (Fig. 14-3). The subject was required to learn the correct response by trial and error.

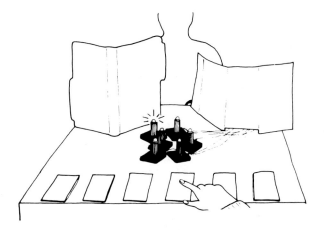

FIG. 14-3. On the spatial conditional associative-learning test, the subject learns the relationship between the six identical response cards arranged horizontally in front of him and the six identical randomly grouped blue lamps. (From Milner: In: *The Neuropsychology of Cognitive Function*, edited by Broadbent and Weiskrantz. The Royal Society, London, 1982; and Petrides: *Neuropsychologia*, with permission.)

The frontal lobe patients were impaired on both the spatial and nonspatial tests; temporal lobe patients with extensive hippocampal removal showed a modality-specific impairment. Right temporal hippocampal pathology impaired the spatial task, whereas left temporal hippocampal pathology affected the nonspatial task. The authors concluded that, because both spatial and nonspatial tests were failed, frontal lobe pathology resulted in general impairment in the use of external cues to guide behavior, not just the deficit in verbal regulation of behavior that Luria had suggested.

Petrides and Milner also examined sequencing. Frontal lobe patients may perform individual tasks yet lose the overall organization. Petrides and Milner (1982) devised a task that theoretically assessed the organization of internally ordered (subjective) sequences. Comparing the performance of frontal lobe damaged patients on this test and the recency tests described in Chapter 12 (which assessed the ability to sequence externally ordered or objective events), the authors concluded that the left frontal area is dominant for programming of voluntary action, i.e., in the programming of self-initiated and self-ordered behavior, whereas the right frontal area was dominant for external ordering (Milner, 1982; Petrides and Milner, 1982).

The clinical value of these experimental procedures remains to be determined. Standardization and validation would be necessary before any firm conclusions could be drawn. These procedures are important, however, as attempts to isolate and test the executive functions of the frontal lobes.

SUMMARY

Anticipation, goal selection, planning, monitoring, and use of feedback—these are specific functions of the executive system. Disorders of the executive functions, if present after focal brain damage, appear to be maximal after frontal lobe damage, suggesting that the frontal lobe is the executive center. This chapter has highlighted the gradual progression toward the more specific assessment of these executive functions.

Although welcome, these aspects also highlight the existing deficiencies. Standard psychological tests are normally insensitive to the effects of frontal lobe damage unless careful analysis of the process of task completion is done. Current tests and observations developed remain too broad; although a number of levels of the executive system are theorized (Lezack, 1976/1983; Lhermitte et al., 1972; Luria, 1973a, 1966/1980; Walsh, 1978), planning is still frequently assessed as a general function, with only infrequent consideration of the heterogeneity and diversity of symptoms and localization within the frontal lobes. Shallice (1982) even suggested that successful group analyses of such functionally distinct deficits are virtually impossible and that reliance on individual case studies remains the methodology of choice. So far very few theories, even those from cognitive psychology, have been used as guides for devising frontal tests. The frontal lobes remain an uncharted frontier (Goldman-Rakic, 1984b).

A review of our knowledge of localization and a formulation of brain organization in Chapter 15 introduces a discussion of proposed theories of frontal activity.

15

Localization of Frontal Lobe Functions

The issue of localization of function automatically initiates a debate on the very nature of brain organization and function. The validity of this controversy is acknowledged, but for this chapter the reported observations of focal frontal damage that produces behavioral changes are presented through a historical review and clinical summary. Many localization details have been presented in earlier chapters and are not repeated.

ISSUES IN LOCALIZATION

Luria (1973a) suggested that one purpose of neuropsychology was to aid in the localization of function. Thus knowledge of the relationship between observed signs and symptoms reflecting damage to specific brain areas can assist in making a diagnosis. With the advent of increasingly sophisticated procedures, however, this clinical purpose assumes diminishing importance. A second purpose subserved by localization concerns theory. Localizing information can be crucial for confirmation or denial of theories of brain-behavioral relations and the functional organization of the brain. This use of localization produces controversy, polarized into opposing camps of localizationists and holists (Kertesz, 1983; Meyer, 1974). Although the holists now accept the cerebral localization of some primary functions (sensory and motor) and the extreme localizationalist ideas proposed during the last century have been considerably modified, many disagreements remain in the characterization of the higher-order cognitive functions (Head, 1926).

A major stumbling block is definitional. Few authors define a brain function. Is it a complete, complex act or the smallest unit of the act? Should the function present after brain damage be defined by the remaining behavior, by absent or impaired behavior, or by some combination? Does performance after a lesion reflect the remaining intact brain structures, the impaired brain areas, or both? What is to be localized? Jackson (1878) stated that a lesion can be localized, but not a function. One hundred years later, Laurence and Stein (1978) stated: "While it would be foolhardy to deny that lesions produce highly consistent behavioral and physiological effects, this does not mean the effects produced represent the functioning of the structure prior to damage" (p. 398). The obvious lesson is that localization attempts cannot by themselves be viewed as a means of specifying the function of a particular brain area.

Brain lesions in humans do not respect the posited functional boundaries, a difficulty described in Chapter 3. A brain lesion not only affects pathways connecting to the focally damaged area but also nearby, totally nonconnected pathways. As many investigators have noted, comparison with animal research, where specific functional subdivisions can be lesioned, is difficult (Iverson, 1973; Mishkin et al., 1969; Oscar-Berman, 1975, 1978; Rosenkilde, 1979; Rosvold, 1972).

Another problem concerns measurement of both the lesion and the behavior. Although some advances in quantification of brain damage have been made (Galaburda and Mesulam, 1983; Kertesz, 1983; Naeser, 1983), the mere measurement of structural damage as a correlate of function appears to be insufficient (Benson, Metter, Kuhl, et al., 1983b). Inadequacies of test measurement, both what and how a function is measured, plague investigation and assessment of frontal lobe function. Results can be achieved in various ways: "The greater the generality, the less likely it is that it is a highly localizable function" (Laurence and Stein, 1978, p. 396). Localization of function to frontal lobes appears particularly dangerous, as most frontal functions are among the most general of all cerebral activities.

Even if the deficiencies of lesion and behavior measurement could be surmounted, many barriers to localization would remain. One is age. In children, there are differential stages of development for different brain areas (see Chapter 2). Similar lesions appear to have more devastating effects in older than younger patients (Hamlin, 1970; Levin, Benton, and Grossman, 1982; Levinson and Meyer, 1965; Porteus and Diamond, 1962; Smith, 1960). Some even suggest that behavior in normal aging individuals resembles, in some respects, that in patients with frontal lobe damage (Albert and Kaplan, 1980). Only careful analysis can distinguish some features of performance of the elderly from those of the frontal lobe patient (Nelson, 1976).

The size of the lesion is an important variable. Jarvie (1954) claimed that no constant relationship existed between the size of the frontal lobe lesion and the degree of disinhibition, but most research suggests a relation of size and deficit. In psychosurgery, smaller leukotomy lesions were not as effective as the full operation (Greenblatt and Solomon, 1966), and residual deficits after topectomy were more likely if the lesions were larger (Smith, 1964). In general, for the frontal lobes, the larger the lesion, the greater the degree of impairment (Shure and Halstead, 1958; Warren, 1964). Luria (1973a, 1966/1980) continually stressed that the frontal lobe syndrome was most notable with "massive" frontal lobe pathology. Moreover, involvement of other areas might be necessary to obtain a full frontal lobe behavioral syndrome, and milder frontal lobe deficits could be compensated (Luria, 1966, 1966/1980, 1969).

Variations based on the effect of different etiologies cannot be discounted (see Chapter 3), and differences between men and women must be considered (Levinson and Meyer, 1965, McGlone, 1980). Duration since frontal damage is important (Goldman, 1974; Goldman and Galkin, 1978), particularly with the possibility of recovery over time (Milner, 1964; Osmond, 1971). Individual differences in terms of skills, past experiences, brain organization and reorganization, and premorbid motivation affect measurements of behavior (Finger and Stein, 1982; Isseroff, Leveton, Freeman, et al., 1976; Will and Rosenzweig, 1976).

Some issues are more directly related to concepts associated with recovery. Effects from one lesion may be categorized as primary or secondary, proximal or distal, residual or transient (Finger and Stein, 1982). Diaschisis refers to effects remote from the actual site of the lesion. Skinhoj (1965) reported bilateral reductions in blood flow after a unilateral lesion to the contralateral (intact) hemisphere. Temporary catecholamine disturbance has been reported in fairly widespread intact areas of rat brain after focal lesions in one hemisphere (Robinson and Bloom, 1978; Robinson, Bloom, and Battenberg, 1977; Robinson, Shoemaker, Schlumpf, et al., 1975). Hypometabolism has been demonstrated in distant, structurally intact areas following discrete aphasia-producing lesions (Metter et al., 1984a). The time of testing functional changes in relation to lesion onset is crucial to the interpretation of structural measures.

Yet another potential factor is supersensitivity, a state following injury where remaining neurons become more efficient (Finger and Stein, 1982). The possibility of spontaneous reorganization or substitution of an intact brain zone for the damaged area deserves consideration (Laurence and Stein, 1978). The patient may spontaneously, or through therapy, learn strategies of compensation leading to entirely different ways to achieve the desired goal.

Reasons for dispute concerning the effects of local lesions on brain function are obvious (Phillips, Zeki, and Barlow, 1984). Attributing a specific behavior to a focal brain area cannot be our contention. On the other hand, lesions affecting a specific area usually produce a relatively coherent pattern of behavioral changes. These alterations and their interactions deserve continued investigation, and the acquisition of localizing knowledge remains clinically and theoretically important.

ISSUES OF ORGANIZATION

The role of the frontal lobes in brain functioning can be understood only in terms of organization of the entire brain. Many theories of brain organization have been postulated, derived from directed research and focused primarily on limited aspects, such as left hemisphere/right hemisphere separation and integration, or the neuroanatomical/behavioral correlates of functional systems, such as sensory-perception, memory, or language. Almost invariably, the frontal lobes, despite their obvious neuroanatomical interconnections with many brain areas, have not been included in the interpretations offered. There has been a great accumulation of knowledge, however, information that provides a basic structure for an integrated view of brain functioning that includes the influence of the frontal lobes.

With this approach the brain can be considered to have a series of *organized integrated fixed functional systems*, each system representing a broad functional entity, such as language or memory, as well as the more basic systems such as sensory-perception and motor effector patterns. The system can be considered fixed in that in the normal adult human the function and its relation to neuroanatomical areas remains relatively constant across individuals and relatively unchanging within individuals. Organized implies that the system consists of different components that play separate but integral parts in the successful functioning of the entire system. Thus a lesion in a specific area of the language system influences language as a general function, but the characteristics of the impairment may well be specific to that region. Integrated connotes several facts: First, it is necessary that the different components of a system be consistently connected so that they can work together to produce the function (e.g., language); second, areas in both hemispheres as well as selected subcortical neural structures and the interconnecting pathways are all important to the system. There is both lateralized and hierarchical integration; third, integration should not be viewed in a strict connectionistic manner. Although pathways exist, they connect "centers," which may well function in a fashion of spreading excitation. Finally, although not a part of these basic systems per se, the prefrontal cortex is associated with each system in an organizational, controlling manner above and beyond the inherent organization of the system itself. The integration of anterior brain functions to the more posterior and subcortical systems represents an important organizational factor.

Language is a good example of an organized integrated fixed functional system. The integrated activity of diverse cerebral areas within the left hemisphere has been well described (Benson, 1979; Benson and Geschwind, 1971; Geschwind, 1974). The role of right hemisphere areas in language function has been described more recently (Gazzaniga et al., 1984; Ross, 1981; Zaidel, 1982) and the contribution of subcortical structures is being outlined (Alexander and LoVerme, 1980; Damasio et al., 1982; Naeser et al., 1982). Geschwind's (1965) monograph on disconnection syndromes demonstrated the importance of the connecting pathways to language functions. Finally, the supervisory role of the frontal lobe has been emphasized (see Chapter 11). A lesion in a single part of the system disturbs language function, but the quality of the disturbance varies depending on the particular area damaged. As the frontal lobes are connected to every system, damage to the frontal lobes affects each system but the features are generalized, reflecting only the input of the frontal lobes.

Behavioral research has focused on individual functions. This has produced artificial and somewhat untrue characterizations of brain activity. Nevertheless, most of these studies are sufficiently advanced that views of overall integration must recognize certain functional systems. Among the behavioral systems to be considered here are attention, visual-spatial skill, memory, language, cognition, motor response patterns, as well as autonomic and emotional functions. Obviously, there is considerable overlap in these functions, the divisions representing academic interests, not necessarily discrete anatomical or psychological systems. Nevertheless, these divisions have developed a considerable background of data and, in the main, are primarily posterior brain functions.

FRONTAL LOBE LOCALIZATION

The behavioral patterns reported after damage to the frontal lobes are now reviewed, stressing separation of frontal from nonfrontal involvement. Within the frontal lobe, three divisions are considered: anterior-posterior; dorsal-lateral/orbital-medial; left-right. More exact anatomical localization must await improved research techniques.

Frontal Lobe Versus Nonfrontal Lobe

Reliable indices of frontal lobe damage have been difficult to demonstrate. It was once stated (Meyer, 1960) that no function could be localized to the frontal lobes, and that focal frontal damage did not produce a specific behavioral problem. Reitan (1964) found no neuropsychological differences that differentiated patients with frontal and nonfrontal lesions. Differences observed in individual case studies (Ackerly and Benton, 1947; Harlow, 1868) were not easily demonstrated in formal investigations (Scherer et al., 1957).

Certain behavioral patterns are relatively consistent in patients with frontal lobe damage, however. Perhaps the most obvious is the "frontal personality" (see Chapters 7 and 8) but despite striking behavioral descriptions (e.g., Blumer and Benson, 1975; Harlow, 1868) little objective research pertains to the frontal personality (Damasio and Van Hoesen, 1983; Stuss and Benson, 1983a). Although some information may be gained from use of tests designed for and validated on psychiatric populations (e.g., MMPI), interpretations based on these limited techniques suggest that frontal damage produces no alteration. The crucial signs of frontal personality disturbance remain unsubstantiated by such experimental methods.

Motor abilities represent important indices of frontal function. Even when paresis is absent, patients with frontal damage may show impairment on contrasting motor tests (Drewe, 1975a), replication of motor sequences (Luria, 1969), and replication of complex limb gestures (Kolb and Milner, 1981). Oral apraxia may follow left premotor area lesions (Geschwind, 1967, 1975), anterior corpus callosum section may produce a unilateral ideomotor apraxia (Geschwind, 1967, 1975; Heilman, 1979a), and medial frontal cortex disturbance can cause magnetic apraxia (Denny-Brown, 1958). Absence of these deficits does not exclude frontal lobe damage, however. Leukotomized patients performed perfectly on a series of frontal motor tests (Benson and Stuss, 1982) despite large frontal lesions. Greater specificity, both behavioral and anatomical, is required, perhaps imitating the research used in the animal literature (e.g., Deuel, 1977).

One neurological sign suggesting frontal pathology is anosmia. The olfactory tract lies on the orbital surface of the frontal lobes and is easily damaged by frontal lobe pathology. In addition, deficits in olfactory discrimination and preference can suggest pathology in pathways involving the dorsal-medial nucleus of the thalamus and part of the frontal cortex (Eichenbaum, Shedlack, and Eckman, 1980; Potter and Butters, 1980; Sapolsky and Eichenbaum, 1980). Anosmia most often reflects a peripheral sensory disorder, however, an olfactory nerve lesion without frontal lobe involvement.

Deviation of conjugate eye movement has been interpreted as a frontal lobe sign (Daroff and Hoyt, 1971) but not an absolute indication (Adams and Victor, 1977/1981). DeRenzi et al. (1982) suggested that the frontal eye findings are based on studies of patients with large lesions and claimed that conjugate gaze paresis is seldom present if pathology is confined to the prerolandic area. They proposed that right conjugate gaze paresis indicates right parietal localization and that a large left middle cerebral artery lesion is normally associated with conjugate deviation to the left. Refined observations are needed.

Chapter 11 suggests that the speech and language syndromes, particularly when correlated with physical findings, offer information for localization of frontal pathology. A persistent Broca aphasia indicates involvement of Broca's area plus deep and posterior extensions (Altemus, Roberson, Fisher, et al., 1976; Benson, 1979; Kertesz et al., 1977). A "little Broca" aphasia reflects more selective involvement of Broca's area (Mohr et al., 1978). Combined neurological, neuroradiological, and language evaluation of transcortical motor aphasia suggests separation of the supplementary motor area from pathology anterior and superior to Broca's area (Freedman et al., 1984), and differentiation of lower motor from lower premotor zones has been suggested on the basis of motor language deficit (Tonkonogy and Goodglass, 1981).

Although such reports are important, awareness of limitations is necessary. The CT scan does not delineate precise boundaries and "... reliance of structurally oriented localization procedures for correlation with aphasia phenomenology may be misleading" (Benson et al., 1983b, p. 128).

Verbal fluency, the generation of word lists, is used for separating frontal from nonfrontal pathology, but only when the patient is not aphasic or does not have generalized brain disturbance (Bruyer and Tuyumbu, 1980; Milner, 1964; Perret, 1974; Ramier and Hécaen, 1970; Taylor, 1979). To date, studies have not been able to localize word list generation difficulties within the frontal lobe, although dorsal-lateral and medial areas appear to be most relevant.

Other positive signs suggesting prefrontal dysfunction have been detailed, and six broad, yet relatively specific deficits secondary to prefrontal damage can be proposed (Stuss and Benson, 1984):

1. Deficit in the ordering or handling of sequential behaviors
2. Impairment in establishing or changing a set
3. Impairment in maintaining a set, particularly in the presence of interference
4. Decreased ability to monitor personal behavior
5. Dissociation of knowlege from the direction of response
6. Altered attitudes

Although apparently specific to focal frontal lobe damage, these signs cannot be used to exclude other brain area dysfunction. It is difficult to dissociate focal frontal disturbance from diffuse brain damage (Robinson et al., 1975). With advancing age, "A diffuse loss of neurons might handicap the victims in such general mental skills as flexible problem solving, the ability to change sets and entertain improbable outcomes as possibilities, as well as to focus, maintain and then adaptively detach attention in a task" (Kinsbourne, 1977a, p. 227). This description strongly resembles the behavior described following frontal lobe damage but also reflects the disorder affecting wider, overlapping brain areas.

Despite the relatively large size of the frontal lobes, determination that specific behavioral disturbance is based on focal frontal lobe pathology has proved remarkably difficult.

Anterior-Posterior Differences

Distinctions have been suggested concerning specific deficits *within* the frontal lobe, based on a rostral-caudal difference. In general, the more caudal (posterior) the pathology, the greater the deterioration. Anterior psychosurgery lesions produced personality changes, but if the lesion was more posterior other deficits were superimposed (LeBeau, 1952, 1954; Petrie, 1952a,b; Riddle and Roberts, 1978). Similar anterior-posterior differences were noted in the behavioral results following topectomy (Hamlin, 1970; Smith, 1960, 1964). The plane of leukotomy excision became a crucial consideration in eliciting maximum behavioral alteration with minimal neurological deficit (Brain and Strauss, 1955).

Except for psychosurgery, little attention has been paid to frontal lobe anterior-posterior differences. Milner (1963) suggested that anterior lesions impaired the ability to shift from one sorting mode to another more than posterior lesions. Luria (1965, 1969) separated frontal motor actions into two types: (1) posterior frontal or medial-basal frontal lesions, extending deep to the subcortical motor areas, that produced compulsive repetition of a movement once initiated; (2) more anterior lesions that did not show this motor perseveration.

Anterior-posterior differences are notable in the analysis of speech and other fine motor movements (see Chapters 5 and 11). It is suggested that pathology in the motor strip results in impaired articulation, whereas more anterior pathology affects the kinetic melody of speech causing difficulty in the transition from one element of articulation to the next (Luria, 1969). Again, additional data are necessary for this to be an accepted localization.

Anterior-posterior differences were suggested using the Porteus Maze test in topectomy research. The more posterior a topectomy lesion, the greater the postoperative decrement in performing the Porteus Maze (Riddle and Roberts, 1978). These differences may actually reflect surface divisions, however, with the superior dorsal lesions lying more posterior and the orbital lesions more anterior.

The relevance of anterior-posterior differences in frontal pathology to the observed behavior is suggestive but remains unsettled.

Dorsal-Lateral/Orbital/Medial Differences

Another possibly relevant localization differentiation centers on the three cortical surfaces described in Chapter 2: dorsal-lateral, orbital, and medial. Terms used to define these areas are inconsistent, and the use of an anatomical label does not exclude pathology involving another area. Interpretation is further complicated by cortical versus white matter considerations and by involvement of neuroanatomical connections.

Baker et al. (1970) suggested two parallel frontal-limbic-hypothalamic midbrain circuits: a medial frontal/cingulate/hippocampal unit and an orbital frontal/temporal/amygdala unit. Different effects on mood and behavior were postulated based on the severing of either or both of the units, and it was postulated that bimedial leukotomy was effective in relation to the destruction of these pathways.

The effects of frontal disconnection on behavioral functions can be estimated by correlating the location of frontal damage as demonstrated by computed tomography (CT) scan with performance on psychological tests (Stuss et al., 1983). In general, low frontal white matter pathways connect to orbital-medial zones, whereas more superior white matter tracts connect with dorsal-lateral cortex. Performance on a test of abstraction correlated positively with lesion sites higher in the frontal lobes ($r = 0.89$) and negatively with the lower sites ($r = -0.50$). These results suggest differential involvement of the frontal lobes in some cognitive functions and imply that white matter pathway connections are significant in localization research.

Language evaluation appears to provide relatively specific information, even when the clinical aphasic syndromes are excluded. The dorsal-lateral cortex was reported to be the most sensitive area for verbal fluency (Milner, 1963, 1964), with the inferior dorsal-lateral cortex anterior to area 44 (Broca's area) most affected (Milner, 1964; Taylor, 1979). Hécaen and Ruel (1981), however, found no significant differences in localization of the lesion within the dorsal-lateral cortex. Other dorsal-lateral areas have been implicated, including the supplementary motor area (Alexander and Schmitt, 1980), the zones anterior and superior to Broca's area (TCMA zones) (Freedman et al., 1984), and the central (rolandic) area (Taylor, 1979). In contrast, patients with focal white matter lesions maximal in lower orbital zones performed within normal limits on language tests (Stuss and Benson, 1983b). Kaczmarek (1984) suggested that the left dorsal-lateral frontal cortex is important for sequential organization and the left orbital frontal lobe for direction of a narrative through monitoring. Another feature that may reflect a dorsal-lateral/orbital frontal difference concerns verbal regulation of behavior. Luria suggested that a deficit in this ability, although not always present (Cicerone et al., 1983; Drewe, 1975b), implied dorsal-lateral frontal pathology, particularly on the left (Luria, 1960, 1966, 1967, 1969).

Control of certain motor functions also appears to be localizing within the frontal lobes. Patients with medial pathology tend to be slow, lethargic, and apathetic, and to lack initiative and spontaneity. In contrast, patients with lateral convexity and lateral orbital pathology tend to be restless, hyperkinetic, explosive, and impulsive (Blumer and Benson, 1975; Goldstein, 1944; Kleist, 1934b; Lishman, 1968). In addition, many of Luria's frontal motor tests including "go/no-go," two- and three-step motor sequences, finger-tapping, "conflicting" motor tasks, and three loop drawings as well as articulation problems and difficulties in transition of articulations were not impaired in patients with focal orbital frontal white matter lesions but can be seen with dorsal convexity damage (Benson and Stuss, 1982; Luria, 1966/1980, 1973a; Luria and Homskaya, 1964; Luria et al., 1964).

There are apparently no demonstrable deficits in IQ on the basis of orbital frontal pathology (Luria, 1969; Stuss et al., 1982a, 1983). When IQ impairment has been reported following frontal lesions, the pathology has almost always involved the dorsal-lateral regions (Girgis, 1971; Malmo, 1948; Petrie, 1952b; Smith and Kinder, 1959). Even this is unusual and may reflect more widespread pathology.

Assessment of the "executive" functions of the frontal lobes also suggests differences based on the surface most involved. With control of cortical mass involved, greater losses were recorded on the Porteus Maze test after superior forebrain ablation than orbital topectomy (Porteus and Diamond, 1962; Smith, 1960; Smith Kinder, 1959), results that may also be interpreted as an anterior-posterior difference.

Abnormal results on the Wisconsin Card Sorting Test (WCST) are maximal with, if not specific to, dorsal-lateral frontal lesions (Milner, 1963, 1964, 1971). Even without surgery, patients with dorsal-lateral epileptogenic lesions performed worse than those with foci in the orbital frontal or temporal lobes. Within the dorsal-lateral cortex, the critical area apparently lies outside the inferior frontal cortex (the area most sensitive to verbal fluency) (Milner, 1963; Taylor, 1979), but this is not the only area affected. Stuss et al. (1982a, 1983) reported impaired performance on the WCST in patients with orbital frontal leukotomy lesions, and Drewe (1974) suggested that the critical area was medial, not dorsal-lateral. Mishkin (1964), using monkeys and a task at least superficially similar to the card sorting test, demonstrated greater deficits with orbital than dorsal-lateral frontal lesions; Passingham (1972), using a test of nonreversal shifts in monkeys, reported greater impairment after orbital-lateral lesions.

Part of the difficulty stems from localization of the pathology. Many of Milner's dorsal-lateral patients also had involvement of medial cortex (Milner, 1963). Her use of "medial" (Milner, 1964) may be different from Drewe's (1974) use of the term, and the white matter lesions of Stuss et al.'s leukotomy patients may affect cortical areas not identified on CT scan.

Further difficulty stems from the definition of what is measured. For example, orbital frontal white matter lesions primarily affected maintenance of correct response (Stuss et al., 1983), whereas dorsal-lateral pathology increased perseverative errors (Milner, 1963).

Confabulation has been postulated as a frontal lobe sign. A spectacular case is Phineas Gage, who regaled others "with the most fabulous recitals of his wonderful feats and hairbreadth escapes, without any foundation except in his fancy" (Harlow, 1868, p. 340). Pathology involved bilateral mesial frontal cortex. Instances of confabulation following anterior communicating artery aneurysms (Lindqvist and Norlen, 1966; Talland et al., 1967) also suggest damage maximal to mesial-orbital frontal areas. Most clinical reports of confabulation suggest maximum involvement in mesial frontal areas (Kapur and Coughlan, 1980; Luria, 1973a; Luria, Homskaya, Blinkov, et al., 1967; Stuss et al., 1978). Many of the reported patients, however, had involvement of other brain areas, including nonfrontal regions. We know of no reports of confabulation secondary to dorsal-lateral frontal pathology.

That mesial/orbital-frontal limbic zones are important in personality changes other than confabulation has been repeatedly suggested. Virtually all early clinical reports stressing dramatic personality changes secondary to frontal lobe damage documented pathology in mesial-orbital frontal areas (Harlow, 1868; Welt, 1888). The behavioral alteration is compatible with proposed neuroanatomical connections between the limbic system and orbital-medial areas (Livingston, 1969, 1977; Nauta, 1971; Stuss and Benson, 1983a) and with animal research on specific behavioral changes defined as emotional (Markowska and Lukaszewska, 1980; Mora, Avrith, Phillips, et al., 1979; Mora, Avrith, and Rolls, 1980). Other areas are also important, however. Kleist (1934b) divided personality changes after frontal lobe damage into orbital (facetious, restless, puerile, irritable, amoral, and euphoric) and convexity (decreased mental and motor initiative, slowness, apathy, and indifference). Similar divisions were noted by others (Faust, 1955, 1960; Spreen, 1956; Walch, 1956), and Blumer and Benson (1975) labeled these two types as pseudopsychopathic and pseudodepressed (pseudoretarded). Damasio and Van Hoesen (1983) reported disturbances in drive, memory, and social behavior after pathology in mesial or orbital frontal extensions of the limbic cortex, disorders not found after focal lateral frontal lesions.

A more precise differentiation may be possible. Eslinger and Damasio (1985) described a patient with bilateral orbital and lower mesial frontal pathology who had superior psychometric IQ and performed well on the "frontal" tests administered but who nevertheless lacked motivation and had impaired implementation of goal-directed behavior in real life. They suggested that these findings were distinct from the symptoms following superior mesial or dorsal-lateral frontal pathology.

In summary, evidence for differences in function based on pathology in either the medial, orbital, or dorsal-lateral frontal cortex apparently exists but must be evaluated with caution and deliberation. Most of the evidence is indirect, dependent on interpretation of complex functions.

Left-Right Differences

In parallel with the debate on localization of any function to the frontal lobes comes the question of the laterality of frontal lobe function. Early authors, even those who advocated specific frontal lobe functions, could not elicit obvious hemispheric differences (Feuchtwanger, 1923; Jefferson, 1937; Kolodny, 1929; Rylander, 1939). The general conclusion was that "personality and the association and sympathies of mental processes are bilaterally represented and that their expression is the simultaneous product of both frontal lobes" (Stookey et al., 1941, p. 163). In recent years, however, some suggestions of hemispheric differences have been described in proverb interpretation, verbal learning, and time orientation (Benton, 1968). Grafman, Vance, Weingartner, et al. (1985a) proposed a laterality-cortical surface interaction for mood states, with right orbital frontal lobe patients exhibiting increased anxiety and depression and left dorsal-lateral lobe patients revealing increased hostility. Left–right differences in mood have been reported, left anterior lobe patients being depressed more than any other patients. Within the right hemisphere, posterior lobe patients were more depressed than anterior lobe patients, who appeared cheerful and apathetic (Robinson et al., 1984). That these effects relate to lesion size and/or extension into other cortical areas is possible. In many instances, the impairment is minimal with unilateral frontal pathology and much more significant with bilateral damage.

Sensory-motor abilities appear to be good lateralizing signs. Crowne et al. (1981) reported that unilateral frontal eye field lesions in the macaque monkey result in marked contralateral neglect. Despite these claims, the work by Deuel and Collins (1984) suggests that conjugate gaze paresis and unilateral inattention may be not only frontal but also thalamic. Motor deficits, particularly of strength and speed of a single limb, have obvious hemispheric differences. Certain tests of apraxia and hand posture appear to be most impaired after left hemisphere damage. Complex tests using motor responses are less differentiating; for example, there appears to be no left–right differences on "go/no-go" tasks (Drewe, 1975a).

The generation of word lists may suggest unilateral frontal lobe specificity. Impaired verbal fluency occurs after either left or right frontal pathology (Benton, 1968; Ramier and Hécaen, 1970), but it is more severe with left involvement (Hécaen and Ruel, 1981; Milner, 1964; Perret, 1974; Ramier and Hécaen, 1970). Damage to the left frontal lobe impairs the ability to generate lists of words beginning with a specific letter (Milner, 1964) but apparently not in semantic categories (Newcombe, 1969). Bilateral damage is either equivalent to the left hemisphere results (Benton, 1968) or falls between the right and left hemisphere scores (Hécaen and Ruel, 1981). Similarly, design fluency deficit (i.e., ease of production of drawings) appears maximum in patients with right frontal or frontal-central pathology (Jones-Gotman and Milner, 1977). Deficits in word generation can occur in disorders with nonfrontal pathology (e.g., aphasia and dementia) (Benson, 1979), and design fluency impairment is reported after lesions in several cortical areas (Jones-Gotman and Milner, 1977). It is not a specific frontal lateralizing sign.

Hebb (1939) stated that the left frontal area is no more important in cognitive abilities than the right unless language and speech areas are involved; and Black (1976), testing patients with frontal lobe damage from penetrating brain wounds, found no verbal versus nonverbal differences. Others, however, suggested that left frontal lobe patients have lower IQ scores than those with right frontal lobe lesions (Busch, 1940; McFie and Piercy, 1952a,b), and Luria (1969) stated that "intellectual impairment," if present, was maximum with bilateral pathology or massive lesions of the dominant (left) hemisphere and difficult to elicit with right frontal lesions. Smith (1966), comparing left and right frontal lobe patients, found a tendency for the left frontal lobe patients to be more impaired. There was no overall IQ difference between frontal lobe patients and control subjects, but there was if the frontal lobe subjects were divided into left (IQ=86.25) or right (IQ=103.5).

A basic rule in visual-perceptual and visual-constructive abilities is that if deficits are obvious after frontal damage at all they are greater with right-sided damage, presumably reflecting the spatial characteristics of the tests (Benson and Barton, 1970; Benton, 1968; Black and Strub, 1976; Brown, 1985; Corkin, 1965; Ettlinger, Teuber, and Milner, 1975; Milner, 1971; Taylor, 1979). Analysis of the procedure of performance suggests that the deficit is one of control, problems of following rules, indecision about beginning, disorganized gestalt, and intrusions or distortions of details (Kaplan, 1983; Milner, 1963; Taylor, 1979). Certain tests for visual-perceptual and visual-constructive disorders do not fit this pattern. Perception of reversible figures is impaired with either left or right frontal damage (Cohen, 1959; Teuber, 1964), personal orientation is most impaired for left frontal lobe patients (Semmes et al., 1963; Teuber, 1964), and the importance of left anterior regions in processing even simple visual stimuli has been emphasized (Kim et al., 1984).

One of the better localizing findings reported in recent literature concerns recency memory tests (see Chapter 12) (Ettlinger et al., 1975; Milner, 1971, 1974, 1982; Petrides and Milner, 1982). Left frontal lobe patients were most impaired on measures of verbal recency and right frontal lobe patients on nonverbal versions. Right frontal lobe patients were also impaired on the verbal recency tests, but left frontal lobe patients were not impaired on the nonverbal test. It was suggested that the right frontal lobe, impaired for both verbal and nonverbal tasks, played a dominant role in monitoring the sequence of externally ordered events. In contrast, tests of programming of internally ordered events revealed that the left frontal lobe patients were impaired on both verbal and nonverbal tasks, whereas the right frontal lobe patients were deficient only on the nonverbal tasks.

The Wechsler Adult Intelligence Scale (WAIS) Picture Arrangement subtest is frequently reported to be more impaired with right frontal lobe pathology. Right frontal lobe patients tend to leave the picture in the order presented (Ettlinger et al., 1975; McFie, 1969; McFie and Piercy, 1952a,b; Smith, 1966). Whether a true asymmetry exists is uncertain, as no results on a verbal counterpart are available.

One early report of Weigl's color-form sorting test stressed the importance of the dominant hemisphere, particularly the left frontal area (McFie and Piercy, 1952a). Early WCST research demonstrated no significant difference between left and right frontal lobe patients (Milner, 1963), but the groups were not fully equal. Others have reported that deficits in card sorting are more frequent and more lasting after left frontal than right frontal lobe damage (Drewe, 1974; Ettlinger et al., 1975; Milner, 1971; Taylor, 1979). One study suggested a relatively greater importance for the right frontal area in this test (Robinson et al., 1980). Shallice (1982) reported a left frontal lobe function for general programming.

In summary, asymmetry of function between left and right frontal lobes, when it can be demonstrated, primarily follows the known material specificity.

SUMMARY

A review of the "localization of function" in the frontal lobes suggests two groups of conclusions. The first concerns general concepts of localization.

1. Behavioral function per se cannot be localized to any specific area of the frontal lobe. Nevertheless, behavioral effects following damage to specific areas are relatively consistent; study of such lawful behavioral changes represents a worthwhile scientific endeavor.

2. A theory of "organized, integrated fixed functional systems" can be proposed. The study of frontal lobe function appears to focus on the study of the brain's control of these organized functions.

The second set of conclusions relates to the present state of knowledge of behavioral changes after frontal brain damage.

1. Some behavioral changes appear to differentiate frontal from nonfrontal lobe damage provided careful dissociation of function is carried out.

2. Differences based on anterior or posterior frontal lobe damage have been described but are not reliably characterized.

3. Differences depending on maximum pathology in dorsal-lateral, orbital, or medial frontal cortical areas have been suggested but may reflect differences in connections as well.

4. Differences based on left versus right frontal lobe involvement can be delineated but primarily reflect the verbal/visual-spatial and other reported general differences of the two hemispheres.

These observations emphasize both the unity and the diversity of frontal lobe functioning.

16

Theories of Frontal Lobe Function

A select group of the major theories offered during the past several decades to explain the functions of the prefrontal cortex are reviewed in this chapter. To start, most of the basic concepts of frontal function presented by earlier investigators (see Chapter 1) have been accepted, providing a base for additional modeling. The theories presented in this chapter are more recent and have been selected for their innovative features; however, these reviews are inadequate and cannot be considered to represent fully the ideas of the selected investigators.

PRIBRAM: FEEDBACK SYSTEM

In Pribram's view, the brain systems associated with problem-solving could be divided into two neuroanatomical areas (Pribram, 1960). The more posterior system is involved with the search to delineate the basic problem, a differentiating behavior. After the search is completed, intentional behavior is commanded by the more anterior (frontal) system. In a later formulation (Pribram and Melges, 1969) he described the posterior convexity connection as participatory, involved in automatic processing, whereas the frontal limbic connection was preparatory, important for episodic processing.

A key promise of Pribram's basic theory is that behavior cannot be explained by the classic reflex arc (Miller, Gallanter, and Pribram, 1960). A far more complex monitoring system is required, with the feedback loop acting as a fundamental process. Miller et al. postulated a test–operate–test–exit (TOTE) system. They posited that a state of incongruity exists between the organism and the stimulus resulting in a testing operation that continues until the incongruity is resolved. Feedback from the results of the testing is used for comparison, not as reinforcement. Feedback is knowledge (information, control) in the form of instructions and acts to assist control. The TOTE system is an organizing, coordinating unit, not a simple reflex.

The TOTE unit, as described, is the most fundamental unit for behavior. Larger operational units are possible, composed of multiple TOTE units, each with its own feedback loop. This organizational structure provides two main properties: Planning is a hierarchical process controlling both the construction of tasks to be performed and the sequence of operations to be carried out; this is followed by an operation phase, subserving both the action to be done and the actual operation.

Action by the organism is an external representation of a neuroprogram in the brain (Pribram, 1967).

The TOTE system can be outlined as a fourfold division of brain function. There are external and internal representations, each of which can be divided into two. The external representation is divided into the sensory modalities and their association areas. The internal representation consists of the limbic systems and the frontal association areas. Basic information for discrimination, the external representation, is formed into plans and sequences by the limbic and subcortical processing units. The frontal regions store the plans while awaiting implementation. It is postulated that behavioral plans are formulated in posterior regions and transferred to frontal regions.

The factor of context was added later (Pribram, 1973). Pribram postulated that behavior at any moment depends on the context of events, providing information for sequential behavior. He described "flexible noticing orders" that allow focus on specific action and inhibition of unnecessary behaviors. With frontal lobe damage, behavior lacks context due to inappropriate or absent schedules or routines, resulting in impaired behavior and planning. If external flexible noticing orders are imposed, such as markers or cues, performance may be improved to near-normal levels (Pribram and Tubbs, 1967). On this basis Pribram hypothesized that "the frontal cortex is especially concerned in structuring context-dependent behaviors" (Pribram, 1973, p. 308), a function of higher-order control (Pribram, 1973; Brody and Pribram, 1978).

TEUBER: COROLLARY DISCHARGE

Teuber's theory of frontal lobe function (1964, 1966, 1972) represented a radical change. Historically, neuroscientists had always considered that brain function began in the posterior sensory regions. Teuber postulated that the reverse might be a better explanation; by demonstrating how anterior anticipatory processing acts on posterior sensory processing, he emphasized the influence of the motor system on sensory function.

Teuber postulated that a corollary or anticipatory discharge travels from motor to sensory areas to prepare the sensory structures for the anticipated change of voluntary action. The most obvious clinical example is voluntary eye movement. Normally, the environment never appears to move; when the eye ball is moved passively, however, the environment appears to relocate. The reason hypothesized for this consistency in vision is that the visual-sensory mechanism has been prepared to expect the change of position by knowledge of the frontal oculomotor discharge. The frontal lobes are crucial for adjusting one's reactions to one's actions. More precisely: "every 'voluntary' movement has two neural correlates: a stream of impulses to the effectors and a simultaneous 'corollary discharge' to central receptor structures, presetting the latter for those predictable changes of input that will be the consequences of the particular motor input" (Teuber, 1964, p. 439). The simple stimulus-response postulate is inadequate, as the prediction of incoming stimuli and the presetting of sensory mechanisms are relevant to the reaction.

Teuber proved this postulate in two ways. First, he provided more than ample negative evidence by the lack of specificity of disturbance on tests such as critical flicker fusion, sorting tests, general intelligence, memory, and attention. However, he demonstrated selective frontal lobe dysfunction on four tests: (1) visual search; (2) the rod and frame (Aubert) task of judgment of visual and postural verticality; (3) perception of reversals and ambiguous perspectives; (4) personal orientation. All tests were dependent on the control of movement, but, as Teuber noted, it was not the movement per se but the anticipation of change and the distinction of internal movement from external movement that were the relevant factors.

To effect an anticipatory function, the frontal lobes must monitor external stimuli, first by feedback from the external stimuli and next by feed-forward, anticipating and predicting the consequences of a selected motor act. Described in another manner, active voluntary movements require at least two sets of signals. The first is a downward signal to effector areas (frontal to motor). The second is a simultaneous signal (frontal to posterior) to preset the sensory system for the anticipated effects of the voluntary act. The corollary discharge depends on the integrity of the frontal lobes and the basal ganglia (Teuber, 1966).

Teuber's theory has altered the attitude of investigators to the functioning of the frontal lobes. The original concept of the frontal lobe as an effector, an active voluntary agent, remains important, but additional functions have been demonstrated.

NAUTA: NEUROANATOMICAL BASIS

The theory proposed by Nauta (1971, 1973) may be viewed as an integration and extension of Teuber's theory, but its creative source was neuroanatomy, not psychological tests. On reviewing the neuroanatomy of the frontal lobes, Nauta was impressed by two interlocking observations. First, he noted that the frontal lobe has strong reciprocal relationships with the two great functional zones: (1) the visual, auditory, and somatosensory zones via the parietal and temporal association cortices; (2) the telencephalic limbic system, including subcortical areas that monitor the internal milieu and provide information for affective and motivational responses. The second observation is that the frontal lobes, with their major frontal-limbic associations, represent the major, if not the only, neocortical representation of the limbic system.

The strong reciprocal connections of the frontal lobes with virtually every cerebral area suggests that the frontal lobes can function as both an effector and a sensor. As an effector, the frontal lobe programs, plans, and modulates. Thus the frontal lobe damaged patient can adequately describe what he senses but cannot plan or modulate his behavior. The sensor aspect of the frontal lobes is involved in perceptual processing. Indeed, the frontal lobes comprise the only area of neocortex that allows the convergence of information from both internal (visceral, endocrine, etc.) and all external (including olfactory) sources.

Nauta presented a neuroanatomical rationale for the presetting of the exteroceptive processing mechanisms, accomplished by the frontal efferent connections with the temporal and inferior parietal areas. Teuber's theory is extended, however, in that the presetting or corollary discharge would exist for interoceptive information as well. The frontal-limbic connections allow behavioral anticipation and foresight. Thus an individual planning a behavior could examine a number of alternative strategies, with the conclusion based on verification of the possible affective responses associated with each possible strategy. Such a course is suggested by phrases such as "the mere thought of doing such a thing makes me ill."

Nauta (1971) postulated that the two major corollary discharges, interoceptive and exteroceptive, provide temporal stability of behavior by establishing a "temporal sequence of affective reference points serving as 'navigational markers' and providing, by their sequential order, at once the general course and the temporal stability of complex goal-directed forms of behavior" (p. 183). This provides an internal "testing ground" of possible behaviors for certain circumstances, enabling an individual to preview possible affective consequences. Frontal lobe patients display flatness of affect, socially inappropriate behavior, and difficulty in foreseeing the outcome of an action.

Nauta's theory then follows the tradition of Pribram and Teuber but solidifies it by adding a neuroanatomical basis. A rational neuroanatomical foundation has been offered for the flexible, guided behavior of humans.

DAMASIO: ANATOMICAL-FUNCTIONAL MODEL

A second, somewhat similar, anatomical-functional model was sketched by Damasio (1979). Three basic factors underlie his model. First, the guiding principle of behavior is preservation of an individual's equilibrium. Second, the general functions of the frontal lobes are to judge and regulate ongoing external perception and, based on this perception, to plan the appropriate response. The third concerns the basic neuroanatomical organization that underlies these functions. Damasio viewed the latter as threefold: (1) reciprocal connections with the reticular activating system and the limbic system; (2) reciprocal connections with the posterior sensory association cortices; (3) reciprocal connections to both cortical and subcortical motor systems.

Against this background Damasio postulated that a stimulus-response network requires the analysis and comparison that the frontal lobes provide. The frontal lobes not only decide how the sensory information should be analyzed but also how to respond most appropriately to accomplish the most beneficial immediate and long-term benefits.

The frontal lobes compute sensation and organize responses based on a set of stabilizing goals accomplished through a series of gating mechanisms. First, a lower system gating is performed by the hypothalamic nuclei. This system is relevant for the evaluation of pleasure/pain and the motivational loading of the particular stimulus, based on past experience, present motivational states, and so on. This lower gating system is almost automatic in operation. Complex information, either stimulus or response, that requires evaluation of both external and internal rules and postulation of goals demands participation of the frontal lobes. This represents a higher-order gating system involved more in learning than mere inherited past behaviors. "It is the ability to handle hyper-complex environmental contingencies in the framework of the individual's own history, and in the perspective of his desired future course, that distinguishes frontal-lobe operation" (Damasio, 1979, p. 371). He also stated that, as learning becomes consolidated, more of the action programs can be carried out by nonfrontal areas. Thus the relative preservation of IQ after frontal lobe damage may be explained.

Although Damasio's theoretical presentation is not as detailed as those described previously, it makes good use of current knowledge of neuroanatomy and neuropsychology to postulate behavioral theories.

FUSTER: TEMPORAL INTEGRATION OF BEHAVIOR

Fuster (1980, 1981) directly addressed the problem of unity and diversity and frontal lobe syndromes. Although, at one level it appears that lesions in specific areas result in specific deficits, these same lesions appear to produce more general problems, suggesting that they might also be part of a superordinate function. Thus there may be both homogeneity and heterogeneity in frontal lobe function, depending on the definition of the function. Fuster posited that the most characteristic function of the prefrontal lobe is temporal structuring of behavior with three subordinate functions: anticipation, provisional memory, and control of interference.

The function of the frontal lobe is to form a temporal framework for any behavior (cognitive or motor) that has a unifying purpose or goal, provided the situation is novel and complex and that these factors exceed a certain critical level. Only if these qualifications are met are the services of the frontal lobes required. The most critical factor demanding the function of the frontal lobes is time; the frontal lobes are necessary to bridge temporal discontiguities. In Fuster's view, behavior represents complex temporal gestalts with each part important not in itself but in relation to each other and to the overall goal. Maintenance of this temporal gestalt is an important frontal function. Interference can distort or pervert the temporal gestalt. The frontal lobes function to avert interfering stimuli through inhibitory protection. On the basis of animal experimentation this control of interference appears to be a function of the ventral and medial frontal lobes.

Two symmetrical functions are very important as subordinate functions of the temporal structuring of behavior. The first can be termed prospective and includes anticipation, preparation, foresight, or set. The frontal cortex, using past experience, enables preparation for anticipated events on the way to achievement of goals. The second function is retrospective; it is called provisional memory by Fuster, who described it as that holding of information until the goal is attained. Provisional memory is not equivalent to the use of short-term memory as a learning function. Both the prospective and retrospective functions have been localized by Fuster to the dorsal-lateral frontal cortex.

The concept of purpose is important in Fuster's view. If behavior is conceptualized as a hierarchical order of temporally structured units of varying duration and complexity, then the hierarchy of units is dependent on the establishment of a purpose or goal. Involvement of the frontal lobes is in direct proportion to establishment of a purpose and to the need for temporal continuity. Finally, the frontal lobes are important in the initiation, intention, motivation, and vigor by which complex behaviors are developed. It is this aspect that has led to the notion of "executive" functions of the frontal lobes. Such activity is not merely motor but, in Fuster's eyes, includes all aspects, such as perception and cognition.

Fuster's ideas are based to a large extent on animal work, but they have obvious carryover to human behavior. His theory is important because it addresses the question of unity and diversity of frontal lobe function, and it stresses the importance of the temporal integration of behavior.

SHALLICE: INFORMATION-PROCESSING MODEL

Shallice, noting that most theories of cognitive psychology present only one selection or general executive component (e.g., Shiffrin and Schneider, 1977), proposed a more detailed model of cognitive function (1978, 1982). His concept is best understood as consisting of four components: (1) cognitive units; (2) schemas; (3) contention scheduling; (4) supervisory attentional system (SAS). The cognitive units are brain functions related to specific anatomical systems, the domain of contemporary neuroanatomy and neuropsychology (e.g., language, visual-spatial). Schemas are behavioral activities above and beyond the cognitive units. They are behaviors that demand integration of multiple cognitive units for their accomplishments. Even though goal-oriented, schemas are usually routine, learned, rehearsed, highly specialized programs for controlling such overlearned skills as making breakfast or driving home from work. Although often complex, they are standard and routine. Schemas may be considered to have hierarchies, so that higher-order schemas might include lower-order schemas and subroutines in an overall behavior.

Contention scheduling is the selection of appropriate schemas for combinations of routine behaviors by triggers activated by sensory perception or the output of other schemas. It is primarily important for relatively rapid, routine selection based on specific rules. Stopping for groceries or at the drycleaner on the trip home from work may demand contention scheduling.

Finally, the purpose of the fourth level, the SAS, is to handle nonroutine goal achievement in a slow but flexible manner. The SAS operates under two circumstances: (1) when contention scheduling fails; (2) when there is no known solution, as when only weakly activated schemas are evoked.

Shallice's theory appears to fit many examples from daily life. For routine tasks, contention scheduling is adequate. Thus a person may drive home and not truly be aware of his behavior. The SAS can rest or deal with other information, and contention schemas correctly handle the routine behaviors. "Capture errors" may occur (Norman, 1981). A strong trigger might activate contention scheduling and lead to an incorrect response. The SAS, not monitoring the routine behavior, would be unaware until later. Thus while driving to a specific destination and passing the regular turnoff to work, the strong trigger of the sign for the turnoff might elicit inappropriate behavior. Behaviorally, this is described as being preoccupied or distracted.

Shallice's theory can also predict abnormal behavior based on brain lesions. He postulated that the SAS is a frontal function. Following frontal damage, contention scheduling remains effective, and routine overlearned tasks are performed efficiently. However, planning, handling novel situations, and making changes for new situations become impaired. Two possible responses occur with frontal lobe damage. Perseveration of behavior occurs because strong environmental triggers continue to elicit a dominant action schema and the patient cannot shift behaviors. On the other hand, when triggers are weak or absent, any new input captures the contention scheduling procedures and the patient is distractible and responds randomly.

Shallice's theory is firmly entrenched in cognitive psychology and information-processing theories. As such, it is more readily verified through current psychological assessment.

LURIA: CLINICAL/ANATOMICAL/ NEUROPSYCHOLOGICAL THEORY

It is in the theory proposed by Luria that the frontal lobes take on the greatest prominence, reflecting both his conceptualization of the organization of the human brain and the importance that he placed on the planning and design formulation characteristics of human behavior.

Luria (1973a) postulated three principal functional units of the brain. The first unit regulates wakefulness and mental tone; the second receives, analyzes, and stores information; and the third programs, regulates, and verifies mental activity. Each unit is hierarchical with at least three cortical levels organized into its system. The first cortical level handles reception (or transmission) of information to and from the periphery. The second zone processes and prepares programs. The third carries out the most complex forms of mental activity for the particular unit.

These three distinct functional units have different neuroanatomical representation. Unit 1 provides optimal levels of cortical tone, without which both physical and mental activity becomes slowed and/or inadequate (psychomotor retardation, hypomania). The neuroanatomical basis is in the subcortex, particularly the reticular activating system. The reticular activating system of the brainstem receives its most general influences from the orbital and medial frontal cortex through the thalamic nuclei and brainstem. Thus *the higher levels of the cortex, participating directly in the formation of intentions and plans, recruit the lower systems of the reticular formation of the thalamus and brainstem*, thereby modulating their work and making possible the most complex forms of conscious activity" (Luria, 1973a, p. 60). This most basic unit of Luria's hierarchy, important for regulation of tone, is influenced to the greatest extent by the frontal cortex.

Unit 2 is located in the posterior portion of the brain and consists of the visual, auditory, and parietal cortical regions and their connections. It is hierarchically organized, with primary zones, secondary association cortices, and tertiary overlapping zones for complex and gnostic activities.

Finally, unit 3 is located in the frontal lobes, anterior to the precentral gyrus. This unit acts primarily as an efferent motor function in contrast to the afferent, sensory action of the second.

Although all three units work in concert, the frontal lobe appears to be the directive controlling force. The higher mental processes of planning and regulating are formed and take place through language. The frontal lobes do not just create programs; they also evaluate them via feedback. By interconnecting with virtually all parts of the cerebral cortex, the reticular activating system, the brainstem, and the limbic system, *"the tertiary portions of the frontal lobes are in fact a super-structure above all other parts of the cerebral cortex, so that they perform a far more universal function of general regulation of behaviour* than that performed by the posterior associative unit, or, in other words, the tertiary areas of the second functional unit" (Luria, 1973a, p. 89). With this statement, Luria placed the prefrontal cortex at the pinnacle of brain function.

Luria's theory resembles a number of subsequent attempts by investigators to formalize practical, workable models of mental functions. Most of these models are based on logical analysis of behavior, not anatomical function. Lhermitte et al. (1972) postulated four steps in any complex behavior: (1) analysis of information; (2) establishment of plans or programs; (3) execution of the programs, including successive initiation and selection of steps and ongoing monitoring and control; (4) comparison of the final results to the initial goal. Walsh (1978), Lezak (1982, 1976/1983), and others have postulated similar theories; indeed, these four steps were presented by Polya (1945) and described by Miller et al. (1960) as important general theoretical steps.

Luria's theory is considerably more specific in anatomical functional correlations. A critical point in Luria's theory is the emphasis on the importance of the frontal lobes through its integrative hierarchical role with other units of the brain. His descriptions of frontal function, however, although clinically accurate, remain general. Although emphasizing the importance of the frontal lobes in many brain functions, Luria does not emphasize correlation of these activites with localized frontal functions.

SUMMARY

The advancement of scientific knowledge of brain–behavior relationships builds on astute clinical observation, innovative and meticulous research with different methodologies, and creative conceptualization of the meaning of the first two. This chapter has summarized recent theories of frontal lobe functioning. These are the cornerstone of the theory proposed by the authors in the final chapter.

17

A Behavioral Anatomical Theory

Based on the combination of clinical/anatomical observations and neuropsychological tests reported in this volume, the authors propose a theoretical explanation of the influence of the frontal lobe on mental activity. Although this theory most strongly reflects behavioral aspects, it is formulated with an understanding and appreciation of the early theories of frontal lobe function as outlined in Chapter 1 and the more recent postulations summarized in Chapter 16. With little exception, the previous postulations have been found to be correct yet limited, each emphasizing one or more aspects of frontal lobe functioning but falling short of a complete explanation. A more comprehensive view of the role of the frontal lobes seems possible.

In this chapter we present our understanding of frontal lobe functioning, a conceptualization clearly rooted in the validity of previous theories but utilizing the experience and knowledge gained in preparing this review. We formulate a more comprehensive view of frontal functioning but recognize that this presentation is also premature and incomplete. The frontal lobes retain many mysteries.

Before our theory of the effect of prefrontal cortex on brain activity can be considered, two major facets of general brain function, pertinent to all theories, must be presented and discussed. These are a review of general brain functioning and a profile of the major psychological systems of the brain. Both facets must be firmly established in order to appreciate the effects of the frontal lobes.

GENERAL THEORETICAL BASIS OF BRAIN FUNCTION

The position of the frontal lobes in brain activity was clearly outlined during the last century and has been modified and sharpened in subsequent years (Bianchi, 1895; Fulton, 1952). The original proposals emphasized that the posterior portions of the cerebral hemispheres specialized in sensory reception and analysis of sensory data, whereas the anterior parts of the brain, specifically the frontal lobes, carried out the motor, executive activities (Meynert, 1884). Although elementary, this basic posterior/anterior division of duties offered a solid basis for the analysis of brain functioning. It was generally accepted that the frontal lobes acted as a gathering point for accumulated sensory data, using this information to initiate the final common pathway for motor response. It was also assumed that the sensory data underwent further analysis and interpretation in the frontal lobes prior to activating the final common pathway. The exact activities that made up this process remained conjectural.

The theories of frontal lobe function offered during the past several decades represent a considerable advance over this early view, particularly in proposing specific roles for the prefrontal cortex in overall mental function. Although often couched in the selective jargon of a particular approach (e.g., information theory, neuroanatomical connections), these theories, individually and together, offer reasonable conjectures concerning prefrontal function. In their own approaches, each theory emphasizes the regulatory, monitoring activity and the ability to anticipate and control behavior that are routinely suggested for the frontal lobes. Certain of the important advances are selectively highlighted below as examples of how the basis for expansion was formed.

Teuber (1964), by boldly emphasizing the importance of the action of the anterior brain on the posterior brain, set the stage for interpretation of the coordinated functioning of the entire brain from the viewpoint of anticipation, action, and decision. An active, organizing, monitoring, and testing function for the frontal lobes was proposed by Pribram and colleagues (Miller et al., 1960; Pribram, 1967, 1973), and a possible neuroanatomical basis for the seemingly pervasive role of the frontal lobes was suggested by Nauta (1971, 1973) and refined by others (e.g., Damasio, 1979; Goldman-Rakic, 1984b). The neuroanatomical presentations utilized a more global picture of how frontal lobe connections influenced observed function.

Logical analysis of behavioral changes after frontal lobe damage has led to subdivisions of the specific characteristics of complex behavior (e.g., Lezak, 1976/ 1983; Lhermitte et al., 1972; Milner, 1964; Milner and Petrides, 1984; Walsh, 1978) or attempts to explain how a complex goal is achieved (Fuster, 1980). The most complete theory of frontal function appears to be that of Luria (1966/1980, 1970a, 1973a). First, the role of the frontal lobes is seen against the background of all brain function, including mental tone and the reception, analysis, and storage of information. These two major functional aspects of brain activity are intimately connected with the third unit, one that programs mental activities. The prefrontal cortex is acknowledged as the key for this third function, and specific prefrontal activities—planning, monitoring, regulating, and changing—are described.

Purely psychological theories such as the hierarchy of mental activities proposed by Shallice (1982) gain meaning in light of this functional/anatomical background. Shallice's cognitive units and schemas would represent the routine handling of sensory information, and his contention scheduling would represent the routine, overlearned responses to complex sensory stimuli. His final system, the supervisory attentional system, would represent an active overview of brain activities including the response to and modulation of novel stimuli, a prefrontal function. Taken together, the correlation of psychological theories with the neuroanatomically based formulations leads toward a rational theory of overall brain function and highlights the role of the frontal lobes.

ORGANIZED INTEGRATED FIXED FUNCTIONAL SYSTEMS

In addition to the concepts of how the brain functions, described above, consideration of how the brain is organized is needed to understand the role of the frontal lobes in brain–behavior relations. Most investigations of frontal lobe functioning (including that presented in this volume) concentrate on the effects the frontal lobes play on a number of functional systems as they carry out complex mental activities.

It was postulated in Chapter 15 that the brain could be considered to have a number of *organized integrated fixed functional systems.* These functional systems include a number of recognized neural activities, such as sensory and motor functions, emotion, language, memory, visual-spatial ability, attention, and even general cognitive abilities. The functional systems can be graphically presented in relation to overall behavior (Fig. 17-1). Whether this list is sufficient and whether there is a hierarchy within these systems remain uncertain. Future clarification should alter and improve this list. Moreover, although each system is usually described as independent, the brain acts as an integrated unit; many interlocked activities make up these functional systems, and separation of the systems is automatically artificial. Nevertheless, a great deal of clinical and laboratory research in both neuropsychology and neurobehavior has demonstrated abnormalities within the individual systems following brain damage and represents a valid approach to brain investigation. For instance, research applied to individual systems has led to considerable understanding of the brain's role in complex functions such as language and memory.

In many respects, the concept of functional systems outlined in Fig. 17-1 represents the first two functional units suggested by Luria. It is emphasized, however, that different functional systems exist within these two units and can be defined and studied behaviorally and neuroanatomically. The functional systems are viewed as "posterior," at least in relation to the prefrontal brain, which plays a supervisory, executive role. Each functional system has direct and reciprocal connections with frontal cortex. The basic activities of a functional system may not be disturbed by frontal lobe damage, but control of the function may be altered. Indeed, the major demonstration presented in many sections of this volume is that *frontal lobe pathology causes only indirect disturbances to many functional systems.* As a corollary, frontal lobe function cannot be adequately assessed by study of language,

POSTERIOR/BASAL FUNCTIONAL SYSTEMS

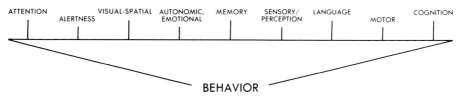

FIG. 17-1. Various organized integrated fixed functional systems hypothesized to be based, in relation to the frontal lobes, in more posterior/basal brain regions.

memory, or other functional system alone. The functional systems, however, because of the considerable accumulation of knowledge concerning their activities, provide the basis for most behavioral studies including the effects of frontal abnormality. It must be recognized that this is indirect, not direct, evidence. Interpretation of frontal function based on abnormalities in the fixed systems remains limited and unsatisfactory. Nevertheless, the individual functional systems remain the basic structures for study of brain function. Their position in the entire picture must be acknowledged.

A BEHAVIORAL/ANATOMICAL APPROACH

Against this background, the authors' theory of frontal lobe functions can be presented. Three separate divisions of frontal lobe functions are proposed; conceptually they are hierarchical and progressively more abstract. Behavioral attributes whose functions overlap but that are conceptually separable are presented. Although not truly syndromes, they can be grouped in this manner, as has been done by Eslinger and Damasio (1985). We prefer to use broader, less clinical terms, such as unit, system, function, or division for the separate frontal lobe functions, as clinical, neuropsychological, and neuroanatomical data are used to define them.

Frontal (Anterior) Functional Systems

In parallel with the posterior functional systems, at least two anterior counterparts can be proposed. These can be designated: (1) sequence, set, and integration; (2) drive, motivation, and will. These systems appear to be anatomically distinct in that their major neuroanatomical base lies in the more caudal regions of frontal lobes. Each of the frontal functional systems is intimately linked with other functional systems. Damage in distant areas can affect the results of any observations or tests used to monitor and identify these systems. Nonetheless, rather pure examples of their disturbance can be seen in the presence of intact posterior functional systems, and when this is observed frontal damage is present. Sequence, set, and integration appear to be most strongly dependent on intact lateral (dorsal and orbital) frontal convexity regions. Drive and motivation appear to be dependent on medial frontal structures. Although having the characteristics of the functional systems described in Chapter 15, these two systems appear to be superordinate in their relationship to the others. Figure 17-2 illustrates this relationship and suggests an increasing complexity to brain functions.

Sequence, Set, and Integration

Starting with the dramatic early clinical descriptions, considerable evidence has been presented that the ability to maintain and organize bits of information in meaningful sequences is dependent, to a considerable extent, on intactness of the frontal lobes. Albert (1972) stressed the importance of frontal sequencing to language functions. Milner and Petrides (Milner, 1982; Petrides and Milner, 1982)

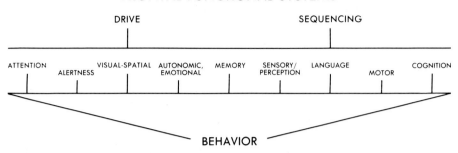

FIG. 17-2. Sequencing and drive, two functions closely allied with the frontal lobes, appear to have a superordinate role in relation to the posterior/basal functional systems.

noted that focal damage to the frontal convexity interfered with the maintenance of the order of one's responses. Fuster (1980) emphasized sequencing ability in his theory of frontal function, stressing temporal integration of behavior as an important function of the dorsal-lateral convexity of the frontal lobe. He suggested that the temporal structuring of behavior could be subdivided into three subordinate functions—anticipation, provisional memory, and control of interference—each important for maintaining a sequence.

Two other functions are closely allied with sequencing and are hypothesized to be strongly dependent on this ability. Both reflect a greater degree of executive control and, as such, reflect additional prefrontal activity. The human brain not only handles multiple bits of information in sequence but can extract crucial elements from such a series. This allows identification of the relevant information and correlation with or progression to another series of information bits. The ability to extract the key data from multiple bits of information and to form this material into sets of related information is a uniquely human attribute, an essential factor in all higher human mental functioning. Set formation allows the production of new, more complex information from available sequences of data.

Beyond the formation of sets lies a related but more complicated mental function, the ability to extract chosen bits from a number of related or unrelated sets of information and to integrate these data into novel knowledge (information) or into an understanding of a complex situation. Although dependent on many nonfrontal activities, particularly the availability of the memory stores that make up the individual's fund of knowledge, the integration of information from diverse sources, both old and novel, into new information appears to be dependent on intact frontal cortex. The ability to integrate data ranks high among the important mental advances of the human.

In summary, one group of significant behavioral control functions that appear to be dependent on the prefrontal cortex concerns the ability to organize and maintain related information in fixed sequence, the establishment of related sets of this information, and the integration of these data with other information to form novel or meaningful interpretations. Prefrontal damage, by limiting one or more of these functions, produces a shallow mentation.

Drive, Motivation, and Will

Another consistently described behavioral finding in frontal lobe damaged humans is a functional alteration best described as a change in drive. The most common alteration is apathy, a decrease in activity. The apathetic patient is unable (or slow) to initiate movements that can be carried out readily after some prompting initiates the activity. The opposite alteration, excessive drive, apparently based on decreased ability to inhibit actions, also appears to reflect frontal abnormality. The two major personality types described in Chapter 8—pseudoretarded and pseudo-psychopathic—feature altered drive states emanating from frontal dysfunction. A growing body of evidence links the medial sagittal frontal structures, particularly the cingulate gyrus and the supplementary motor area, with the initiation of both motor and mental activities. Damage in this area almost routinely decreases the initiation of activity. Conversely, a fair amount of evidence suggests that orbital frontal abnormality can produce a decrease in the ability to inhibit drive, a tendency to act without adequate mental control. The ubiquity of abnormal drive in frontal lobe damaged patients and the fact that the abnormality covers a spectrum of behaviors suggest that drive is best considered a separate frontal lobe function with an obvious effect on the functioning of the posterior systems.

Two other factors, motivation and will, are closely allied with drive and are often found to be impaired after frontal lobe damage. Whether they deserve separate consideration is uncertain. Motivation is closely associated with drive, but, to most, the term reflects a greater degree of intellectual control. Where drive represents a basic energizing force, motivation suggests some mental (intellectual) control of this force. Will is rarely discussed in neurological or neuropsychological parlance, but only slight introspection indicates that a close linkage between human will and the factors of drive and motivation is entirely reasonable. Will is a term used almost exclusively in philosophy/theology/psychiatry at present and, as such, is given metaphysical connotations. Nevertheless, human will represents a brain activity, one that can be altered by focal damage, and appears to be strongly linked to the functions of drive and motivation (Feuchtwanger, 1923). Human will appears to be a frontal function and, inasmuch as it is based on drive, seems to be dependent on medial frontal structures. The connotation of mental control, however, suggests the effects of other frontal regions also.

In summary, two units of mental activity that bear a resemblance to the better-established posterior functional systems have been described. One, the ability to handle information in sequences and to combine bits of this information with other material, appears to be a lateral frontal convexity function. The second, drive and its related functions, appears more dependent on medial frontal structures. Both of these frontal functional systems appear to interact, but as superordinates, with the posterior functional systems.

EXECUTIVE FUNCTION

A second, apparently independent, level of frontal lobe functioning can now be postulated. The executive function represents many of the important activities that are almost universally attributed to the frontal lobes which become active in nonroutine, novel situations that require new solutions. These behavioral characteristics have been described by many authors and include at least the following: anticipation, goal selection, preplanning (means–end establishment), monitoring, and use of feedback (if–then statements). Each of these represents a separate and experimentally testable frontal lobe function. Figure 17-3 illustrates the relationship of executive functions to the previously described functional systems.

The executive functions of the frontal lobe as presented here are analogous to most of the theoretical concepts of control presented earlier. First, the frontal lobe primarily carries out nonroutine control. Second, this control can be defined and studied only by means of the divisions of executive function as outlined above.

Most early theories of brain functioning focused on the activities of the posterior functional systems. Although this approach was of value, a control process capable of providing conscious direction to the activity of the functional systems was obviously necessary to explain the human ability to process information. The concept of control provides an explanation of how the basic operations of a system are to be used, and in what order, to achieve a specified goal within the given limitations of time and space (Newell, 1977).

The prefrontal cortex is the anatomical basis for the function of control. This statement is based on the information presented in the previous chapters and appears in all theories discussing the control of mental functioning and consciousness. The frontal lobes are imperative at the time a new activity is being learned and active control is required; after the activity has become routine, however, these activities can be handled by other brain areas, and frontal participation is no longer demanded

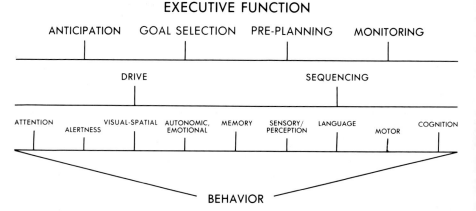

FIG. 17-3. Executive control functions, called into action in nonroutine or novel situations, provide conscious direction to the functional systems for efficient processing of information.

(Damasio, 1979; Shallice, 1982). This concept has been dramatically supported by positron emission tomography (PET) studies demonstrating that overlearned motor acts such as writing the signature require only subcortical activity, whereas a newly acquired act of a similar nature demands frontal participation (Mazziotta, 1985).

Historically, consciousness, control, and mental functioning have been perceived in three ways (Carr, 1979). The first is a mental blackboard, or primary memory, referring to readily available information kept in one's mind for immediate use. The second is an internal programmer or executive decision-maker, reflected in models that focus on goal establishment and attainment. Finally, the third postulated means of interpreting consciousness or control reflects attention as the selectivity of relevant information. The latter two concepts, executive controller or information selector, are closely related (Carr, 1979; Carr and Bacharach, 1976). All three approaches have been linked with frontal lobe functioning.

The view of the frontal lobe as a *deus ex machina* control mechanism is inadequate, as it does not state how the control is used (Newell, 1977). Merely to label the frontal lobes as the executive function does not do justice to the activities under consideration. First, there appear to be different types of control, and these appear, at least partly, to be hierarchichal (Carver and Scheier, 1982; Powers, 1973a,b). The lowest level would include functions such as control of the appropriate muscles. In this manner control would refer to the automatic, routine control used by the posterior functional systems. Superordinate control levels, such as those described for the frontal lobes, might be labeled principle control, program control, and sequence control.

A hypothetical example has been given by Carver and Scheier (1982) to illustrate different types of control. A young business woman, writing a report for her superiors, would have a basic principle guiding her report preparation; for example, it should be readable. The preparation, rearrangement, and rewriting would all be organized according to this PRINCIPLE CONTROL. To achieve the goal derived from principle control, PROGRAM CONTROL would be necessary; a series of "if–then" decisions would be established to evaluate if change is needed, to determine how it should be done, and eventually to carry it out. To make such changes effectively, however, the actions must be performed in proper order. The establishment and monitoring of order can be called SEQUENCE CONTROL. These types of control, derived from information-processing theories, parallel the frontal executive functions described above.

Clinical examples can be given to support these concepts of executive control. For example, control of visceral phenomena, including such activities as anticipation, initiation, execution, and inhibition of autonomic nervous system activity, can be noted. Most such activities are overlearned and governed at a subcortical level; frontal involvement is not needed. Visceral acts can be novel, however, demanding frontal participation in their organization. A well-known example is pavlovian conditioning, the autonomic response to a conditioning signal that depends on higher level control until sufficiently overlearned. The various stress control techniques, including biofeedback, offer current examples of cognitive control of visceral functions. Clinical evidence suggests that frontal damage disturbs the acquisition of new visceral activities and can disturb the control of already learned visceral activities. Thus although usually unconsciously formed, a frontal control function for visceral activities seems probable.

The control functions of the prefrontal cortex became more and more obvious in the chapters of this volume. Although clearly a factor in the chapters that described frontal influence on such posterior functional systems as sensory/perception and motor functions, frontal control became paramount in the chapters discussing language, memory, and cognition, reflecting the greater complexity of the functions.

The ability to take the information extracted from other, higher brain systems, verbal and nonverbal, and to anticipate, select goals, experiment, modify, and otherwise act on this information to produce novel responses represents the ultimate mental activity; all available data indicate that these executive functions are prefrontal activities. The frontal lobes perform the supervisory, attentional tasks suggested by Shallice, the planning and design formulation proposed by Luria, the establishment of goals postulated by Damasio, and the executive function of Fuster, Lhermitte, Milner, and others.

SELF-AWARENESS AND SELF-CONSCIOUSNESS

Yet another pinnacle of mental functioning is the attribute called self-awareness or self-consciousness, a recognized human quality that has been seriously discussed and debated for centuries. Consciousness (or, better, self-consciousness or self-reflectiveness), that attribute of the human which not only allows awareness of the self but also realizes the position of this self within the social milieu, has long been a topic of philosophy, theology, and psychology. Only recently have neuroscientists and information-processing theorists become interested. Magoun and Moruzzi (Magoun, 1963; Moruzzi and Magoun, 1949) established a neural basis for awakeness; in so doing they clearly demonstrated that this represents only a portion of the conscious state. The brainstem reticular system was demonstrated to be crucial for overall awakeness. Although consciousness (awakeness) represents a necessary condition for self-consciousness, multiple observations clearly demonstrated that the mesencephalic reticular substance was not responsible for this attribute. Many investigators had delved into the question of human consciousness; Freud (1933) established the presence of an unconscious state but made no attempt to locate the function within the brain. More recent cognitive theorists discuss another form of self-consciousness, the "knowing about knowing," using terms such as metacognition, metamemory, and metatheory. This introspection is thought to be the basis of intelligent behavior, as it implies organized and deliberate acquisition and use of knowledge, as well as the maintenance and generalization of facts and strategies (Brown, 1978; Cavanaugh and Borkowski, 1980). The characteristics stressed by the metapsychologists closely resemble those attributed to prefrontal functions.

Some tentative suggestions have been made concerning the neural basis of self-consciousness. Jaynes (1976) postulated that consciousness is a relatively recent human acquisition that developed when the mental functions of the two cerebral hemispheres became separate; most specifically, he linked the origin of self-consciousness with the left hemisphere becoming dominant for language. Human consciousness, in this view, would be a function of the left hemisphere. Others, however, particularly Sperry (1985), did not agree, believing the right hemisphere to be fully conscious of its own deeds and thoughts but unable to express this competency in language. Popper and Eccles (1977) and Eccles (1979) have discussed and described the conscious self, proclaiming it the highest of mental activities. Although they listed a number of probably important neuroanatomical areas, including the prefrontal cortex, they refrained from localizing consciousness.

Tulving (1985) reported three kinds or systems of memory, each characterized by a specific type of consciousness. The third, episodic memory or memory for events, is characterized by self-knowing. Tulving described a patient who, following closed head injury, had relatively intact language skills, general knowledge, and sense of objective time but whose subjective time was severely disturbed, resulting in a loss of conscious awareness and greatly impaired past and future contemplation. Tulving, based on Ingvar's (1979) blood flow work and theory of the frontal lobe as the basis of memory of the future, suggested a relationship of autonoetic (self-knowing) consciousness to the frontal lobes.

A strong argument can be made for self-consciousness as a function of the prefrontal area of the human brain. One striking finding in some (but not all) frontally damaged patients is an apparent decrease in normal self-awareness. Variously described as shallowness of interest, loss of self-concern, impairment of self-monitoring, and so on, this alteration suggests prefrontal dysfunction to the experienced clinician. A fair amount of evidence links self-awareness to the executive control functions just discussed. Self-awareness is necessary for controlling, via a feedback loop, the perceived discrepancy between a present state and a mental comparison (Carver and Scheier, 1982). Without this ability, there would be decreased self-regulation, a frequently observed phenomenon after frontal lobe damage. Self-awareness is easily retranslated as "awareness of self," a key attribute of the "self" discussed by Popper and Eccles (1977). It can be suggested that many additional mental functions are included in self and self-consciousness, but self-awareness is a key factor. A strong link between the disturbed self-awareness of the frontal lobe damaged patient and the conscious awareness of self discussed by many investigators appears plausible. Figure 17-4 illustrates our conception of the hierarchical divisions of frontal functions, superimposed on each other and on the posterior functional systems. Self-awareness and executive functions, although routinely interfunctional, appear to be separable and are so indicated in the diagram. It seems appropriate that one of the newest areas of the brain phylogenetically, the prefrontal lobes, would be crucial for the highest and most clearly human of mental activities.

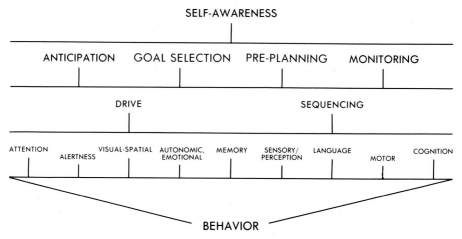

FIG. 17-4. Self-awareness, or self-consciousness, is hypothesized to be the highest attribute of the frontal lobes.

SUMMARY

The arbitrary division of frontal lobe function into different hierarchical functions presented here can only be interpreted as part of an integrated model of brain functioning. The different functions of the brain do not work in isolation. When a new mental activity or preference is formed, it represents an amalgam of many nervous system attributes, actively derived from a process of trial against many relevant systems. The integration of autonomic and somatic nervous system elements, the correlation of visceral and emotional facets with verbal and nonverbal somatic information, provides an advanced level of mental control. Before establishment of a new "final-common-pathway," the pros and cons of the activity have been "discussed," "argued," and "tested" by the integrative capability of the prefrontal cortex. Even following establishment of a new response pattern, the effects are monitored by prefrontal lobes, and, if potentially adverse results can be anticipated, are discontinued or modified.

The control activity of the prefrontal lobes is superimposed on other, equally essential brain activities, as suggested in Fig. 17-4. Each of the three levels of frontal lobe functioning is exhibited most clearly by its influence on the functioning of the posterior systems; each must be interpreted in light of total brain functioning.

The human prefrontal cortex attends, integrates, formulates, executes, monitors, modifies, and judges all nervous system activities. Most individual mental functions, those carried out by the posterior systems, can be maintained without prefrontal participation, but the responses are automatic and the qualities that make a well-rounded human are clearly deficient. In this mechanical functioning, the posterior functional systems and even some parts of the frontal functional systems, resemble the activities postulated for advanced generations of computers by the more ardent advocates of artificial intelligence (Hofstadter and Dennette, 1982). The mental abilities attributed to the higher levels of prefrontal activity, however, are clearly beyond current computer potentials.

Although not the seat of "intelligence" demonstrated by formal IQ tests, the prefrontal lobes are essential for the highest of mental activities, those demanding control of intelligence. Moreover, in the role of "I," the consciousness of self, the prefrontal structures bridge the gap between the complex, multi-integrated response mechanisms that make up the brain and the free-willed, independently thinking entity called the mind. The mind–brain dichotomy is more clearly expressed and loses sharp differentiation with study of prefrontal functioning. Investigation of these functions are difficult and easily lead to erroneous simplifications. Nevertheless, it is through understanding the influence of prefrontal brain structures on mental activity that the true essence of humanness will be approached. The frontal lobes are the key to the highest human functions.

Appendix: Northampton VA Leukotomy Study Publications

1. Benson, D. F., and Stuss, D. T. (1982): Motor abilities after frontal leukotomy. *Neurology (NY)*, 32:1353–1357.
2. Benson, D. F., Stuss, D. T., Naeser, M. A., Weir, W. S., Kaplan, E. F., and Levine, H. (1981): The long-term effects of prefrontal leukotomy. *Arch. Neurol.*, 38:165–169.
3. Naeser, M. A., Levine, H. L., Benson, D. F., Stuss, D. T., and Weir, W. S. (1981): Frontal leukotomy size and hemispheric asymmetries on computerized tomographic scans of schizophrenics with variable recovery. *Arch. Neurol.*, 38:30–37.
4. Stuss, D. T., and Benson, D. F. (1983): Emotional concomitants of psychosurgery. In: *Neuropsychology of Human Emotion*, edited by K. M. Heilman and P. Satz, pp. 111–140. Guilford Press, New York.
5. Stuss, D. T., and Benson, D. F. (1983): Frontal lobe lesions and behavior. In: *Localization in Neuropsychology*, edited by A. Kertesz, pp. 429–454. Academic Press, New York.
6. Stuss, D. T., and Benson, D. F. (1984): Neuropsychological studies of the frontal lobes. *Psychol. Bull.*, 95:3–28.
7. Stuss, D. T., Benson, D. F., Clermont, R., Della Malva, C. L., Kaplan, E. F., and Weir, W. S. (1986): Language functioning after bilateral prefrontal leucotomy. *Brain Lang.*, 28, 66–70.
8. Stuss, D. T., Benson, D. F., Kaplan, E. F., Della Malva, C. L., and Weir, W. S. (1984): The effects of prefrontal leucotomy on visuoperceptive and visuoconstructive tests. *Bull. Clin. Neurosci.*, 49: 43–51.
9. Stuss, D. T., Benson, D. F., Kaplan, E. F., Weir, W. S., and Della Malva, C. (1981): Leucotomized and nonleucotomized schizophrenics: Comparison on tests of attention. *Biol. Psychiatry*, 16:1085–1100.
10. Stuss, D. T., Benson, D. F., Kaplan, E. F., Weir, W. S., Naeser, M. A., Lieberman, I., and Ferrill, D. (1983): The involvement of orbitofrontal cerebrum in cognitive tasks. *Neuropsychologia*, 21:235–248.
11. Stuss, D. T., Kaplan, E. F., and Benson, D. F. (1982): Long-term effects of prefrontal leucotomy: Cognitive functions. In: *Neuropsychology and Cognition*, Vol. II, edited by R. N. Malatesha and L. C. Hartlage, pp. 252–271. Martinus Nijhoff, The Hague.
12. Stuss, D. T., Kaplan, E. F., Benson, D. F., Weir, W. S., Chiulli, S., and Sarazin, F. F. (1982): Evidence for the involvement of orbitofrontal cortex in memory functions: An interference effect. *J. Comp. Physiol. Psychol.*, 16:913–925.
13. Stuss, D. T., Kaplan, E. F., Benson, D. F., Weir, W. S., Naeser, M. A., and Levine, H. L. (1981): Long-term effects of prefrontal leucotomy: An overview of neuropsychologic residuals. *J. Clin. Neuropsychol.*, 3:13–32.

References

Ackerly, S. (1935): Instinctive, emotional and mental changes following prefrontal lobe extirpation. *Am. J. Psychiatry*, 92:717–729.

Ackerly, S. S. (1964): A case of paranatal bilateral frontal lobe defect observed for thirty years. In: *The Frontal Granular Cortex and Behavior*, edited by J. M. Warren and K. Akert, pp. 192–215. McGraw-Hill, New York.

Ackerly, S. S., and Benton, A. L. (1947): Report of a case of bilateral frontal lobe defect. *Res. Publ. Assoc. Res. Nerv. Ment. Dis.*, 27:479–504.

Adams, K. M. (1980a): In search of Luria's battery: A false start. *J. Consult. Clin. Psychol.*, 48:511–516.

Adams, K. M. (1980b): An end of innocence for behavioral neurology? Adams replies. *J. Consult. Clin. Psychol.*, 48:522–524.

Adams, R. D., and Victor, M. (1977/1981): *Principles of Neurology*, 2nd Ed. McGraw-Hill, New York.

Aimard, G., Devic, M., Lebel, M., Trouillas, P., and Boisson, D. (1975): Agraphi pure (dynamique?) d'origine frontale: A propos d'une observation. *Rev. Neurol. (Paris)*, 131:505–512.

Akert, K. (1964): Comparative anatomy of frontal cortex and thalamofrontal connections. In: *The Frontal Granular Cortex and Behavior*, edited by J. M. Warren and K. Akert, pp. 373–444. McGraw-Hill, New York.

Alajouanine, Th., Lhermitte, F., Cambier, J., Rondot, P., and Lefebvre, J. P. (1959): Perturbations dissociées de la motricité facio-bucco-pharyngée avec aphémie dans un ramollissement sylvien profond partiel. *Rev. Neurol. (Paris)*, 100:493–498.

Albert, M. L. (1972): Auditory sequencing and left cerebral dominance for language. *Neuropsychologia*, 10:245–248.

Albert, M. L. (1973): A simple test of visual neglect. *Neurology (NY)*, 23:658–664.

Albert, M. L., Feldman, R. G., and Willis, A. L. (1974): The 'subcortical dementia' of progressive supranuclear palsy. *J. Neurol. Neurosurg. Psychiatry*, 37:121–130.

Albert, M. L., Goodglass, H., Helm, N. A., Rubens, A. B., and Alexander, M. P. (1981): *Clinical Aspects of Dysphasia*. Springer-Verlag, New York.

Albert, M. L., and Hécaen, H. (1971): Relative movement perception following unilateral cerebral damage. *Trans. Am. Neurol. Assoc.*, 96:200–202.

Albert, M. S., and Kaplan, E. F. (1980): Organic implications of neuropsychological deficits in the elderly. In: *New Directions in Memory and Aging*, Proceedings of the George A. Talland Memorial Conference, edited by L. W. Poon, J. Fozard, L. Cermak, D. Arenberg, and L. W. Thompson, pp. 403–432. Lawrence Erlbaum, Hillsdale, New Jersey.

Alexander, G. E. (1982): Functional development of frontal association cortex in monkeys: Behavioral and electrophysiological studies. *Neurosci. Res. Program Bull.*, 20:471–479.

Alexander, M. P. (1982): Traumatic brain injury. In: *Psychiatric Aspects of Neurologic Disease* Vol. II, edited by D. F. Benson and D. Blumer, pp. 219–249. Grune & Stratton, New York.

Alexander, M. P. (1984): Frontal language disorders. Presented to the Neurobehavioral Seminar, UCLA School of Medicine.

Alexander, M. P., and Freedman, M. (1984): Amnesia after anterior communicating artery aneurysm rupture. *Neurology (NY)*, 34:752–757.

Alexander, M. P., and LoVerme, S. R., Jr. (1980): Aphasia after left hemispheric intracerebral hemorrhage. *Neurology (NY)*, 30:1193–1202.

Alexander, M. P., and Schmitt, M. A. (1980): The aphasia syndrome of stroke in the left anterior cerebral artery territory. *Arch. Neurol.*, 37:97–100.

Alexander, M. P., Stuss, D. T., and Benson, D. F. (1979): Capgras syndrome: A reduplicative phenomenon. *Neurology (NY)*, 29:334–339.

Allen, J. H., and Meacham, W. F. (1966): Colloidal barium sulfate as radiologic marker in surgical treatment of cavitary brain lesions. *Radiology*, 87:683–687.

Altemus, L. R., Roberson, G. H., Fisher, C. M., and Pessin, M. (1976): Embolic occlusion of the superior and inferior divisions of the middle cerebral artery with angiographic-clinical correlation. *AJR*, 126:576–581.

American Psychiatric Association (1952): *Diagnostic and Statistical Manual of Mental Disorders (DSM-1)*. American Psychiatric Association Press, Washington, D.C.

Angelergues, R., Hécaen, H., and de Ajuriaguerra, J. (1955): Les troubles mentaux au cours des tumeurs du lobe frontal; à propos de 80 observations dont 54 avec troubles mentaux. *Ann. Med. Psychol. (Paris)*, 113:577–642.

Anton, G. (1899): Ueber die Selbstwahrnehmungen der Herderkrankungen des Gehirns durch den Kranken bei Rindenblindheit und Rindentaubheit. *Arch. Psychiatr. Nervenkr.*, 32:86–127.

A Psychiatric Glossary, 5th Ed. (1980). American Psychiatric Association, Washington, D.C.

Arnot, R. (1952): A theory of frontal lobe function. *Arch. Neurol. Psychiatry*, 67:487–495.

Arnsten, A. F. T., and Goldman-Rakic, P. S. (1984): Selective prefrontal cortical projections to the region of the locus coeruleus and raphe nuclei in the rhesus monkey. *Brain Res.*, 306:9–18.

Arrigoni, G., and De Renzi, E. (1964): Constructional apraxia and hemispheric locus of lesion. *Cortex*, 1:170–197.

Arseni, C., and Botez, M. I. (1961): Speech disturbances caused by tumours of the supplementary motor area. *Acta Psychiatr. Scand.*, 36:279–99.

Asarnow, R. F., Steffy, R. A., MacCrimmon, D. J., and Cleghorn, J. M. (1978): An attentional assessment of foster children at risk for schizophrenia. In: *The Nature of Schizophrenia*, edited by L. C. Wynne, R. L. Cromwell, and S. Matthysee, pp. 339–358. Wiley, New York.

Astruc, J. (1971): Corticofugal connections of area 8 (frontal eye field) in Macaca mulatta. *Brain Res.*, 33:241–256.

Atack, E. A., and Suranyi, L. (1975): Respiratory inhibitory apraxia. *Can. J. Neurol. Sci.*, 2:37–43.

Auburtin, E. (1863): Considérations sur les localisations cérébrales, et en particulier sur le siège de la faculté du langage articulé. *Gaz. Hebd.*, 318–321, 348–351, 397–402, 455–458.

Ausman, J. I., French, L. A., and Baker, A. B. (1974): Intracranial neoplasms. In: *Clinical Neurology*, edited by A. B. Baker and L. H. Baker, Chap. 14. Harper & Row, Philadelphia.

Babinski, J. (1914): Contribution à l étude des troubles mentaux dans l'hémiplégie organique cérébrale (Anosognosie). *Rev. Neurol. (Paris)*, 27:845–848.

Babinski, J. (1918): Anosognosie. *Rev. Neurol. (Paris)*, 25:365–367.

Bachman, D. L., and Albert, M. L. (1984): The dopaminergic syndromes of dementia. In: *Cerebral Ageing and Degenerative Dementias*, edited by G. Pilleri and F. Tagliavini. *Brain Pathology, Vol. 1*, pp. 91–119. Brain Anatomy Institute, Bern, Switzerland.

Bailey, H. R., Dowling, J. L., and Davies, E. (1977): Cingulotractotomy and related procedures for severe depressive illness (studies in depression: IV). In: *Neurosurgical Treatment in Psychiatry, Pain, and Epilepsy*, edited by W. H. Sweet, S. Obrador, and J. G. Martin-Rodriquez, pp. 229–251. University Park Press, Baltimore.

Bailey, P. (1933): *Intracranial Tumours*. Charles C Thomas, Springfield, Illinois.

Baker, E. F. W., Young, M. P., Gauld, D. M., and Fleming, J. F. R. (1970): A new look at bimedial prefrontal leukotomy. *Can. Med. Assoc. J.*, 102:37–41.

Baker, H. L., Campbell, J. K., Houser, D. W., Reese, P. F., Sheedy, P. F., Holman, C. B., and Kurland, R. L. (1974): Computer-assisted tomography of the head. *Mayo Clin. Proc.*, 49:17–27.

Balint, R. (1909): Die seelenlahmung des "Schauens." *Monatsschr. Psychiatr. Neur.*, 1:25:51–81. Referenced in Hécaen, H., and Albert, M. (1978): *Human Neuropsychology*. Wiley, New York.

Ballantine, H. T., Cassidy, W. L., Flanagan, N. B., and Marino, R. (1967): Stereotaxic anterior cingulotomy for neuropsychiatric illness and intractable pain. *J. Neurosurg.*, 26:488–495.

Bannon, M. J., and Roth, R. H. (1983): Pharmacology of mesocortical dopamine neurons. *Pharmacol. Rev.*, 35:53–68.

Barbas, H., and Mesulam, M-M. (1981): Organization of afferent input to subdivisions of area 8 in the rhesus monkey. *J. Comp. Neurol.*, 200:407–431.

Barbas, H., and Pandya, D. N. (1982): Cytoarchitecture and intrinsic connections of the prefrontal cortex of the rhesus monkey. *Neurosci. Abstr.*, 8:268.3.

Barbas, H., and Pandya, D. N. (1984): Topography of commissural fibers of the prefrontal cortex in the rhesus monkey. *Exp. Brain Res.*, 55:187–191.

Barbizet, J. (1971): Rôle du lobe frontal dans les conduites mnésiques. *Presse Med.*, 79:2033–2037.

Barkley, R. A. (1977): A review of stimulant drug research with hyperactive children. *J. Child Psychol. Psychiatry*, 18:137–165.

Barton, M., Maruszewski, M., and Urrea, D. (1969): Variation of stimulus context and its effect on word-finding ability in aphasics. *Cortex*, 5:351–365.

Bastian, H. C. (1898): *Aphasia and Other Speech Defects*. H. K. Lewis, London.

Battersby, W. S., Bender, M. B., Pollack, M., and Kahn, R. L. (1956): Unilateral spatial agnosia (inattention) in patients with cerebral lesions. *Brain*, 79:68–93.

Batuyev, A. S. (1969): The frontal lobes and the processes of synthesis in the brain. *Brain Behav. Evol.*, 2:202–212.

Bear, D. M. (1983): Hemispheric specialization and the neurology of emotion. *Arch. Neurol.*, 40:195–202.

Bell, D. (1968): Speech functions of the thalamus inferred from the effects of thalamotomy. *Brain*, 91:619–638.

Belyi, B. (1979): The syndrome of aspontaneity in tumors of the frontal lobes. *J. Neuropathol. Psychiatr. (Moscow)*, 7:833–992 [original in Russian].

Bennett, T. L. (1975): The electrical activity of the hippocampus and processes of attention. In: *The Hippocampus, Vol. 2: Neurophysiology and Behavior*, edited by R. L. Isaacson and K. H. Pribram, pp. 71–99. Plenum, New York.

Benson, D. F. (1977): The third alexia. *Arch. Neurol.*, 34:327–331.

Benson, D. F. (1978): Amnesia. *South. Med. J.*, 71:1221–1228.

Benson, D. F. (1979): *Aphasia, Alexia, and Agraphia*. Churchill Livingstone, New York.

Benson, D. F. (1984): New developments in diagnosis—CAT, PET, and NMR. *Psychiatr. Ann.*, 14:192–197.

Benson, D. F. (1984): The neurology of emotion. *Bull. Clin. Neurosci.*, 49:23–42.

Benson, D. F., and Barton, M. I. (1970): Disturbances in constructional ability. *Cortex*, 6:19–46.

Benson, D. F., and Blumer, D. (1982): Amnesia: A clinical approach to memory. In: *Psychiatric Aspects of Neurologic Disease*, Vol. II, edited by D. F. Benson and D. Blumer, pp. 251–278. Grune & Stratton, New York.

Benson, D. F., Brown, J., and Tomlinson, E. B. (1971): Varieties of alexia: Word and letter blindness. *Neurology (NY)*, 21:951–957.

Benson, D. F., Gardner, H., and Meadows, J. C. (1976): Reduplicative paramnesia. *Neurology (NY)*, 26:147–151.

Benson, D. F., and Geschwind, N. (1967): Shrinking retrograde amnesia. *J. Neurol. Neurosurg. Psychiatry*, 30:457–461.

Benson, D. F., and Geschwind, N. (1971): Aphasia and related cortical disturbances. In: *Clinical Neurology*, edited by A. B. Baker and L. H. Baker, Chap. 8. Harper & Row, New York.

Benson, D. F., and Geschwind, N. (1975): Psychiatric conditions associated with focal lesions of the central nervous system. In: *American Handbook of Psychiatry, Vol. 4: Organic Disorders and Psychosomatic Medicine*, 2nd Ed., edited by S. Arieti and M. Reiser, pp. 208–243. Basic Books, New York.

Benson, D. F., Kuhl, D. E., Hawkins, R. A., Phelps, M. E., Cummings, J. L., and Tsai, S. Y. (1983a): The fluorodeoxyglucose 18F scan in Alzheimer's disease and multi-infarct dementia. *Arch. Neurol.*, 40:711–714.

Benson, D. F., Lemay, M., Patten, D. H., and Rubens, A. B. (1970): Diagnosis of normal-pressure hydrocephalus. *N. Engl. J. Med.*, 283:609–615.

Benson, D. F., Marsden, D. C., and Meadows, J. C. (1974): The amnesic syndrome of posterior cerebral artery occlusion. *Acta Neurol. Scand.*, 50:133–145.

Benson, D. F., Metter, E. J., Kuhl, D. E., and Phelps, M. E. (1983b): Positron-computed tomography in neurobehavioral problems. In: *Localization in Neuropsychology*, edited by A. Kertesz, pp. 121–139. Academic Press, New York.

Benson, D. F., Sheremata, W., Bouchard, R., Segarra, H. M., Price, D., and Geschwind, N. (1973): Conduction aphasia: A clinico-pathological study. *Arch. Neurol.*, 28:339–346.

Benson, D. F., and Stuss, D. T. (1982): Motor abilities after frontal leukotomy. *Neurology (NY)*, 32:1353–1357.

Benson, D. F., Stuss, D. T., Naeser, M. A., Weir, W. S., Kaplan, E. F., and Levine, H. (1981): The long-term effects of prefrontal leukotomy. *Arch. Neurol.*, 38:165–169.

Benton, A. (1977): The amusias. In: *Music and the Brain*, edited by M. Critchley and R. Henson, pp. 378–397. Charles C Thomas, Springfield, Illinois.

Benton, A. L. (1967): Constructional apraxia and the minor hemisphere. *Confin. Neurol.*, 29:1–16.

Benton, A. L. (1968): Differential behavioral effects in frontal lobe disease. *Neuropsychologia*, 6:53–60.

Benton, A. L., Elithorn, A., Fogel, M. L., and Kerr, M. (1963): A perceptual maze test sensitive to brain damage. *J. Neurol. Neurosurg. Psychiatry*, 26:540–544.

Benton, A. L., Hamsher, K. de S., Varney, N. R., and Spreen, O. (1983): *Contributions to Neuropsychological Assessment: A Clinical Manual.* Oxford University Press, New York.

Benton, A. L., and Joynt, R. J. (1960): Early descriptions of aphasia. *Arch. Neurol.*, 3:205–222.

Ben-Yishay, Y., Diller, L., Gerstman, L., and Haas, A. (1968): The relationship between impersistence, intellectual function and outcome of rehabilitation in patients with left hemiplegia. *Neurology (NY)*, 18:852–861.

Ben-Yishay, Y., Haas, A., and Diller, L. (1967): The effects of oxygen inhalation on motor impersistence in brain-damaged individuals: A double-blind study. *Neurology (NY)*, 17:1003–1010.

Berger, P. A. (1981): Biochemistry and the schizophrenias: Old concepts and new hypotheses. *J. Nerv. Ment. Dis.*, 169:90–99.

Berlin, L. (1955): Compulsive eye opening and associated phenomena. *Arch. Neurol. Psychiatry*, 73:597–601.

Berlyne, N. (1972): Confabulation. *Br. J. Psychiatry*, 120:31–39.

Bianchi, L. (1895): The functions of the frontal lobes. *Brain*, 18:497–522.

Bianchi, L. (1922): *The Mechanism of the Brain and the Functions of the Frontal Lobes.* William Wood, New York.

Bingley, T., Leksell, L., Meyerson, B. A., and Rylander, G. (1977): Long term results of stereotactic anterior capsulotomy in chronic obsessive-compulsive neurosis. In: *Neurosurgical Treatment in Psychiatry, Pain, and Epilepsy*, edited by W. H. Sweet, S. Obrador, and J. G. Martin-Rodriquez, pp. 287–299. University Park Press, Baltimore.

Bizzi, E. (1968): Discharge of frontal eye field neurons during saccadic and following eye movements in unanesthetized monkeys. *Exp. Brain Res.*, 6:69–80.

Bizzi, E., and Schiller, P. H. (1970): Single unit activity in the frontal eye fields of unanesthetized monkeys during eye and head movements. *Exp. Brain Res.*, 10:150–158.

Bjorklund, A., Divac, I., and Lindvall, O. (1978): Regional distribution of catecholamines in monkey cerebral cortex, evidence for a dopaminergic innervation of the primate prefrontal cortex. *Neurosci. Lett.*, 7:115–119.

Black, F. W. (1976): Cognitive deficits in patients with unilateral war-related frontal lobe lesions. *J. Clin. Psychol.*, 32:366–372.

Black, F. W., and Bernard, B. A. (1984): Constructional apraxia as a function of lesion locus and size in patients with focal brain damage. *Cortex*, 20:111–120.

Black, F. W., and Strub, R. L. (1976): Constructional apraxia in patients with discrete missile wounds of the brain. *Cortex*, 12:212–220.

Black, F. W., and Strub, R. L. (1978): Digit repetition performance in patients with focal brain damage. *Cortex*, 14:12–21.

Blakemore, C. B. (1967): Personality and brain damage. In: *The Biological Basis of Behavior*, edited by H. J. Eysenck. Charles C Thomas, Springfield, Illinois.

Blinkov, S. M., and Glazer, I. I. (1968): *The Human Brain: A Quantitative Handbook.* Basic Books/Plenum Press, New York.

Blum, G. S. (1953): *Psychoanalytic Theories of Personality.* McGraw-Hill, New York.

Blumer, D. (1982): Chronic pain as a psychobiologic phenomenon: The pain-prone disorder. In: *Psychiatric Aspects of Neurologic Disease*, Vol. II, edited by D. F. Benson and D. Blumer, pp. 179–192. Grune & Stratton, New York.

Blumer, D., and Benson, D. F. (1975): Personality changes with frontal and temporal lobe lesions. In: *Psychiatric Aspects of Neurologic Disease*, Vol. I, edited by D. F. Benson and D. Blumer, pp. 151–170. Grune & Stratton, New York.

Blustein, J., and Seeman, M. V. (1972): Brain tumors presenting as functional psychiatric disturbances. *Can. Psychiatr. Assoc. J.*, 17:59–63.

Bogen, J. E. (1969): The other side of the brain: II. An appositional mind. *Bull. Los Angeles Neurol. Soc.*, 34:135–162.

Bogen, J. E. (1979): The callosal syndrome. In: *Clinical Neuropsychology*, edited by K. M. Heilman and E. Valenstein, pp. 308–359. Oxford University Press, New York.

Boll, T. J. (1981): The Halstead-Reitan neuropsychology battery. In: *Handbook of Clinical Neuropsychology*, edited by S. B. Filskov and T. J. Boll, pp. 577–607. Wiley, New York.

Boll, T. J., and Reitan, R. M. (1973): Effect of age on performance of the trail-making test. *Percept. Mot. Skills*, 36:691–694.

Bond, M. (1984): The psychiatry of closed head injury. In: *Closed Head Injury. Psychological, Social and Family Consequences*, edited by N. Brooks, pp. 148–178. Oxford University Press, Oxford.

Bonhoeffer, K. (1904): Die Korsakowsche symptomenkomplex in Seinen beziehungen zu den verschiedenen Krankheitsformen. *Allg. Z. Psychiatr.*, 61:744–752.

Bonhoeffer, K. (editor) (1934): *Handbuch der Artzlichen Erfahrungen in Weltkriege 1914/1918.* Barth, Leipzig.

Borda, R. P. (1970): The effect of altered drive states on the contingent negative variation (CNV) in rhesus monkeys. *Electroencephalogr. Clin. Neurophysiol.*, 29:173–180.

Borkowski, J. G., Benton, A. L., and Spreen, O. (1967): Word fluency and brain damage. *Neuropsychologia*, 5:135–140.

Botez, M., and Wertheim, N. (1959): Expressive aphasia and amusia following right frontal lesions in a right-handed man. *Brain*, 82:186–203.

Botez, M. I. (1974): Frontal lobe tumours. In: *Handbook of Clinical Neurology, Vol. 17: Tumours of the Brain and Skull*, edited by P. J. Vinken and G. W. Bruyn, pp. 234–280. North Holland, Amsterdam.

Botez, M. I., and Barbeau, A. (1971): Role of subcortical structures and particularly of the thalamus, in the mechanisms of speech and language. *Int. J. Neurol.*, 8:300–320.

Botez, M. I., and Carp, N. (1968): Nouvelles données sur le problème du déclenchement de la parole. *Rev. Roumaine Neurol.*, 5:153–158.

Botez, M. I., Lecours, A. R., and Bérube, L. (1983): Speech and language in the frontal syndrome. In: *Aphasiology*, edited by A. R. Lecours, F. Lhermitte, and B. Bryan, pp. 124–140. Baillière Tindall, London.

Bouillard, J. B. (1825): Recherches cliniques propres à démontrer que la perte de la parole correspond à la lésion des lobules antérieures du cerveau et à confirmer l'opinion de M. Gall sur le siège de l'organe du langage articulé. *Arch. Gen. Med.*, 8:25–45.

Brain, R., and Strauss, E. G. (1955): *Recent Advances in Neurology and Neuropsychiatry*. Churchill, London.

Brain, W. R. (1941): Visual disorientation with special reference to lesions of the right cerebral hemisphere. *Brain*, 64:244–272.

Brickner, R. M. (1936): *The Intellectual Functions of the Frontal Lobes*. Macmillan, New York.

Bricolo, A., Turazzi, S., and Feriotti, G. (1980): Prolonged post-traumatic unconsciousness: Therapeutic assets and liabilities. *J. Neurosurg.*, 52:625–634.

Brion, S., and Jedynak, C.-P. (1972): Troubles du transfert interhémisphérique (callosal disconnection): A propos de trois observations de tumeurs du corps calleux, le signe de la main étrangère. *Rev. Neurol. (Paris)*, 126:257–266.

Brion, S., Pragier, C., Guerin, R., and Teitgen, M. M. C. (1969): Korsakoff syndrome due to bilateral softening of fornix. *Rev. Neurol. (Paris)*, 120:255–262.

Broca, P. (1861a): Perte de la parole: Ramollissement chronique et destruction partielle du lobe antérieur gauche du cerveau. *Paris Bull. Soc. Anthropol.*, 2:235–238.

Broca, P. (1861b): Remarques sur le siège de la faculté du langage articulé, suivi d'une observation d'aphémie. *Bull. Anat. Soc. (Paris)*, 2:330–357.

Broca, P. (1865): Sur la faculté du langage articulé. *Paris Bull. Soc. Anthropol.*, 6:493–494.

Broch, S., and Wiesel, B. (1948): Psychotic symptoms masking the onset in cases of brain tumor. *Med. Clin. North Am.*, 32:759–767.

Brodmann, K. (1909): *Vergleichende Lokalisationslehre der Grosshirnrinde.* Barth, Leipzig.

Brodmann, K. (1914): Physiologie des gerhirn. In: *Die Allgemaine Chirurgie der Gehirnkrankheiten, New Deutsche Chirurgie.* Enke, Stuttgart.

Brody, B. A., and Pribram, K. H. (1978): The role of the frontal and parietal cortex in cognitive processing. *Brain*, 101:607–633.

Brown, A. L. (1978): Knowing when, where, and how to remember: A problem of metacognition. In: *Advances in Instructional Psychology*, Vol. I, edited by R. Glasser. Lawrence Erlbaum, Hillsdale, New Jersey.

Brown, J. (1958): Some tests of the decay theory of immediate memory. *Q. J. Exp. Psychol.*, 10:12–21.

Brown, J. W. (1972): *Aphasia, Apraxia, and Agnosia. Clinical and Theoretical Aspects.* Charles C Thomas, Springfield, Illinois.

Brown, J. W. (1985): Frontal lobe syndromes. In: *Handbook of Clinical Neurology, Vol. 45: Clinical Neuropsychology*, edited by J. A. M. Frederiks, pp. 23–41. Elsevier, Amsterdam.

Brown, R. M., Crane, A. M., and Goldman, P. S. (1979): Regional distribution of monoamines in the cerebral cortex and subcortical structures of the rhesus monkey: Concentrations and in vivo synthesis rates. *Brain Res.*, 168:151–167.

Brown, R. M., and Goldman, P. S. (1977): Catecholamines in neocortex of rhesus monkeys: Regional distribution and ontogenetic development. *Brain Res.*, 124:576–580.

Brozoski, T. J., Brown, R. M., Rosvold, H. E., and Goldman, P. S. (1979): Cognitive deficit caused by regional depletion of dopamine in prefrontal cortex of rhesus monkey. *Science*, 205:929–932.

Bruce, C. J., and Goldberg, M. E. (1984): Physiology of the frontal eye fields. *Trends Neurosci.*, 7:436–441.

Bruetsch, W. L. (1975): Neurosyphilitic conditions: General paralysis, general paresis, dementia paralytica. In: *American Handbook of Psychiatry*, 2nd Ed., Vol. IV, edited by S. Arieti, pp. 135–151. Basic Books, New York.

Brunner, R. J., Kornhuber, H. H., Seemuller, E., Suger, G., and Wallesch, C.-W. (1982): Basal ganglia participation in language pathology. *Brain Lang.*, 16:281–299.

Bruyer, R., and Tuyumbu, B. (1980): Fluence verbale et lésions du cortex cérébral: Performances et types d'erreurs. *Encephale*, 6:287–297.

Buchsbaum, M. S., Ingvar, D. H., Kessler, R., Waters, R. N., Cappelletti, J., van Kammen, D. P., King, A. C., Johnson, J. L., Manning, R. G., Flynn, R. W., Mann, L. S., Bunney, W. E., and Sokoloff, L. (1982): Cerebral glucography with positron tomography. *Arch. Gen. Psychiatry*, 39:251–259.

Buffery, A. W. H. (1967): Learning and memory in baboons with bilateral lesions of frontal or inferotemporal cortex. *Nature*, 214:1054–1056.

Bull, J. (1965): Localization of cerebral lesions by radioactive isotopes and ultrasound. *Proc. R. Soc. Med.*, 58:1051–1053.

Busch, E. (1940): Physical symptoms in neurosurgical disease. *Acta Psychiatr. Scand.*, 15:257–290.

Butter, C. M., Mishkin, M., and Mirsky, A. F. (1968): Emotional responses toward humans in monkeys with selective frontal lesions. *Physiol. Behav.*, 3:213–215.

Butter, C. M., Mishkin, M., and Rosvold, H. E. (1963): Conditioning and extinction of a food rewarded response after selective ablations of frontal cortex in rhesus monkeys. *Exp. Neurol.*, 7:65–75.

Butter, C. M., and Snyder, D. R. (1972): Alterations in aversive and aggressive behaviors following orbital frontal lesions in rhesus monkeys. *Acta Neurobiol. Exp. (Warsz)*, 32:525–565.

Butter, C. M., Snyder, D. R., and McDonald, J. (1970): Effects of orbital frontal lesions on aversive and aggressive behaviors in rhesus monkeys. *J. Comp. Physiol. Psychol.*, 72:132–144.

Butters, N. (1984): Alcoholic Korsakoff's syndrome: An update. *Semin. Neurol.*, 4:226–244.

Butters, N., and Barton, M. (1970): Effects of parietal lobe damage on the performance of reversible operations in space. *Neuropsychologia*, 8:205–214.

Butters, N., Barton, M., and Brody, B. A. (1970): Role of the right parietal lobe in the mediation of cross-modal associations and reversible operations in space. *Cortex*, 6:174–190.

Butters, N. T., and Cermak, L. S. (1975): Some analyses of amnesic syndromes in brain-damaged patients. In: *The Hippocampus*, Vol. 2, edited by R. L. Isaacson and K. H. Pribram, pp. 377–409. Plenum Press, New York.

Butters, N., Samuels, I., Goodglass, H., and Brody, B. (1970): Short-term visual and auditory memory disorders after parietal and frontal lobe damage. *Cortex*, 6:440–459.

Butters, N., Soeldner, C., and Fedio, P. (1972): Comparison of parietal and frontal lobe spatial deficits in man: Extrapersonal vs personal (egocentric) space. *Percept. Mot. Skills*, 34:27–34.

Bychowski, Z. (1920): Uber das Fehlen der Wahrnekmung der eigenen Blindheit bei zwei Kriegsver-
letzen. *Neurol. Centralbl.*, 106:354–357. Referenced in Hécaen, H., and Albert, M. (1978): *Human
Neuropsychology*, Wiley, New York.

Caine, E. D., Hunt, R. D., Weingartner, H., and Ebert, M. H. (1978): Huntington's dementia: Clinical
and neuropsychological features. *Arch. Gen. Psychiatry*, 35:377–384.

Cameron, N. (1938): Reasoning, regression and communication in schizophrenics. *Psychol. Monogr.*,
No. 221.

Campbell, R. J., and Harlow, H. F. (1945): Problem solution by monkeys following bilateral removal of
the prefrontal areas. V. Spatial delayed reactions. *J. Exp. Psychol.*, 35:110–126.

Canavan, A. G. M. (1983): Stylus-maze performance in patients with frontal-lobe lesions: Effects of
signal valency and relationship to verbal and spatial abilities. *Neuropsychologia*, 21:375–382.

Cannon, W. B. (1927): The James-Lange theory of emotion: A critical examination and an alternative
theory. *Am. J. Psychol.*, 34:106–124.

Caplan, L. R., and Zervas, N. T. (1978): Speech arrest in a dextral with a right mesial frontal astrocytoma. *Arch. Neurol.*, 35:252–253.

Caramazza, A., and Berndt, R. S. (1978): Semantic and syntactic processes in aphasia: A review of the
literature. *Psych. Bull.*, 85:898–918.

Carlsson, A. (1978): Antipsychotic drugs, neurotransmitters, and schizophrenia. *Am. J. Psychiatry*,
135:165–173.

Carpenter, M. B., and Sutin, J. (1983): *Human Neuroanatomy*. Williams & Wilkins, Baltimore.

Carr, T. H. (1979): Consciousness in models of human information processing: Primary memory,
executive control and input regulation. In: *Aspects of Consciousness, Vol. 1: Psychological Issues*,
edited by G. Underwood and R. Stevens, pp. 123–153. Academic Press, New York.

Carr, T. H., and Bacharach, V. R. (1976): Perceptual tuning and conscious attention: Systems of input
regulation in visual information processing. *Cognition*, 4:281–302.

Carver, C., and Scheier, M. F. (1982): Self-awareness and the self-regulation of behavior. In: *Aspects
of Consciousness, Vol. 3: Awareness and Self-Awareness*, edited by G. Underwood, pp. 235–266.
Academic Press, New York.

Cavanaugh, J. C., and Borkowski, J. G. (1980): Searching for metamemory–memory connections: A
developmental study. *Dev. Psychol.*, 16:441–453.

Cermak, L. S., and Butters, N. (1972): The role of interference and encoding in the short-term memory
deficits of Korsakoff patients. *Neuropsychologia*, 10:89–95.

Chambers, W. R. (1955): Neurosurgical conditions masquerading as psychiatric diseases. *Am. J. Psychiatry*, 112:387–389.

Chance, M. R. A. (1980): An ethological assessment of emotion. In: *Emotion: Theory, Research and
Experience*, edited by R. Plutchik and H. Kellerman, pp. 81–111. Academic Press, New York.

Chapman, J. (1966): The early symptoms of schizophrenia. *Br. J. Psychiatry*, 112:225–251.

Chapman, L. F., and Wolff, H. G. (1959): The cerebral hemispheres and the highest integrative functions
of man. *Arch. Neurol.*, 1:357–424.

Chavis, D. A., and Pandya, D. N. (1976): Further observations on corticofrontal connections in the
rhesus monkey. *Brain Res.*, 117:369–386.

Chédru, F., and Geschwind, N. (1972): Writing disturbances in acute confusional states. *Neuropsychologia*, 10:343–353.

Chi, J. G., Dooling, E. C., and Gilles, F. H. (1977): Gyral development of the human brain. *Ann.
Neurol.*, 1:86–93.

Chorover, S. L., and Cole, M. (1966): Delayed alternation performance in patients with cerebral lesions.
Neuropsychologia, 4:1–7.

Christensen, A-L. (1975): *Luria's Neuropsychological Investigation*. Spectrum, New York.

Chusid, J. G. (1970): *Correlative Neuroanatomy and Functional Neurology*. Lange, Los Altos, California.

Chusid, J. G., Sugar, O., and French, J. D. (1948): Corticocortical connections of the cerebral cortex
lying within the arcuate and lunate sulci of the monkey (Macaca mulatta). *J. Neuropathol. Exp.
Neurol.*, 7:439–446.

Cicerone, K. D., Lazar, R. M., and Shapiro, W. R. (1983): Effects of frontal lobe lesions on hypothesis
sampling during concept formation. *Neuropsychologia*, 21:513–524.

Cicone, M., Wapner, W., and Gardner, H. (1980): Sensitivity to emotional expressions and situations
in organic patients. *Cortex*, 16:145–158.

Cleckley, H. (1964): *The Mask of Sanity*, 4th Ed. Mosby, St. Louis.

Cogan, D. G., and Adams, R. D. (1953): A type of paralysis of conjugate gaze (ocular motor apraxia). *Arch. Ophthalmol.*, 50:434–442.

Cohen, L. (1959): Perception of reversible figures after brain injury. *Arch. Neurol. Psychiatry*, 81:765–775.

Conrad, K. (1954): New problems of aphasia. *Brain*, 77:491–509.

Conte, H. R. (1975): A Circumplex Model for Personality Traits. Ph.D. dissertation, New York University.

Corkin, S. (1964): Somesthetic Function after Focal Cerebral Damage in Man. Ph.D. thesis, McGill University.

Corkin, S. (1965): Tactually-guided maze learning in man: Effects of unilateral cortical excisions and bilateral hippocampal lesions. *Neuropsychologica*, 3:339–351.

Corsellis, J. A. N. (1976): Ageing and the dementias. In: *Greenfield's Neuropathology*, edited by W. Blackwood and J. A. N. Corsellis, pp. 796–848. Edward Arnold, London.

Corsi, P. M. (1972): Human Memory and the Medial Temporal Region of the Brain, pp. 1–78. Ph.D. thesis, McGill University.

Costa, L. D. (1975): The relation of visuospatial dysfunction to digit span performance in patients with cerebral lesions. *Cortex*, 11:31–36.

Costa, L. D., Vaughan, H. G., Jr., Levita, E., and Farber, N. (1963): Purdue pegboard as a predictor of the presence and laterality of cerebral lesions. *J. Consult. Phychol.*, 27:133–137.

Courville, C. B. (1937): *Pathology of the Central Nervous System*, Part 4. Pacific Publishers, Mountain View, California.

Coyle, J. T. (1982): Development of neurotransmitters in the neocortex. *Neurosci. Res. Prog. Bull.*, 20:479–491.

Critchley, M. (1930): The anterior cerebral artery and its syndromes. *Brain*, 53:120–165.

Critchley, M. (1953): *The Parietal Lobes*. Hafner, New York.

Critchley, M. (1957): Observations on anosodiaphoria. *Encephale*, 46:540–546.

Critchley, M. (1970): Preface. In: Luria, A. R.: *Traumatic Aphasia: Its Syndromes, Psychology, and Treatment*. Basic Books, New York.

Crosby, E. C., Humphrey, T., and Lauer, E. W. (1962): *Correlative Neuroanatomy of the Nervous System*. Macmillan, New York.

Crown, S. (1951): Psychological changes following prefrontal leucotomy: A review. *J. Ment. Sci.*, 97:49–83.

Crowne, D. P. (1983): The frontal eye field and attention. *Psychol. Bull.*, 93:232–260.

Crowne, D. P., Yeo, C. H., and Russell, I. S. (1981): The effect of unilateral frontal eye field lesions in the monkey: Visual-motor guidance and avoidance behavior. *Behav. Brain Res.*, 2:165–187.

Cummings, J. L. (1982): Cortical dementias. In: *Psychiatric Aspects of Neurologic Disease*, Vol. II, edited by D. F. Benson and D. Blumer, pp. 93–121. Grune & Stratton, New York.

Cummings, J. L., and Benson, D. F. (1983): *Dementia: A Clinical Approach*. Butterworth, Boston.

Curtis, B. A., Jacobsen, S., and Marcus, E. M. (1972): *An Introduction to the Neurosciences*. Saunders, Philadelphia.

Damasio, A. R. (1979): The frontal lobes. In: *Clinical Neuropsychology*, edited by K. M. Heilman and E. Valenstein, pp. 360–412. Oxford University Press, New York

Damasio, A. R., and Benton, A. L. (1979): Impairment of hand movements under visual guidance. *Neurology (NY)*, 29:170–174.

Damasio, A. R., Damasio, H., and Chui, H. C. (1980): Neglect following damage to frontal lobe or basal ganglia. *Neuropsychologia*, 18:123–132.

Damasio, A. R., Damasio, H., Rizzo, M., Varney, N., and Gorsh, F. (1982): Aphasia with nonhemorrhagic lesions in the basal ganglia and internal capsule. *Arch. Neurol.*, 39:15–20.

Damasio, A. R., and Van Hoesen, G. W. (1980): Structure and function of the supplementary motor area. *Neurology (NY)*, 30:359.

Damasio, A. R., and Van Hoesen, G. W. (1983): Emotional disturbances associated with focal lesions of the limbic frontal lobe. In: *Neuropsychology of Human Emotion*, edited by K. M. Heilman and P. Satz, pp. 85–110. Guilford Press, New York.

Darley, F. L., Aronson, A. E., and Brown, J. R. (1975): *Motor Speech Disorders*. Saunders, Philadelphia.

Daroff, R. B., and Hoyt, W. F. (1971): Supranuclear disorders of ocular control systems in man: Clinical, anatomical, and physiological correlations. In: *The Control of Eye Movements*, edited by P. Bach-Y-Rita, C. C. Collins, and J. E. Hyde, pp. 175–235. Academic Press, New York.

Darwin, C. (1892/1965): *The Expression of Emotions in Man and Animals*. University of Chicago Press, Chicago.

Davenport, C. B., and Muncey, E. B. (1916): Huntington's chorea in relation to heredity and eugenics. *Am. J. Insanity*, 73:195–222.

Davitz, J. R. (1969): *The Language of Emotion*. McGraw-Hill, New York.

Dax, M. (1836): Lésions de la moitié gauche de l'encéphale coincidant avec l'oubli des signes de la pensée. Paper presented in Montpelier (published in *Gaz. Hebd.*, 2nd series, 1865).

DeAjuriaguerra, J., Hécaen, H., and Angelergues, R. (1960): Les apraxies: Variétés cliniques et latéralisation lésionnelle. *Rev. Neurol. (Paris)*, 102:566–594.

DeAjuriaguerra, J., and Tissot, R. (1969): The apraxias. In: *Handbook of Clinical Neurology, Vol. 4: Disorders of Speech, Perception and Symbolic Behavior*, edited by P. J. Vinken and G. W. Bruyn, pp. 48–66. North Holland, Amsterdam.

Dejerine, J. (1914/1977): *Sémiologie des Affections du Système Nerveux*, Vol. II, 3rd Ed., Masson, Paris.

DeJong, R. N. (1979): *The Neurologic Examination*. 4th Ed. Harper & Row, Hagerstown, Maryland.

Delaney, R. C., Rosen, A. J., Mattson, R. H., and Novelly, R. A. (1980): Memory function in focal epilepsy: A comparison of non-surgical unilateral temporal lobe and frontal lobe samples. *Cortex*, 16:103–117.

Delisle, M., Stuss, D. T., and Picton, T. W. (1985): Event-related potentials to feedback in a concept-formation task. *Electroencephalogr. Clin. Neurophysiol. [Suppl.] (in press)*.

DeLong, M. R., Georgopoulos, A. P., and Crutcher, M. D. (1983): Cortico-basal ganglia relations and coding of motor performance. In: *Neural Coding of Motor Performance*, edited by J. Massion, J. Paillard, W. Schultz, and M. Wiesendanger, pp. 30–40. Springer-Verlag, Berlin.

DeMille, R. (1962): Intellect after lobotomy in schizophrenia: A factor analytic study. *Psychol. Monogr.*, 76:1–18.

Denny-Brown, D. (1951): The frontal lobes and their functions. In: *Modern Trends in Neurology*, edited by A. Feiling, pp. 13–89. Butterworth, London.

Denny-Brown, D. (1958): The nature of apraxia. *J. Nerv. Ment. Dis.*, 126:9–32.

Denny-Brown, D. (1963): The physiological basis of perception and speech. In: *Problems of Dynamic Neurology*, edited by L. Halpern, pp. 30–62. Hebrew University Hadassah Medical School, Jerusalem.

Denny-Brown, D., and Banker, B. Q. (1954): Amorphosynthesis from left parietal lesion.*Arch. Neurol. Psychiatry*, 71:302–313.

Denny-Brown, D., Meyer, J. S., and Horenstein, S. (1952): The significance of perceptual rivalry resulting from parietal lesion. *Brain*, 75:433–471.

DeRenzi, E., Colombo, A. Faglioni, P., and Gibertoni, M. (1982): Conjugate gaze paresis in stroke patients with unilateral damage: An unexpected instance of hemispheric asymmetry. *Arch. Neurol.*, 39:482–486.

DeRenzi, E., Faglioni, P., Lodesani, M., and Vecchi, A. (1983): Performance of left brain-damaged patients on imitation of single movements and motor sequences, frontal and parietal-injured patients compared. *Cortex*, 19:333–343.

DeRenzi, E., Motti, F., and Nichelli, P. (1980): Imitating gestures: A quantitative approach to ideomotor apraxia. *Arch. Neurol.*, 37:6–10.

DeRenzi, E., and Nichelli, P. (1975): Verbal and non-verbal short-term memory impairment following hemispheric damage. *Cortex*, 11:341–354.

DeRenzi, E., Pieczuro, A., and Vignolo, L. A. (1966): Oral apraxia and aphasia. *Cortex*, 2:50–73.

Desmedt, J. E., and Noel, P. (1973): Average cerebral evoked potentials in the evaluation of lesions of the sensory nerves and of the central somatosensory pathway. In: *New Developments in Electromyography and Clinical Neurophysiology*, Vol. 2, edited by J. E. Desmedt, pp. 352–371. Karger, Basel.

Deuel, R. K. (1977): Loss of motor habits after cortical lesions. *Neuropsychologia*, 15:205–215.

Deuel, R. K., and Collins, R. C. (1983): Recovery from unilateral neglect. *Exp. Neurol.*, 81:733–748.

Deuel, R. K., and Collins, R. C. (1984): The functional anatomy of frontal lobe neglect in the monkey: Behavioral and quantitative 2-deoxyglucose studies. *Ann. Neurol.*, 15:521–529.

DiChiro, G., Reames, P. M., and Matthews, W. B., Jr. (1964): RISA-ventriculography and RISA-cisternography. *Neurology (NY)*, 14:185–191.

Distel, H., and Fries, W. (1982): Contralateral cortical projections to the superior colliculus in the macaque monkey. *Exp. Brain Res.*, 48:157–162.

Doehring, D. G., and Reitan, R. M. (1962): Concept attainment of human adults with lateralized cerebral lesions. *Percept. Mot. Skills*, 14:27–33.

Donald, A. G., Still, C. N., and Pearson, J. M., Jr. (1972): Behavioral symptoms with intracranial neoplasm. *South. Med. J.*, 65:1006–1009.

Dorland's Illustrated Medical Dictionary, 25th Ed. (1974): Saunders, Philadelphia.

Doty, R. W. (1973): Ablation of visual areas in the central nervous system. In: *Handbook of Sensory Physiology*, Vol. VII/3, edited by R. Jung, pp. 483–541. Springer-Verlag, Berlin.

Drachman, D. A., and Arbit, J. (1966): Memory and the hippocampal complex. II. Is memory a multiple process? *Arch. Neurol.*, 15:52–61.

Drewe, E. A. (1974): The effect of type and area of brain lesion on Wisconsin Card Sorting Test performance. *Cortex*, 10:159–170.

Drewe, E. A. (1975a): Go–no-go learning after frontal lobe lesions in humans. *Cortex*, 11:8–16.

Drewe, E. A. (1975b): An experimental investigation of Luria's theory on the effects of frontal lobe lesions in man. *Neuropsychologia*, 13:421–429.

DSM-III. Diagnostic and Statistical Manual of Mental Disorders (Third Ed.) (1980): American Psychiatric Association, 1980.

Duara, R., Grady, C., Haxby, J., Ingvar, D., Sokoloff, L., Margolin, R. A., Manning, R. G., Cutler, N. R., and Rapaport, S. I. (1984): Human brain glucose utilization and cognitive function in relation to age. *Ann. Neurol.*, 16:702–713.

Dupui, Ph., Güell, A., Bessoles, G., Géraud, G., and Bès, A. (1984): Cerebral blood flow in aging: Decrease of hyperfrontal distribution. In: *Monographs in Neural Sciences*, edited by M. M. Cohen, pp. 131–138. Karger, Basel.

Eccles, J. C. (1979): *The Human Mystery*, Springer-Verlag, Berlin.

Ehrenwold, G. (1931): Anosognosie und depersonalization. *Nervenarzt*, 4:681–688.

Eichenbaum, H., Shedlack, K. J., and Eckman, K. W. (1980): Thalamocortical mechanisms in odor-guided behavior. I. Effects of lesions of the mediodorsal thalamic nucleus and frontal cortex on olfactory discrimination in the rat. *Brain Behav. Evol.*, 17:255–275.

Eie, N. (1954): Macroscopical investigations of twenty-nine brains subjected to frontal leukotomy with some observations on clinico-pathological correlations. *Acta Psychiatr. Neurol. Scand. [Suppl.]*, 90:3–40.

Elithorn, A. (1964): Intelligence, perceptual integration and the minor hemisphere syndrome. *J. Neurol. Neurosurg. Psychiatry*, 2:327–332.

Emson, P. C., and Koob, G. F. (1978): The origin and distribution of dopamine-containing afferents to the rat frontal cortex. *Brain Res.*, 142:249–267.

Enoch, M. D., and Trethowan, W. H. (1979): *Uncommon Psychiatric Syndromes*, 2nd Ed. Year Book, Chicago.

Eslinger, P. J., and Damasio, A. R. (1985): Severe disturbance of higher cognition following bilateral frontal lobe ablation: Patient EVR. *Neurology (NY)*, 35:1731–1741.

Ethelberg, S. (1951): On changes in circulation through the anterior cerebral artery: A clinico-angiographical study. *Acta Psychiatr. Neurol. Scand. [Suppl.]*, 75:3–211.

Ettlinger, G., Teuber, H.-L., and Milner, B. (1975): The seventeenth international symposium of neuropsychology. *Neuropsychologia*, 13:125–133.

Evarts, E. V., Kimura, M., Wurtz, R. H., and Hikosaka, O. (1984): Behavioral correlates of activity in basal ganglia neurons. *Trends Neurosci.*, 7:447–453.

Exner, S. (1881): *Untersuchungen uber die Lokalisation der Funktionen in der Grosshirnrinde des Menschen*. Braumuller, Vienna.

Eysenck, H. J. (1947): *Dimensions of Personality*. Kegan-Paul, London.

Eysenck, H. J. (1952): *The Scientific Study of Personality*. Macmillan, New York.

Eysenck, H. J. (1967): *The Biological Basis of Behavior*. Charles C Thomas, Springfield, Illinois.

Fabbri, W. (1956): Leucotomia transorbitaria di Fiamberti e rispetto della personalita individuale nei silievi psycometrici con il test di Porteus. *Note e Rivista di Psichiatria*, 311–332. Referenced in Walsh, K. W. (1978): *Neuropsychology: A Clinical Approach*. Churchill Livingstone, Edinburgh.

Fano (1895): *Arch Italiennes de Biologie*. Referenced in Bianchi, L. (1922): *The Mechanism of the Brain and the Functions of the Frontal Lobes*. William Wood, New York.

Faust, C. (1955): Zur symptomatik Frischer und alter Stirnhirnverletzungen. *Arch. Psychiatr. Neurol.*, 193:78–97.

Faust, C. (1960): Die psychischen Storungen nach Hirntraumen: Akute traumatische Psychosen und psychische Spatfolgen nach Hirnverletzungen. In: *Psychiatrie der Gegenwart*, Vol. II, edited by H. W. Gruhle, B. R. Jung, W. Mayer-Gross, and M. Muller, pp. 552–645. Springer, Berlin.

Feldman, M. J., and Drasgow, J. (1960): *The Visual-Verbal Test Manual*. Western Psychological Services, Beverley Hills, California.

Ferrier, D. (1874): The localization of function in the brain. *Proc. R. Soc. Lond. [B]*, 22:229–232.

Ferrier, D. (1875): Experiments on the brain of monkeys. No. 1. *Proc. R. Soc.*, 23:409–430.

Ferrier, D. (1886): *The Functions of the Brain*. Smith, Elder, London.

Feuchtwanger, E. (1923): Die Funktionen des Stirnhirns ihre Pathologie und Psychologie. *Monogr. Ges. Neurol. Psychiatr.*, 38:1–193.

Finan, J. L. (1942): Delayed response with pre-delay reinforcement in monkeys after the removal of the frontal lobes. *Am. J. Psychol.*, 55:202–214.

Finger, S., and Stein, D. G. (1982): *Brain Damage and Recovery. Research and Clinical Perspectives*. Academic Press, New York.

Fisher, C. M. (1965): Lacunes: Small, deep cerebral infarcts. *Neurology (NY)*, 15:774–784.

Fisher, C. M. (1975): The anatomy and pathology of the cerebral vasculature. In: *Modern Concepts of Cerebrovascular Disease*, edited by J. S. Meyer, pp. 1–42. Spectrum, New York.

Fisher, M. (1956): Left hemiplegia and motor impersistence. *J. Nerv. Ment. Dis.*, 123:201–218.

Fitzgerald P. G., and Picton, T. W. (1983): Event-related potentials recorded during the discrimination of improbable stimuli. *Biol. Psychol.*, 17:241–276.

Flechsig, P. (1896): *Gehirn und Seele*. Viet, Leipzig.

Flechsig, P. (1905): Hirnpathologie und Willenstheorie: Atti del Congresso Interno di Psicologia. Quoted in Bianchi, L. (1922) *The Mechanism of the Brain and the Functions of the Frontal Lobes*, William Wood, New York.

Fleurens, P. (1824): *Recherches Expérimentales sur les Propriétés et les Fonctions du Système Nerveux dans les Animaux Vertébrés*. Crevat, Paris (2nd Ed., 1842). Quoted in Bianchi, L. (1922): *The Mechanism of the Brain and the Functions of the Frontal Lobes*. William Wood, New York.

Foerster, O. (1931): The cerebral cortex in man. *Lancet*, 2:309–312.

Foerster, O. (1936a): Motorische felder und bahnen. In: *Handbuch der Neurologie*, Vol. 6, edited by O. Bumke and O. Foerster, pp. 1–357. Julius Springer, Berlin.

Foerster, O. (1936b): The motor cortex in man in the light of Hughlings Jackson's doctrines. *Brain*, 59:135–159.

Fog, T. (1965): The topography of plaques in multiple sclerosis with special reference to cerebral plaques. *Acta Neurol. Scand. [Suppl. 15]*, 41:9–161.

Fogel, M. L. (1967): Picture description and interpretation in brain-damaged patients. *Cortex*, 3:433–438.

Foix, C. (1928): Aphasies. In: *Nouveau Traité de Médecine*, Vol. 18, edited by G. Roger, F. Widal, and P. J. Teissier, pp. 135–213. Masson et Cie, Paris.

Forster, E. (1919): Die psychischen Storungen der Hirnverletzten. *Monatsschr. Psychiatr. Neurol.*, 46:61–105.

Frackowiak, R. S. J., Pozzili, C., Legg, N. J., DuBoulay, G. H., Marshall, J., Lenzi, G. L., and Jones, T. (1981): Regional cerebral oxygen supply and utilization in dementia. *Brain*, 104:753–758.

Franz, S. I. (1907): *On the Functions of the Cerebrum of the Frontal Lobes*. Science Press, New York.

Franzen, G., and Ingvar, D. H. (1975a): Abnormal distribution of cerebral activity in chronic schizophrenia. *J. Psychiatr. Res.*, 12:199–214.

Franzen, G., and Ingvar, D. H. (1975b): Absence of activation in frontal structures during psychological testing of chronic schizophrenics. *J. Neurol. Neurosurg. Psychiatry*, 38:1027–1032.

Freedman, A. M., Kaplan, H. I., and Sadock, B. J. (1975): *Comprehensive Textbook of Psychiatry/II*, 2nd Ed. Williams & Wilkins, Baltimore.

Freedman, M., Alexander, M. P., and Naeser, M. A. (1984): The anatomical basis of transcortical motor aphasia. *Neurology (NY)*, 34:409–417.

Freedman, M., and Oscar-Berman, M. (1986): Bilateral frontal lobe disease and selective delayed response deficits in humans. *Behav. Neurosci.*, 100:337–342.

Freeman, W. (1949): Recent techniques in psychosurgery: Transorbital leucotomy: deep frontal cut. *Proc. R. Soc. Med. [Suppl.]*, 42:8–12.

Freeman, W. (1971): Frontal lobotomy in early schizophrenia: Long follow-up in 415 cases. *Br. J. Psychiatry*, 119:621–624.

Freeman, W., and Watts, J. W. (1942): *Psychosurgery*. Charles C Thomas, Springfield, Illinois.

Freeman, W., and Watts, J. M. (1944): Behavior and the frontal lobes. *NY Acad. Sci.*, 6:284–310.

Freeman, W., and Watts, J. W. (1950): *Psychosurgery in the Treatment of Mental Disorders and Intractable Pain*, 2nd Ed. Charles C Thomas, Springfield, Illinois.

French, J. D. (1952): Brain lesions associated with prolonged unconsciousness. *A.M.A. Arch. Neurol. Psychiatry*, 68:727–740.

Freud, S. (1933): New Introductory lectures on psychoanalysis. In: *Standard Edition of the Works of Sigmund Freud*, Vol. 22, Hogarth, London.

Fritsch, G. T., and Hitzig, E. (1870): Uber die electrische Erregbarkeit des Grosshirns. *Arch. Anat. Physiol. Physiol. Abt.*, 37:300–332.

Fulton, J. F. (1934): Forced grasping and groping in relation to the syndrome of the premotor area. *Arch. Neurol. Psychiatry*, 31:221–235.

Fulton, J. F. (1952): *The Frontal Lobes and Human Behavior*. Charles C Thomas, Springfield, Illinois.

Fulton, J. F., and Ingraham, F. D. (1929): Emotional disturbances following experimental lesions of the base of the brain (pre-chiasmal). *Am. J. Physiol.*, 90:353.

Fulton, J. F., and Jacobsen, C. F. (1935): The functions of the frontal lobes: A comparative study in monkeys, chimpanzees and man. *Adv. Mod. Biol. (Moscow)*, 4:113–123.

Fuster, J. M. (1980): *The Prefrontal Cortex. Anatomy, Physiology, and Neuropsychology of the Frontal Lobe*. Raven Press, New York.

Fuster, J. (1981): Prefrontal cortex in motor control. In: *Handbook of Physiology—The Nervous System, Vol. II: Motor Control*, edited by V. B. Brooks, pp. 1149–1178. American Physiological Society, Bethesda.

Fuster, J. M. (1984): Behavioral electrophysiology of the prefrontal cortex. *Trends Neurosci.*, 7:408–414.

Fuster, J. M., and Bauer, R. H. (1974): Visual short-term memory deficit from hypothermia of frontal cortex. *Brain Res.*, 81:393–400.

Gainotti, G. (1972): Emotional behavior and hemispheric side of the lesion. *Cortex*, 8:41–55.

Gainotti, G., Messerli, P., and Tissot, R. (1972): Qualitative analysis of unilateral spatial neglect in relation to laterality of cerebral lesions. *J. Neurol. Neurosurg. Psychiatry*, 35:545–550.

Galaburda, A. M., and Mesulam, M-M. (1983): Neuroanatomical aspects of cerebral localization. In: *Localization in Neuropsychology*, edited by A. Kertesz, pp. 21–61. Academic Press, New York.

Gall, F. J., and Spurzheim, G. (1809): Recherches sur le système nerveux en général et sur celui du cerveau en particulier. Presented at the Institut de France, Paris.

Gardner, E. (1975): *Fundamentals of Neurology. A Psychophysiological Approach*. Saunders, Philadelphia.

Gazzaniga, M. S. (1970): *The Bisected Brain*. Appleton-Century-Crofts, New York.

Gazzaniga, M. S., Smylie, C. S., Baynes, K., Hirst, W., and McCleary, C. (1984): Profiles of right hemisphere language and speech following brain bisection. *Brain Lang.*, 22:206–220.

Gazzaniga, M. S., and Sperry, R. W. (1967): Language after section of the cerebral commissures. *Brain*, 90:131–138.

Gelmers, H. J. (1983): Non-paralytic motor disturbances and speech disorders: The role of the supplementary motor area. *J. Neurol. Neurosurg. Psychiatry*, 46:1052–1054.

Gerstmann, J. (1930): Zur symptomatologie der Hirnlasionem in uebergangsgbeit der Unteren Parietal und Mittleren Occipitalwindung. *Nervenartz*, 3:691–695.

Gerstmann, J., and Schilder, P. (1926): Uber eine besondere gangstorung bei stirnhirmerkrankung. *Wien. Med. Wochenschr.*, 76:97–102.

Geschwind, N. (1965): Disconnexion syndromes in animals and man. *Brain*, 88:237–294, 585–644.

Geschwind, N. (1967): The apraxias. In: *Phenomenology of Will and Action*, edited by E. W. Straus and R. M. Griffith, pp. 91–102. Duquesne University Press, Pittsburgh.

Geschwind, N. (1970): The organization of language and the brain. *Science*, 170:940–944.

Geschwind, N. (1974): *Selected Papers on Language and the Brain*. Reidel, Boston.

Geschwind, N. (1975): The apraxias: Neural mechanisms of disorders of learned movement. *Am. Sci.*, 63:188–195.

Geschwind, N. (1977): *Lectures in Neurobehavior*. Harvard Medical School, Boston.

Geschwind, N. (1982): Disorders of attention: A frontier in neuropsychology. In: *The Neuropsychology of Cognitive Function*, edited by D. E. Broadbent and L. Weiskrantz, pp. 173–185. The Royal Society, London.

Geschwind, N., and Kaplan, E. (1962): A human cerebral deconnection syndrome. *Neurology (NY)*, 12:675–685.

Ghent, L., Mishkin, M., and Teuber, H. L. (1962): Short-term memory after frontal-lobe injury in man. *J. Comp. Physiol. Psychol.*, 55:705–709.

Gibo, H., Carver, C. C., Rhoton, A. L., Jr., Lenkey, C., and Mitchell, R. (1981): Microsurgical anatomy of the middle cerebral artery. *J. Neurosurg.*, 54:151–169.

Girgis, M. (1971): The orbital surface of the frontal lobe of the brain and mental disorders. *Acta Psychiatr. Scand. [Suppl.]*, 222:1–58.

Girotti, F., Milanese, C., Casazza, M., Allegranza, A., Corridori, F., and Avanzini, G. (1982): Oculomotor disturbances in Balint's syndrome: Anatomoclinical findings and electrooculographic analysis in a case. *Cortex*, 18:603–614.

Glowinski, J., Tassin, J. P. and Thierry, A. M. (1984): The mesocortico-prefrontal dopaminergic neurons. *Trends Neurosci.*, 7:415–418.

Glueck, S., and Glueck, E. T. (1970): *Toward a Typology of Juvenile Offenders. Implications for Therapy and Prevention.* Grune & Stratton, New York.

Godukhin, O. V., Zharikova, A. D., and Novoselov, V. I. (1980): The release of labelled L-glutamic acid from rat neostriatum in vivo following stimulation of frontal cortex. *Neuroscience*, 5:2151–2154.

Goeders, N. E., and Smith, J. E. (1983): Cortical dopaminergic involvement in cocaine reinforcement. *Science*, 221:773–775.

Goldberg, G., Mayer, N. H., and Toglia, J. U. (1981): Medial frontal cortex infarction and the alien hand sign. *Arch. Neurol.*, 38:683–686.

Goldberg, M. E., and Bruce, C. J. (1981): Frontal eye fields in the monkey: Eye movements remap the effective coordinates of visual stimuli. *Soc. Neurosci. Abstr.*, 7:131.

Goldberg, M. E., and Bushnell, M. C. (1981): Behavioral enhancement of visual responses in monkey cerebral cortex. II. Modulation in frontal eye fields specifically related to saccades. *J. Neurophysiol.*, 46:773–787.

Golden, C. J. (1978): *Diagnosis and Rehabilitation in Clinical Neuropsychology.* Charles C Thomas, Springfield, Illinois.

Golden, C. J. (1980): In reply to Adam's "In search of Luria's battery: a false start." *J. Consult. Clin. Psychol.*, 48:517–521.

Golden, C. J. (1981): A standardized version of Luria's neuropsychological tests: A quantitative and qualitative approach to neuropsychological evaluation. In: *Handbook of Clinical Neuropsychology*, edited by S. B. Filskov and T. J. Boll, pp. 608–642. Wiley-Interscience, New York.

Golden, C. J., Osmon, D. C., Moses, J. A., Jr., and Berg, R. A. (1981): *Interpretation of the Halstead-Reitan Neuropsychological Test Battery: A Casebook Approach.* Grune & Stratton, New York.

Goldman, P. S. (1971): Functional development of the prefrontal cortex in early life and the problem of neuronal plasticity. *Exp. Neurol.*, 32:366–387.

Goldman, P. S. (1974): An alternative to developmental plasticity: Heterology of CNS structures in infants and adults. In: *Plasticity and Recovery of Function in the Central Nervous System*, edited by D. Stein, J. J. Rosen, and N. Butters, pp. 149–174. Academic Press, New York.

Goldman, P. S. (1979): Contralateral projections to the dorsal thalamus from frontal association cortex in the rhesus monkey. *Brain Res.*, 166:166–171.

Goldman, P. S., and Galkin, T. W. (1978): Prenatal removal of frontal association cortex in the fetal rhesus monkey: Anatomical and functional consequences in postnatal life. *Brain Res.*, 152:451–485.

Goldman, P. S., and Nauta, W. J. H. (1976): Autoradiographic demonstration of a projection from prefrontal association cortex to the superior colliculus in the rhesus monkey. *Brain Res.*, 116:145–149.

Goldman, P. S., and Nauta, W. J. H. (1977a): An intricately patterned prefronto-caudate projection in the rhesus monkey. *J. Comp. Neurol.*, 171:369–386.

Goldman, P. S., and Nauta, W. J. H. (1977b): Columnar distribution of cortico-cortical fibres in the frontal association, limbic, and motor cortex of the developing rhesus monkey. *Brain Res.*, 122:393–413.

Goldman, P. S., and Rosvold, H. E. (1970): Localization of function within the dorsolateral prefrontal cortex of the rhesus monkey. *Exp. Neurol.*, 27:291–304.

Goldman-Rakic, P. S. (1984a): Modular organization of prefrontal cortex. *Trends Neurosci.*, 7:419–424.

Goldman-Rakic, P. S. (1984b): The frontal lobes: Uncharted provinces of the brain. *Trends Neurosci.*, 7:425–429.

Goldman-Rakic, P. S., Selemon, L. D., and Schwartz, M. L. (1984): Dual pathways connecting the dorsolateral prefrontal cortex with the hippocampal formation and parahippocampal cortex in the rhesus monkey. *Neuroscience*, 12:719–743.

Goldstein, K. (1909): Der makroskopische Hirnbefund in meinem falle von Linksseitiger motorischer Apraxie. *Neurol. Centralblatt*, 28:898–906. Referenced in Hécaen, H. (1981): Apraxias. In: *Handbook of Clinical Neuropsychology*, edited by S. B. Filskov and T. J. Boll, pp. 257–286. Wiley-Interscience, New York.

Goldstein, K. (1917): *Die Transkortikalen Aphasien*. Gustav Fischer, Jena.

Goldstein, K. (1936a): The significance of the frontal lobes for mental performances. *J. Neurol. Psychopathol.*, 17:27–40.

Goldstein, K. (1936b): Modifications of behavior consequent to cerebral lesions. *Psychiatr. Q.*, 10:586–610.

Goldstein, K. (1939): Clinical and theoretic aspects of lesions of the frontal lobes. *Arch. Neurol. Psychiatry*, 41:865–867.

Goldstein, K. (1944): Mental changes due to frontal lobe damage. *J. Psychol.*, 17:187–208.

Goldstein, K. (1948): *Language and Language Disturbances*. Grune & Stratton, New York.

Goldstein, K., and Scheerer, M. (1941): Abstract and concrete behavior; an experimental study with special tests. *Psychol. Monogr.*, 53:1–151.

Goltz. (1884): Zur Physiologie der Grosshirns. *Arch. Psychiatr.*, 15. Referenced in Bianchi, L. (1922): *The Mechanism of the Brain and the Functions of the Frontal Lobes*. William Wood, New York.

Gonen, J. Y. (1970): The use of Wechsler's deterioration quotient in cases of diffuse and symmetrical cerebral atrophy. *J. Clin. Psychol.*, 26:174–177.

Goodglass, H. (1968): Studies in the grammar of aphasics. In: *Developments in Applied Psycholinguistics Research*, edited by S. Rosenberg and J. Koplin, pp. 177–208. Macmillan, New York.

Goodglass, H., and Berko, J. (1960): Agrammatism and inflectional morphology in English. *J. Speech Hear. Res.*, 3:257–267.

Goodglass, H., and Kaplan, E. (1963): Disturbance of gesture and pantomime in aphasia. *Brain*, 86:703–720.

Goodglass, H., and Kaplan, E. (1972): *The Assessment of Aphasia and Related Disorders*. Lea & Febiger, Philadelphia.

Goodglass, H., and Kaplan, E. (1979): Assessment of cognitive deficit in the brain-injured patient. In: *Handbook of Behavioral Neurobiology, Vol. 2: Neuropsychology*, edited by M. S. Gazzaniga, pp. 3–22. Plenum Press, New York.

Goodglass, H., Kaplan, E., Weintraub, S., and Ackerman, N. (1976): The "tip-of-the-tongue" phenomenon in aphasia. *Cortex*, 12:145–153.

Goodglass, H., and Stuss, D. T. (1979): Naming to picture versus description in three aphasic subgroups. *Cortex*, 15:199–211.

Grafman, J., Vance, S. C., Weingartner, H., and Salazar, A. M. (1985a): Specific effects of orbital-frontal brain wounds upon regulation of mood. Submitted.

Grafman, J., Vance, S. C., Weingartner, H., Salazar, A. M., and Amin, D. (1985b): The effects of lateralized frontal lesions upon mood regulation. Presented at the International Neuropsychological Society Meeting, San Diego.

Grafman, J., Weingartner, H., Salazar, A., Vance, S., and Amin, D. (1984): Frontal lobe lesions: Persistent effects upon cognition and behavior. Presented at the International Neuropsychological Society 12th Annual Meeting, Houston.

Grant, D. A., and Berg, E. A. (1948): A behavioral analysis of degree of reinforcement and ease of shifting to new responses in a Weigl-type card-sorting problem. *J. Exp. Psychol.*, 38:404–411.

Gray, J. A. (1970): The psychophysiological basis of introversion-extraversion. *Behav. Res. Ther.*, 8:249–266.

Gray, J. A. (1981): Anxiety as a paradigm case of emotion. *Br. Med. Bull.*, 37:193–197.

Greenblatt, M., Arnot, R., and Solomon, H. (1950): *Studies in Lobotomy*. Grune & Stratton, New York.

Greenblatt, M., and Solomon, H. C. (1966): Studies of lobotomy. *Proc. Assoc. Res. Nerv. Ment. Dis.*, 36:19–34.

Greenfield, J. G. (1958): Infectious diseases of the central nervous system. In: *Neuropathology*, edited by J. G. Greenfield, W. Blackwood, A. Meyer, W. H. McMenemey, and R. M. Norman, pp. 132–229. Edward Arnold, London.

Gronwall, D. M. A., and Sampson, H. (1974): *The Psychological Effects of Concussion.* Auckland University Press, Auckland, N. Z.

Gross, C. G., and Weiskrantz, L. (1962): Evidence for dissociation of impairment on auditory discrimination and delayed response following lateral frontal lesions in monkeys. *Exp. Neurol.,* 5:453–476.

Grossman, M., Shapiro, B. E., and Gardner, H. (1981): Dissociable musical processing strategies after localized brain damage. *Neuropsychologia,* 19:425–433.

Grueninger, W. E., and Pribram, K. H. (1969): Effects of spatial and nonspatial distractors on performance latency of monkeys with frontal lesions. *J. Comp. Physiol. Psychol.,* 68:203–209.

Grünbaum, A. S. F., and Sherrington, C. S. (1903): Observations on the physiology of the cerebral cortex of the anthropoid apes. *Proc. R. Soc. Lond.,* 72:152–155.

Guard, O., Perenin, M. T., Vighetto, A., Giroud, M., Tommasi, M., and Dumas, R. (1984): Syndrome pariétal bilatéral proche d'un syndrome de Balint. *Rev. Neurol. (Paris),* 5:358–367.

Guberman, A., and Stuss, D. (1983): The syndrome of bilateral paramedian thalamic infarction. *Neurology (NY),* 33:540–546.

Guitton, D., Buchtel, H. A., and Douglas, R. M. (1982): Disturbances of voluntary saccadic eye-movement mechanisms following discrete unilateral frontal-lobe removals. In: *Functional Basis of Ocular Motility Disorders,* edited by G. Lennerstrand, D. S. Zee, and E. L. Keller, pp. 497–499. Pergamon Press, Oxford.

Haaland, K. Y., and Delaney, H. D. (1981): Motor deficits after left or right hemisphere damage due to stroke or tumor. *Neuropsychologia,* 19:17–27.

Haaland, K. Y., Porch, B. E., and Delaney, H. D. (1980): Limb apraxia and motor performance. *Brain Lang.,* 9:315–323.

Hakim, S. (1964): Some observations on CSF pressure: Hydrocephalic syndrome in adults with "normal" CSF pressure. Thesis, Javinana University School of Medicine, Bogota, Columbia.

Halstead, W. (1940): Preliminary analysis of grouping behavior in patients with cerebral injury by the method of equivalent and non-equivalent stimuli. *Am. J. Psychiatry,* 96:1263–1294.

Halstead, W. C. (1943): Function of the frontal lobe in man: The dynamic visual field. *Arch. Neurol. Psychiatry,* 49:633.

Halstead, W. C. (1947a): *Brain and Intelligence: A Quantitative Study of the Frontal Lobes.* University of Chicago Press, Chicago.

Halstead, W. C. (1947b): Specialization of behavioral functions and the frontal lobes. *Res. Publ. Assoc. Nerv. Ment. Dis.,* 27:59–66.

Halstead, W. C., Carmichael, H. T., and Bucy, P. C. (1946): Prefrontal lobotomy: A preliminary appraisal of the behavioral results. *Am. J. Psychiatry,* 103:217–228.

Hamlin, R. M. (1970): Intellectual function 14 years after frontal lobe surgery. *Cortex,* 6:299–307.

Hansen, J. C., and Hillyard, S. A. (1980): Endogenous brain potentials associated with selective auditory attention. *Electroencephalogr. Clin. Neurophysiol.,* 49:277–290.

Hanson, M. L. (1983): *Articulation.* Saunders, Philadelphia.

Harlow, H. F., and Settlage, P. H. (1948): Effect of extirpation of frontal areas upon learning performances of monkeys. *Res. Publ. Assoc. Nerv. Ment. Dis.,* 27:446–459.

Harlow, J. M. (1868): Recovery after severe injury to the head. *Publ. Mass. Med. Soc.,* 2:327–346.

Harriman, P. L. (1947): *Dictionary of Psychology.* Philosophical Library, New York.

Hartmann, F. (1907): Beitrage zur Apraxielehre. *Monatsschr. Psychiatr. Neurol.,* 21:97–118, 248–270.

Hausser, C. O., Robert, F., and Giard, N. (1980): Balint's syndrome. *Can. J. Neurol. Sci.,* 7:157–161.

Hayman, M. (1942): Two minute clinical test for measurement of intellectual impairment in psychiatric disorders. *Arch. Neurol. Psychiatry,* 47:454–464.

Head, H. (1922): The diagnosis of hysteria. *Br. Med. J.,* 1:827–829.

Head, H. (1926): *Aphasia and Kindred Disorders of Speech.* Cambridge University Press, London.

Heath, R. G., and Pool, J. L. (1948a): Treatment of psychoses with bilateral ablation of a focal area of the frontal cortex. *Psychosom. Med.,* 10:254–256.

Heath, R. G., and Pool, J. L. (1948b): Bilateral fractional resection of frontal cortex for the treatment of psychoses. *J. Nerv. Ment. Dis.,* 107:411–429.

Hebb, D. O. (1939): Intelligence in man after large removals of cerebral tissue: Report of four left frontal lobe cases. *J. Gen. Psychol.,* 21:73–87.

Hebb, D. O. (1945): Man's frontal lobes: A critical review. *Arch. Neurol. Psychiatry,* 54:10–24.

Hebb, D. O., and Penfield, W. (1940): Human behavior after extensive bilateral removal from the frontal lobes. *Arch. Neurol. Psychiatry,* 44:421–438.

Hécaen, H. (1962): Clinical symptomatology in right and left hemisphere lesions. In: *Interhemispheric Relations and Cerebral Dominance*, edited by V. B. Mountcastle, pp. 215–243. Johns Hopkins Press, Baltimore.

Hécaen, H. (1964): Mental symptoms associated with tumors of the frontal lobe. In: *The Frontal Granular Cortex and Behavior*, edited by J. M. Warren and K. Akert, pp. 335–352. McGraw-Hill, New York.

Hécaen, H. (1972): *Introduction à là Neuropsychologie*. Larousse, Paris.

Hécaen, H. (1981): Apraxias. In: *Handbook of Clinical Neuropsychology*, edited by S. B. Filskov and T. J. Boll, pp. 257–286. Wiley, New York.

Hécaen, H., and Albert, M. L. (1975): Disorders of mental functioning related to frontal lobe pathology. In: *Psychiatric Aspects of Neurologic Disease*, Vol. I, edited by D. F. Benson and D. Blumer, pp. 137–149. Grune & Stratton, New York.

Hécaen, H., and Albert, M. (1978): *Human Neuropsychology*. Wiley, New York.

Hécaen, H., and Angelerques, R. (1966): L'agraphie secondaire aux lésions du lobe frontal. *Int. J. Neurol.*, 5:381–394.

Hécaen, H., de Ajuriaguerra, J., Rouques, L., David, M., and Dell, M. B. (1950): Paralysie psychique du regard de Balint au cours de l'évolution d'une leucoencéphalite type Balo. *Rev. Neurol. (Paris)*, 83:81–104.

Hécaen, H., and Gimeno, A. (1960): L'apraxie idéomotrice unilatérale gauche. *Rev. Neurol. (Paris)*, 102:648–653.

Hécaen, H., and Ruel, J. (1981): Sièges lésionnels intrafrontaux et déficit au test de "fluence verbale." *Rev. Neurol. (Paris)*, 137:277–284.

Heilbrun, A. B. (1958): The digit span test and the prediction of cerebral pathology. *Arch. Neurol. Psychiatry*, 80:228–231.

Heilman, K. M. (1979a): Apraxia. In: *Clinical Neuropsychology*, edited by K. M. Heilman and E. Valenstein, pp. 159–185. Oxford University Press, New York.

Heilman, K. M. (1979b): Neglect and related disorders. In: *Clinical Neuropsychology*, edited by K. Heilman and E. Valenstein, pp. 268–307. Oxford Press, New York.

Heilman, K. M., Pandya, D. P., and Geschwind, N. (1970): Trimodal inattention following parietal lobe ablations. *Trans. Am. Neurol. Assoc.*, 95:259–261.

Heilman, K. M., Rothi, L., and Kertesz, A. (1983a): Localization of apraxia-producing lesions. In: *Localization in Neuropsychology*, edited by A. Kertesz, pp. 371–392. Academic Press, New York.

Heilman, K. M., Rothi, L. J., and Valenstein, E. (1982): Two forms of ideomotor apraxia. *Neurology (NY)*, 32:342–346.

Heilman, K. M., Scholes, R., and Watson, R. T. (1975): Auditory affective agnosia: Disturbed comprehension of affective speech. *J. Neurol. Neurosurg. Psychiatry*, 38:69–72.

Heilman, K. M., Schwartz, H. D., and Watson, R. T. (1978): Hypoarousal in patients with a neglect syndrome and emotional indifference. *Neurology (NY)*, 28:229–232.

Heilman, K. M., and Valenstein, E. (1972): Frontal lobe neglect in man. *Neurology (NY)*, 22:660–664.

Heilman, K. M., and Van den Abell, T. (1980): Right hemisphere dominance for attention: The mechanism underlying hemispheric asymmetries of inattention (neglect). *Neurology (NY)*, 30:327–330.

Heilman, K. M., Watson, R. T., Valenstein, E., and Damasio, A. R. (1983b): Localization of lesions in neglect. In: *Localization in Neuropsychology*, edited by A. Kertesz, pp. 471–492. Academic Press, New York.

Hendrickson, C. W., Kimble, R. J., and Kimble, D. P. (1969): Hippocampal lesions and the orienting response. *J. Comp. Physiol. Psychol.*, 67:220–227.

Heninger, G. R., Charney, D. S., and Sternberg, D. E. (1984): Serotoninergic function in depression. *Arch. Gen. Psychiatry*, 41:398–402.

Henneman, E. (1980a): Organization of the motor systems: A preview. In: *Medical Physiology*, Vol. 1, 14th Ed., edited by V. B. Mountcastle, pp. 669–674. Mosby, St. Louis.

Henneman, E. (1980b): Motor function of the cerebral cortex. In: *Medical Physiology*, Vol. 1, 14th Ed., edited by V. B. Mountcastle, pp. 859–889. Mosby, St. Louis.

Henschen, S. (1926): On the function of the right hemisphere of the brain in relation to the left in speech, music and calculation. *Brain*, 49:110–123.

Hewson, L. R. (1949): Wechsler-Bellevue scale and substitution test as aids in neuropsychiatric diagnosis. *J. Nerv. Ment. Dis.*, 109:158–183, 246–266.

Hier, D. B., Mondlock, J., and Caplan, L. R. (1983): Behavioral abnormalities after right hemisphere stroke. *Neurology (NY)*, 33:337–344.

Hillyard, S. A., and Kutas, M. (1983): Electrophysiology of cognitive processing. *Annu. Rev. Psychol.*, 34:33–61.

Hinde, R. A. (1966/1970): *Animal Behavior. A Synthesis of Etiology and Comparative Psychology.* McGraw-Hill, New York.

Hinsie, L. E., and Campbell, R. J. (1970): *Psychiatric Dictionary*, 4th Ed. Oxford University Press, Toronto.

Hirose, S. (1965): Orbito-ventromedial undercutting—1957–1963: Follow-up study of 77 cases. *Am. J. Psychiatry*, 121:1194–1202.

Hirschi, T. (1969): *Causes of Delinquency.* University of California Press, Berkeley.

Hitzig, P. (1874): *Untersuchen uber das Gehirn.* Hirschwald, Berlin. Quoted in Bianchi, L. (1922): *The Mechanism of the Brain and the Functions of the Frontal Lobes*, William Wood, New York.

Hobbs, G. E. (1963): Brain tumors simulating psychiatric disease. *Can. Med. Assoc. J.*, 88:186–188.

Hofstadter, D. R., and Dennette, D. C. (1982): *The Minds I.* Basic Books, New York.

Holmes, G. (1918): Disturbances of vision by cerebral lesions. *Br. J. Ophthalmol.*, 2:353–384.

Holmes, G. (1921): Palsies of the conjugate ocular movements. *Br. J. Ophthalmol.*, 5:241–250.

Holmes, G. (1931): Mental symptoms associated with brain tumors. *Proc. R. Soc. Med.*, 24:65–76.

Horsley, V., and Schafer, E. A. (1888): Functions of the cerebral cortex. *Philos. Trans. R. Soc. Lond. [B]*, 179:1–45.

Howes, D., and Geschwind, N. (1964): Quantitative studies of aphasic language. In: *Disorders of Communication.*, edited by D. M. Rioch and E. A. Weinstein, pp. 229–244. Williams & Wilkins, Baltimore.

Hunt, T. (1942): Intelligence. In: *Psychosurgery*, edited by W. Freeman and J. W. Watts, pp. 153–164. Charles C Thomas, Springfield, Illinois.

Hunt, W. L. (1949): The relative rates of decline of Wechsler-Bellevue "Hold" and "Don't Hold" tests. *J. Consult. Psychol.*, 13:440–443.

Hutton, E. L. (1943): Results of prefrontal leucotomy. *Lancet*, 1:362–366.

Ingvar, D. (1979): "Hyperfrontal" distribution of the central grey matter flow in resting wakefulness; on the functional anatomy of the conscious state. *Acta Neurol. Scand.*, 60:12–25.

Ingvar, D. H. (1980): Abnormal distribution of cerebral activity in chronic schizophrenia: A neuro-physiological interpretation. In: *Perspectives in Schizophrenia Research*, edited by C. F. Baxter and T. Melnechuck, pp. 107–125. Raven Press, New York.

Ingvar, D. H., and Franzen, G. (1974): Distribution of cerebral activity in chronic schizophrenia. *Lancet*, 2:1484–1486.

Isaac, W., and DeVito, J. L. (1958): Effect of sensory stimulation on the activity of normal and prefrontal-lobectomized monkeys. *J. Comp. Physiol. Psychol.*, 51:172–174.

Isseroff, A., Leveton, L., Freeman, G., Lewis, M. E., and Stein, D. G. (1976): Differences in the behavioral effects of single-stage and serial lesions of the hippocampus. *Exp. Neurol.*, 53:339–354.

Ito, M. (1984): *The Cerebellum and Neural Control.* Raven Press, New York.

Itoh, M., Sasanuma, S., and Ushijima, T. (1979): Velar movements during speech in a patient with apraxia of speech. *Brain Lang.*, 7:227–239.

Iverson, L. L. (1975): Dopamine receptors in the brain. *Science*, 188:1084–1089.

Iverson, S. D. (1973): Brain lesions and memory in animals. In: *The Physiologic Basis of Memory*, edited by J. A. Deutsch, pp. 305–364. Academic Press, New York.

Jackson, H. (1878): Remarks on non-protusion of the tongue in some cases of aphasia. *Lancet*, 1:716. In: Taylor, J., editor (1932): *Selected Writings of Hughlings Jackson*, Vol. II. Hodder & Stoughton, London.

Jackson, J. H. (1864): *Selected Writings of John Hughlings Jackson*, edited by J. Taylor (1956). Basic Books, New York.

Jacobsen, C. F. (1935): Functions of frontal association area in primates. *Arch. Neurol. Psychiatry*, 33:558–569.

Jacobsen, C. F. (1936): Studies of cerebral function in primates. I. The functions of the frontal association areas in monkeys. *Comp. Psychol. Monogr.*, 13:1–60.

Jacobsen, C. F., and Nissen, H. W. (1937): Studies of cerebral function in primates. IV. The effects of frontal lobe lesions on the delayed alternation habit in monkeys. *J. Comp. Psychol.*, 23:101–112.

Jacobson, P. L., and Farmer, T. W. (1979): The "hypernormal" CT scan in dementia: Bilateral isodense subdural hematomas. *Neurology (NY)*, 29:1522–1524.

Jakobson, R. (1964): Towards a linguistic typology of aphasic impairments. In: *Ciba Foundation Symposium on Disorder of Language*. Churchill, London.

James, W. (1890): *Principles of Psychology*, Vols. I and II. Dover, New York.

Janet, P. (1920): *The Major Symptoms of Hysteria*. Macmillan, New York.

Jarvie, H. F. (1954): Frontal lobe wounds causing disinhibition: A study of six cases. *J. Neurol. Neurosurg. Psychiatry*, 17:14–32.

Jarvilehto, T., and Fruhstorfer, H. (1970): Differentiation between slow cortical potentials associated with motor and mental acts in man. *Exp. Brain Res.*, 11:309–317.

Jaynes, J. (1976): *The Origin of Consciousness in the Breakdown of the Bicameral Mind*. Houghton Mifflin, Boston.

Jefferson, G. (1937): Removal of right or left frontal lobes in man. *Br. Med. J.*, 2:199–206.

Jenkner, F. L., and Kutschera, E. (1965): Frontal lobes and vision. *Confin. Neurol.*, 25:63–78.

Jones, E. G., and Powell, T. P. S. (1970): An anatomical study of converging sensory pathways within the cerebral cortex of the monkey. *Brain*, 93:793–820.

Jones-Gotman, M., and Milner, B. (1977): Design fluency: The invention of nonsense drawings after focal cortical lesions. *Neuropsychologia*, 15:653–674.

Joseph, M. H., Frith, C. D., and Waddington, J. L. (1979): Dopaminergic mechanisms and cognitive deficit in schizophrenia. *Psychopharmacology*, 63:273–280.

Jouandet, M., and Gazzaniga, M. S. (1979): The frontal lobes. In: *Handbook of Behavioral Neurobiology, Vol. 2: Neuropsychology*, edited by M. S. Gazzaniga, pp. 25–59. Plenum Press, New York.

Joynt, R. J., Benton, A. L., and Fogel, M. L. (1962): Behavioral and pathological correlates of motor impersistence. *Neurology (NY)*, 12:876–881.

Kaczmarek, B. L. J. (1984): Neurolinguistic analysis of verbal utterances in patients with focal lesions of frontal lobes. *Brain Lang.*, 21:52–58.

Kaplan, E. (1983): Process and achievement revisited. In: *Toward a Holistic Developmental Psychology*, edited by S. Wapner and B. Kaplan, pp. 143–156. Lawrence Erlbaum, Hillsdale, New Jersey.

Kapur, N., and Coughlan, A. K. (1980): Confabulation and frontal lobe dysfunction. *J. Neurol. Neurosurg. Psychiatry*, 43:461–463.

Kemp, J. M., and Powell, T. P. S. (1970): The cortico-striate projection in the monkey. *Brain*, 93:525–546.

Kemp, J. M., and Powell, T. P. S. (1971): The site of termination of afferent fibers in the caudate nucleus. *Philos. Trans. R. Soc. (Lond.)*, 262:413–427.

Kennard, M. A. (1939): Alterations in response to visual stimuli following lesions of frontal lobes in monkeys. *Arch. Neurol. Psychiatry*, 41:1153–1165.

Kennard, M. A., and Ectors, L. (1938): Forced circling movements in monkeys following lesions of the frontal lobes. *J. Neurophysiol.*, 1:45–54.

Kernohan, J. W., and Sayre, G. P. (1952): Tumors of the central nervous system. In: *Atlas of Tumor Pathology*, Armed Forces Institute of Pathology, Washington, D.C.

Kertesz, A. (1979): *Aphasia and Associated Disorders: Taxonomy, Localization and Recovery*. Grune & Stratton, New York.

Kertesz, A. (1983): Issues in localization. In: *Localization in Neuropsychology*, edited by A. Kertesz, pp. 1–20. Academic Press, New York.

Kertesz, A., and Dobrowolski, S. (1981): Right-hemisphere deficits, lesion size and location. *J. Clin. Neuropsychol.*, 3:283–299.

Kertesz, A., Ferro, J. M., and Shewan, C. M. (1984): Apraxia and aphasia: The functional-anatomical basis for their dissociation. *Neurology (NY)*, 34:40–47.

Kertesz, A., Lesk, D., and McCabe, P. (177): Isotope localization of infarcts in aphasia. *Arch. Neurol.*, 34:590–601.

Kertesz, A., Nicholson, I., Cancelliere, A., Kassa, K., and Black, S. E. (1985): Motor impersistence: A right-hemisphere syndrome. *Neurology (NY)*, 35:662–666.

Kety, S. A. (1980): The syndrome of schizophrenia: unresolved questions and opportunities for research. *Br. J. Psychiatry*, 136:421–436.

Kiloh, L., and Osselton, J. W. (1966): *Clinical Electroencephalography*. Butterworth, Washington, D.C.

Kim, Y., Morrow, L., Passafiume, D., and Boller, F. (1984): Visuoperceptual and visuomotor abilities and locus of lesion. *Neuropsychologia*, 22:177–185.

Kimble, D. P., Bagshaw, M. H., and Pribram, K. H. (1965): The GSR of monkeys during orienting and habituation after selective partial ablations of the cingulate and frontal cortex. *Neuropsychologia*, 3:121–128.

Kimura, D. (1963): Right temporal-lobe damage. *Arch. Neurol.*, 8:264–271.

Kimura, D. (1977): Acquisition of a motor skill after left-hemisphere damage. *Brain*, 100:527–542.

Kimura, D. (1982): Left-hemisphere control of oral and brachial movements and their relation to communication. In: *The Neuropsychology of Cognitive Function*, edited by D. E. Broadbent and L. Weiskrantz, pp. 135–149. The Royal Society, London.

King, H. E. (1949): Intellectual function. In: *Selective Partial Ablation of the Frontal Cortex. A Correlative Study of its Effects on Human Psychotic Subjects*, edited by F. A. Mettler, Columbia-Greystone Associates pp. 178–207. Hoeber, New York.

King, W. R. (1949): Ability to abstract. In: *Selective Partial Ablation of the Frontal Cortex: A Correlative Study of its Effects on Human Psychotic Subjects*, edited by F. A. Mettler, Columbia-Greystone Associates, pp. 218–238. Hoeber, New York.

Kinsbourne, M. (1977a): Cognitive decline with advancing age: An interpretation. In: *Aging and Dementia*, edited by W. Lynn Smith and M. Kinsbourn, pp. 217–235. Spectrum, New York.

Kinsbourne, M. (1977b): Hemi-neglect and hemisphere rivalry. *Adv. Neurol.*, 18:41–49.

Kleist, K. (1907): Korticale (innervatorische) Apraxie. *Jaarb. Psychiatr. Neurol.*, 28:46–112.

Kleist, K. (1934a): *Kriegverletzungen des Gehirns in ihrer Bedeutung fur Hirnlokalisation und Hirnpathologie*. Barth, Leipzig.

Kleist, K. (1934b): *Gehirnpathologie*. Barth, Leipzig.

Knight, G. (1964): The orbital cortex as an objective in the surgical treatment of mental illness. *Br. J. Surg.*, 51:114–124.

Knight, R. T. (1984): Decreased response to novel stimuli after prefrontal lesions in man. *Electroencephalogr. Clin. Neurophysiol.*, 59:9–20.

Knight, R. T., Hillyard, S. A., Woods, D. L., and Neville, H. J. (1981): The effects of frontal and temporal-parietal lesions on the auditory evoked potential in man. *Electroecephalogr. Clin. Neurophysiol.*, 52:571–582.

Knopman, D. S., Selnes, O. A., Niecum, M., Rubens, A. B., Yock, D., and Larson, D. (1983) A longitudinal study of speech fluency in aphasia: CT correlates of recovery and persistent nonfluency. *Neurology (NY)*, 33:1170–1178.

Kojima, S., and Goldman-Rakic, P. S. (1982): Delay-related activity of prefrontal neurons in rhesus monkeys performing delayed response. *Brain Res.*, 248:43–49.

Kolb, B., and Milner, B. (1981): Performance of complex arm and facial movement after focal brain lesions. *Neuropsychologia*, 19:491–503.

Kolb, B., and Whishaw, I. Q. (1980): *Fundamentals of Human Neuropsychology*. Freeman, San Francisco.

Kolodny, A. (1929): Symptomatology of tumor of the frontal lobe. *Arch. Neurol. Psychiatry*, 21:1107–1127.

Konorski, J.(1959): A new method of physiological investigation of recent memory in animals. *Bull. Acad. Pol. Sci.*, 7:115–117.

Konorski, J. (1967): Some new ideas concerning the physiological mechanisms of perception. *Acta Biol. Exp. (Warsz.)*, 27:147–161.

Konorski, J., Teuber, H. L., and Zernicki, B., editors (1972): The frontal granular cortex and behavior. *Acta Neurobiol. Exp. (Warsz.)*, 32:1.

Kowalska, D. M., Bachevalier, J., and Mishkin, M. (1984): Inferior prefrontal cortex and recognition memory. *Soc. Neurosci. Abstr.*, 10:385.

Kretschmer, E. (1949): Die orbitalhirn und Zwischenhirnsyndrome nach Schadelbasisfrakturen. *Arch. Psychiatr.*, 182:452–477.

Krieg, W. J. S. (1949): Connections of the cerebral cortex. II. The macaque. C. Frontal areas and subareas. *J. Comp. Neurol.*, 91:467–506.

Krischner, H. S., and Webb, W. G. (1982): Word and letter reading and the mechanism of the third alexia. *Arch. Neurol.*, 39:84–87.

Kuhl, D. E, Metter, E. J., Riege, W. H., and Phelps, M. E. (1982a): Effects of human aging on patterns of local cerebral glucose utilization determined by the 18F fluorodeoxyglucose method. *J. Cereb. Blood Flow Metab.*, 2:163–171.

Kuhl, D. E., Phelps, M. E., Markham, C. H., Metter, E. J., Riege, W. H., and Winter, J. (1982b): Cerebral metabolism and atrophy in Huntington's disease determined by 18 FDG and computed tomographic scan. *Ann. Neurol.*, 12:425–434.

Kuypers, H. G. J. M., and Lawrence, D. G. (1967): Cortical projections to the red nucleus and the brain stem in the rhesus monkey. *Brain Res.*, 4:151–188.

Kuypers, H. G. J. M., Szwarcbart, M. K., Mishkin, M., and Rosvold, H. E. (1965): Occipitotemporal corticocortical connections in the rhesus monkey. *Exp. Neurol.*, 11:245–262.

Lagrange, H., Bertrand, I., and Garcin, R. (1929): Cécité corticale par ramollissement des deux cunes. *Rev. Neurol. (Paris)*, 1:417–427.

Landis, C. (1949): Psychologic changes following topectomy. In: *Selective Partial Ablation of the Frontal Cortex: A Correlative Study of its Effects on Human Psychotic Subjects*, edited by F. A. Mettler, Columbia-Greystone Associates, pp. 306–312. Hoeber, New York.

Langworthy, O. R., and Richter, C. P. (1939): Increased spontaneous activity produced by frontal lobe lesions in cats. *Am. J. Physiol.*, 126:158–161.

Laplane, D., Talairach, J., Meininger, V., Bancaud, J., and Orgogozo, J. M. (1977): Clinical consequences of corticectomies involving the supplementary motor area in man. *J. Neurol. Sci.*, 34:310–314.

Larsen, B., Skinhoj, E., and Lassen, N. A. (1978): Variations in regional cortical blood flow in the right and left hemispheres during automatic speech. *Brain*, 101:193–209.

Lashley, K. S. (1929): *Brain Mechanisms and Language*. University of Chicago Press, Chicago.

Laurence, S., and Stein, D. G. (1978): Recovery after brain damage and the concept of localization of function. In: *Recovery from Brain Damage: Research and Theory*, edited by S. Finger, pp. 369–407. Plenum Press, New York.

Lawrence, D. G., and Kuypers, H. G. (1968): The functional organization of the motor system in the monkey. I. The effects of bilateral pyramidal lesions. II. The effects of the descending brain stem pathways. *Brain*, 91:1–36.

LeBeau, J. (1952): Post-operative syndromes in selective prefrontal surgery. *J. Ment. Sci.*, 98:12–22.

LeBeau, J. (1954): *Psychochirugie et Fonctions Mentales*. Masson et Cie, Paris.

LeBeau, J., and Petrie, A. (1953): A comparison of the personality changes after 1. prefrontal selective surgery for the relief of intractable pain and for the treatment of mental cases, 2. cingulectomy and topectomy. *J. Ment. Sci.*, 99:53–61.

Lecours, A. R., and Lhermitte, F. (1983): Clinical forms of aphasia. In: *Aphasiology*, edited by A. R. Lecours, F. Lhermitte, and B. Bryans, pp. 76–108. Baillière Tindall, London.

Lecours, A. R., Lhermitte, F., and Bryans, B. (1983): *Aphasiology*. Baillière, Tindall, London.

Lee, D. A. (1981): Paul Broca and the history of aphasia: Roland P. Mackay award essay, 1980. *Neurology (NY)*, 31:600–602.

Lehmann, H. E. (1975): Unusual psychiatric disorders and atypical psychoses. In: *Comprehensive Textbook of Psychiatry/II*, 2nd Ed., edited by A. M. Freedman, H. I. Kaplan, and B. J. Sadock. Williams & Wilkins, Baltimore.

Leichnetz, G. R. (1982): Connections between the frontal eye field and pretectum in the monkey: An anterograde/retrograde study using HRP gel and TMB neurohistochemistry. *J. Comp. Neurol.*, 207:394–402.

Leichnetz, G. R., Spencer, R. F., Hardy, S. G. P., and Astruc, J. (1981): The prefrontal corticotectal projection in the monkey: An anterograde and retrograde horseradish peroxidase study. *Neuroscience*, 6:1023–1041.

Leischner, A. (1969): The agraphias. In: *Handbook of Clinical Neurology, Vol. 4: Disorders of Speech, Perception and Symbolic Behaviour*, edited by P. J. Vinken and G. W. Bruyn, pp. 141–180. North Holland, Amsterdam.

Lenneberg, E. (1967): *Biological Foundations of Language*. Wiley, New York.

Lesser, R. P., Lueders, H., Dinner, D. S., Hahn, J., and Cohen, L. (1984): The location of speech and writing functions in the frontal language area: Results of extraoperative cortical stimulation. *Brain*, 107:275–291.

Leventhal, C. M., Baringer, J. R., Arnason, B. G., and Fisher, C. M. (1965): A case of Marchiafava Bignami disease with clinical recovery. *Trans. Am. Neurol. Assoc.*, 90:87–91.

Levin, H. (1973): Motor impersistence in patients with unilateral cerebral disease: A cross-validation study. *J. Consult. Clin. Psychol.*, 41:287–290.

Levin, H. S., Benton, A. L., and Grossman, R. G. (1982): *Neurobehavioral Consequences of Closed Head Injury*. Oxford University Press, New York.

Levin, H. S., and Grossman, R. G. (1978): Behavioral sequelae of closed head injury: A quantitative study. *Arch. Neurol.*, 35:720–727.

Levin, H. S., Grossman, R. G., Rose, J. E., and Teasdale, G. (1979): Long-term neuropsychological outcome of closed head injury. *J. Neurosurg.*, 50:412–422.

Levin, H. S., Madison, C. F., Bailey, C. B., Meyers, C. A., Eisenberg, H. M., and Guinto, F. C. (1983): Mutism after closed head injury. *Arch. Neurol.*, 40:601–606.

Levin, S. (1984a): Frontal lobe dysfunctions in schizophrenia. I. Eye movement impairments. *J. Psychiatr. Res.*, 18:27–55.

Levin, S. (1984b): Frontal lobe dysfunctions in schizophrenia. II. Impairments of psychological and brain functions. *J. Psychiatr. Res.*, 18:57–72.

Levine, D. N., and Mohr, J. P. (1979): Language after bilateral cerebral infarctions: Role of the minor hemisphere in speech. *Neurology (NY)*, 29:927–938.

Levinson, F., and Meyer, V. (1965): Personality changes in relation to psychiatric status following orbital cortex undercutting. *Br. J. Psychiatry*, 111:207–218.

Lewandowsky, M. (1907): Ueber apraxie des lidschlusses. *Berl. Klin. Wochenschr.*, 44:921. Referenced in Fisher, M. (1956): Left hemiplegia and motor impersistence. *J. Nerv. Ment. Dis.*, 123:201–218.

Lewinsohn, P. M., Zieler, J. L., Libet, J., Eyeberg, S., and Nielson, G. (1972): Short-term memory: A comparison between frontal and nonfrontal right- and left-hemisphere brain-damaged patients. *J. Comp. Physiol. Psychol.*, 81:248–255.

Lewis, G. P., Golden, C. J., Moses, Jr., J. A., Osmon, D. C., Purisch, A. D., and Hammeke, T. A. (1979): Localization of cerebral dysfunction with a standardized version of Luria's neuropsychological battery. *J. Consult. Clin. Psychol.*, 47:1003–1019.

Lewis, N. D. C., Landis, C., and King, H. E. (1956): *Studies in Topectomy*. Grune & Stratton, New York.

Lezak, M. D. (1979): Recovery of memory and learning functions following traumatic brain injury. *Cortex*, 15:63–72.

Lezak, M. D. (1982): The problem of assessing executive functions. *Int. J. Psychol.*, 17:281–297.

Lezak, M. D. (1976/1983): *Neuropsychological Assessment*. 2nd Ed. Oxford University Press, New York.

Lhermitte, F. (1983): "Utilization behaviour" and its relation to lesions of the frontal lobes. *Brain*, 106:237–255.

Lhermitte, F., Derouesne, J., and Signoret, J-L. (1972): Analyse neuropsychologique du syndrôme frontal. *Rev. Neurol. (Paris)*, 127:415–440.

Lhermitte, J. (1939): L'image de Notre Corps. Nouvelle Revue Critique, Paris.

Lichtheim, L. (1885): On aphasia. *Brain*, 7:463–484.

Lieberman, A., and Benson, D. F. (1977): Control of emotional expression in pseudobulbar palsy: A personal experience. *Arch. Neurol.*, 34:717–719.

Liepmann, H. (1977): The syndrome of apraxia (motor asymboly) based on a case of unilateral apraxia. In: *Neurological Classics in Modern Translation*, edited by D. A. Rottenberg, and F. H. Hochberg, pp. 155–181. Hafner New York. From *Monatschr. Psychait. Neurol.*, 8:15–44.

Liepmann, H. (1905): Der wertere Krankheitsverlauf bei dem ein Sertig Apraktis den und der Gehirnbefund auf Grund von Serienschmitten. *Monatschr. Psychiatr. Neurol.*, 17:289–311.

Liepmann, H., and Maas, O. (1907): Fall von linksseitger agraphie und apraxie bei rechtsseitiger lahmung. *J. Psychol. Neurol.*, 10:214–227.

Lindqvist, G., and Norlen, G. (1966): Korsakoff's syndrome after operation on ruptured aneurysm of the anterior communicating artery. *Acta Psychiatr. Scand.*, 42:24–34.

Lindvall, O., Bjorklund, A., and Divac, I. (1978): Organization of catecholamine neurons projecting to the frontal cortex in the rat. *Brain Res.*, 142:1–24.

Lindvall, O., Bjorklund, A., Moore, R. Y., and Stenevi, U. (1974): Mesencephalic dopamine neurons projecting to neocortex. *Brain Res.*, 81:325–331.

Lipowski, Z. J. (1980): *Delirium: Acute Brain Failure in Man*. Charles C. Thomas, Springfield, Illinois.

Lipsey, J. R., Robinson, R. G., Pearlson, G. D., Rao, K., and Price, T. R. (1983): Mood change following bilateral hemisphere brain injury. *Br. J. Psychiatry*, 143:266–273.

Lishman, W. A. (1966): Psychiatric disability after head injury: The significance of brain damage. *Proc. R. Soc. Med.*, 59:261–266.

Lishman, W. A. (1968): Brain damage in relation to psychiatric disability after head injury. *Br. J. Psychiatry*, 114:373–410.

Lishman, W. A. (1969): Split minds: A review of the results of brain bisection in man. *Br. J. Hosp. Med.*, 7:477–484.

Lishman, W. A. (1978): *Organic Psychiatry. The Psychological Consequences of Cerebral Disorder*. Blackwell, Oxford.

Livingston, K. E. (1969): The frontal lobes revisited: The case for a second look. *Arch. Neurol.*, 20:90–95.

Livingston, K. E. (1977): Limbic system dysfunction induced by "kindling": Its significance for psychiatry. In: *Neurosurgical Treatment in Psychiatry, Pain, and Epilepsy*, edited by W. H. Sweet, S. Obrador, and J. G. Martin-Rodriguez, pp. 63–75. University Park Press, Baltimore.

Livingston, K. E., and Escobar, A. (1973): Tentative limbic system models for certain patterns of psychiatric disorders. In: *Surgical Approaches in Psychiatry*, edited by L. V. Laitinen and K. E. Livingston, pp. 245–252. University Park Press, Baltimore.

Loeb (1886): Biträge zur Physiologie des Grosshirns. *Pflugers Arch.*, 39. Referenced in Bianchi, L. (1922): *The Mechanism of the Brain and the Functions of the Frontal Lobes*. William Wood, New York.

Logue, V., Durward, M., Pratt, R. T. C., Piercy, M., and Nixon, W. L. B. (1968): The quality of survival after rupture of an anterior cerebral aneurysm. *Br. J. Psychiatry*, 114:137–160.

Long, C. J., Pueschel, K., and Hunter, S. E. (1978): Assessment of the effects of cingulate gyrus lesions by neuropsychological techniques. *J. Neurosurg.*, 49:264–271.

Luciani (1912): *Tratto di Fisiologia*, Vol III. Referenced in Bianchi, L. (1922): *The Mechanism of the Brain and the Functions of the Frontal Lobes*. William Wood, New York.

Lugaro (1908): Presented to the Congress of the Society of Neurology, Naples.

Luria, A. R. (1960): Verbal regulation of behaviour. In: *The Central Nervous System and Behavior, Third Macy Conference*, edited by M. A. B. Brazier, pp. 359–423. Madison Printing Co., Madison, New Jersey.

Luria, A. R. (1965): Two kinds of motor perseveration in massive injury of the frontal lobes. *Brain*, 88:1–10.

Luria, A. R. (1966): *Human Brain and Psychological Processes*. Harper & Row, New York.

Luria, A. R. (1966/1980): *Higher Cortical Functions in Man*. Basic Books, New York.

Luria, A. R. (1967): The regulative function of speech in its development and dissolution. In: *Research in Verbal Behavior and Some Neurophysiological Implications*, edited by K. Salzinger and S. Salzinger, pp. 405–422. Academic Press, New York.

Luria, A. R. (1969): Frontal lobe syndromes. In: *Handbook of Clinical Neurology*, Vol. 2, edited by P. J. Vinken and G. W. Bruyn, pp. 725–757. North Holland, Amsterdam.

Luria, A. R. (1970a): The functional organization of the brain. *Sci. Am.*, 222:66–78.

Luria, A. R. (1970b): *Traumatic Aphasia: Its Syndromes, Psychology and Treatment*. Mouton, The Hague.

Luria, A. R. (1973a): *The Working Brain. An Introduction to Neuropsychology*, translated by B. Haigh. Basic Books, New York.

Luria, A. R. (1973b): The frontal lobes and the regulation of behavior. In: *Psychophysiology of the Frontal Lobes*, edited by K. H. Pribram and A. R. Luria, pp. 3–26. Academic Press, New York.

Luria, A. R., and Homskaya, E. D. (1964): Disturbance in the regulative role of speech with frontal lobe lesions. In: *The Frontal Granular Cortex and Behavior*, edited by J. M. Warren and K. Akert, pp. 353–371. McGraw-Hill, New York.

Luria, A. R., Homskaya E. D., Blinkov, S. M., and Critchley, M. (1967): Impaired selectivity of mental processes in association with a lesion of the frontal lobe. *Neuropsychologia*, 5:105–117.

Luria, A. R., Karpov, B. A., and Yarbuss, A. L. (1966): Disturbances of active visual perception with lesions of the frontal lobes. *Cortex*, 2:202–212.

Luria, A. R., Pribram, K. H., and Homskaya, E. D. (1964): An experimental analysis of the behavioral disturbance produced by a left frontal arachnoidal endothelioma (meningioma). *Neuropsychologia*, 2:257–280.

Luria, A. R., and Tsvetkova, L. S. (1964): The programming of construction activity in local brain injuries. *Neuropsychologia*, 2:95–107.

MacLean, P. D. (1949): Psychosomatic disease and "the visceral brain," recent developments bearing on Papez theory of emotion. *Psychosom. Med.*, 11:338–353.

Magoun, H. W. (1963): *The Waking Brain*. Charles C Thomas, Springfield, Illinois.

Mahoudeau, D., David, M., and Lecoeur, J. (1951): Un nouveau cas d'agraphie sans aphasie, révélatrice d'une tumeur métastatique du pied de la deuxième circonvolution frontale gauche. *Rev. Neurol. (Paris)*, 85:159–161.

Maioli, M. G., Squatrito, S., Galletti, C., Battaglini, P. P., and Sanseverino, E. R. (1983): Cortico-cortical connections from the visual region of the superior temporal sulcus to frontal eye field in the macaque. *Brain Res.*, 265:294–299.

Malamud, N. (1957): *Atlas of Neuropathology*. University of California Press, Berkeley.

Malmo, R. B. (1942): Interference factors in delayed response in monkeys after removal of frontal lobes. *J. Neurophysiol.*,5:295–308.

Malmo, R. B. (1948): Psychological aspects of frontal gyrectomy and frontal lobotomy in mental patients. *Res. Publ. Assoc. Res. Nerv. Ment. Dis.*, 27:537–564.

Malmo, R. B., and Amsel, A. (1948): Anxiety-produced interference in serial rote learning with observations on rote learning after partial frontal lobectomy. *J. Exp. Psychol.*, 38:440–454.

Margolin, D. I. (1978): The hyperkinetic child syndrome and brain monoamines: Pharmacology and therapeutic implications. *J. Clin. Psychiatry*, 39:120–123.

Marie, P. (1906): Révision de la question de l'aphasie. *Sem. Med.*, 26:241–247, 493–500, 565–571.

Marie, P., and Foix, C. (1917): Les aphasies de guerre. *Rev. Neurol. (Paris)*, 24:53–87.

Marino, R., Jr. (1977): Stereotactic anatomy and vascularization of cingulate gyrus and adjacent areas. In: *Neurosurgical Treatment in Psychiatry, Pain, and Epilepsy*, edited by W. H. Sweet, S. Obrador, and J. G. Martin-Rodriquez, pp. 321–332. University Park Press, Baltimore.

Markovitsch, H. J. (1984): The frontal eye fields in mammals: A comment on Crowne. *Psychol. Bull.*, 95:327–331.

Markowska, A., and Lukaszewska, I. (1980): Emotional reactivity after frontomedial cortical neostriatal or hippocampal lesions in rats. *Acta Neurobiol. Exp. (Warsz)*, 40:881–893.

Martin, A. D. (1974): Some objections to the term apraxia of speech. *J. Speech Hear. Disord.*, 39:53–64.

Martin, A. D. (1975): Reply to Aten, Darley, Deal and Johns. *J. Speech Hear. Disord.*, 40:420–422.

Masdeu, J. C. (1980): Aphasia after infarction of the left supplementary motor area. *Neurology (NY)*, 30:359.

Masdeu, J. C., Schoene, W. C., and Funkenstein, H. (1978): Aphasia following infarction of the left supplementary motor area. *Neurology (NY)*, 28:1220–1223.

Maslow, A. R. (1955): The effect of prefrontal lobotomy upon abstract behavior. *J. Clin. Psychol.*, 11:407–409.

Mason, S. T. (1981): Noradrenaline in the brain: Progress in theories of behavioural function. *Prog. Neurobiol.*, 16:263–303.

Mastaglia, F. L., and Cala, L. A. (1980): Computed tomography of the brain in multiple sclerosis. *Trends Neurosci.*, 3:16–20.

Masterton, B., and Skeen, L. C. (1972): Origins of anthropoid intelligence. *J. Comp. Physiol. Psychol.*, 81:423–433.

Mateer, C. (1978): Impairments of nonverbal oral movements after left hemisphere damage: A followup analysis of errors. *Brain Lang.*, 6:334–341.

Mateer, C., and Kimura, D. (1977): Impairment of nonverbal oral movements in aphasia. *Brain Lang.*, 4:262–276.

Mattes, J. A. (1980): The role of frontal lobe dysfunction in childhood hyperkinesis. *Compr. Psychiatry*, 21:358–369.

Mayer-Gross, W. (1936): Further observations on apraxia. *J. Ment. Sci.*, 82:744–762.

Mazziotta, J. (1986): Tracer kinetic studies of cerebral and myocardial function: Positron computed tomography and autoradiography. In: *Principles of PET and Autoradiography in the Study of Cerebral and Myocardial Function*, edited by M. Phelps, J. Mazziotta, and S. Heinz. Raven Press, New York *(in press)*.

McFie, J. (1969): The diagnostic significance of disorders of higher nervous activity: Syndromes related to frontal, temporal, parietal and occipital lesions. In: *Handbook of Clinical Neurology, Vol. 4: Disorders of Speech, Perception and Symbolic Behavior*, edited by P. J. Vinken and G. W. Bruyn, pp. 1–12. North Holland, Amsterdam.

McFie, J., and Piercy, M. F. (1952a): The relation of laterality of lesion to performance on Weigl's Sorting Test. *J. Ment. Sci.*, 98:299–305.

McFie, J., and Piercy, M. F. (1952b): Intellectual impairment with localized cerebral lesions. *Brain*, 75:292–311.

McFie, J., and Thompson, J. A. (1972): Picture arrangement: A measure of frontal lobe function? *Br. J. Psychiatry*, 121:547–552.

McGeer, P. L., and McGeer, E. G. (1977): Possible changes in striatal and limbic cholinergic systems in schizophrenia. *Arch. Gen. Psychiatry*, 34:1319–1323.

McGhie, A., and Chapman, J. (1961): Disorders of attention and perception in early schizophrenia. *Br. J. Med. Psychol.*, 34:103–116.

McGhie, A., Chapman, J., and Lawson, J. S. (1965): The effect of distraction on schizophrenic performance. I. Perception and immediate memory. *Br. J. Psychiatry*, 111:383–390.

McGinty, D. J., and Siegel, J. M. (1983): Sleep states. In: *Handbook of Behavioral Neurobiology, Vol. 6: Motivation*, edited by E. Satinoff and E. Teitelbaum, pp. 105–181. Plenum, New York.

McGlone, J. (1980): Sex differences in human brain asymmetry: A critical survey. *Behav. Brain Sci.*, 3:215–263.

McHugh, P. R., and Folstein, M. F. (1975): Psychiatric syndromes of Huntington's chorea: A clinical and phenomenologic study. In: *Psychiatric Aspects of Neurologic Disease*, Vol. 1, edited by D. F. Benson and D. Blumer, pp. 267–286. Grune & Stratton, New York.

McKay, S., and Golden, C. J. (1979): Empirical derivation of neuropsychological scales for localization of brain damage using the Luria-Nebraska Neuropsychological test Battery. *Clin. Neuropsychol.*, 1:1–5.

McMenemey, W. H. (1958): The dementias and progressive diseases of the basal ganglia. In: *Neuropathology*, edited by J. G. Greenfield, W. Blackwood, A. Meyer, W. H. McMenemey, and R. M. Norman, pp. 475–528. Edward Arnold, London.

McReynolds, P. (1960): Anxiety, perception and schizophrenia. In: *The Etiology of Schizophrenia*, edited by D. D. Jackson, pp. 248–292. Basic Books, New York.

Medina, R. F., Pearson, J. S., and Buchstein, H. F. (1954): The long term evaluation of prefrontal lobotomy in chronic psychotics. *J. Nerv. Ment. Dis.*, 119:23–30.

Meichenbaum, D., and Cameron, R. (1973): Training schizophrenics to talk to themselves: A means of developing attentional controls. *Behav. Ther.*, 4:515–534.

Meichenbaum, D., and Goodman, J. (1971): Training impulsive children to talk to themselves: A means of developing self-control. *J. Abnorm. Psychol.*, 77:115–126.

Mercer, B., Wapner, W., Gardner, H., and Benson, D. F. (1977): A study of confabulation. *Arch. Neurol.*, 34:429–433.

Messimy, R. (1948): Faits expérimentaux et cliniques, concernant les fonctions des lobes préfrontaux. *Ann. Med.*, 49:69–85.

Mesulam, M-M. (1981): A cortical network for directed attention and unilateral neglect. *Ann. Neurol.*, 10:309–325.

Mesulam, M. M., and Geschwind, N. (1978): On the possible role of neocortex and its limbic connections in the process of attention and schizophrenia: Clinical cases of inattention in man and experimental anatomy in monkey. *J. Psychiatr. Res.*, 14:249–259.

Mesulam, M. M., Waxman, S. G., Geschwind, N., and Sabin, T. D. (1976): Acute confusional states with right middle cerebral artery infarctions. *J. Neurol. Neurosurg. Psychiatry*, 39:84–89.

Metter, E. J., Riege, W. H., Hanson, W. R., Phelps, M. E., and Kuhl, D. E. (1984): Local cerebral metabolic rates of glucose in movement and language disorders from positron tomography. *Am. J. Physiol.*, 246:R897–R900.

Mettler, F. A., editor, Columbia-Greystone Associates (1949): *Selective Partial Ablation of the Frontal Cortex: A Correlative Study of Its Effects on Human Psychotic Subjects*. Hoeber, New York.

Mettler, F. A. (1952): *Psychosurgical Problems*. Blakiston, Philadelphia.

Meyer, A. (1974): The frontal lobe syndrome, the aphasias and related conditions: A contribution to the history of cortical localization. *Brain*, 97:565–600.

Meyer, A., and Beck, E. (1954): *Prefrontal Leucotomy and Related Operations*. Oliver & Boyd, London.

Meyer, G., McElhaney, M., Martin, W., and McGraw, C. P. (1973): Stereotactic cingulotomy with results of acute stimulation and serial psychological testing. In: *Surgical Approaches in Psychiatry*, edited by L. V. Laitinen and K. E. Livingston, pp. 39–58. University Park Press, Baltimore.

Meyer, J. S., and Barron, D. W. (1960): Apraxia of gait: A clinicophysiological study. *Brain*, 83:261–284.

Meyer, V. (1960): Psychological effects of brain damage. In: *Handbook of Abnormal Psychology: An Experimental Approach*, edited by H. J. Eysenck, pp. 529–565. Basic Books, New York.

Meynert, T. (1884): *Psychiatrie Klinik der Erkrankungen des Vordeshirns Erst Halfe*. Braumuller, Vienna.

Miller, G. A., Galanter, E. H., and Pribram, K. H. (1960): *Plans and the Structure of Behavior*. Holt, Rinehart, & Winston, New York.

Milner, A. D., Foreman, N. P., and Goodale, M. A. (1978): Go-left go-right discrimination performance and distractibility following lesions of prefrontal cortex or superior colliculus in stumptail macaques. *Neuropsychologia*, 16:381–390.

Milner, B. (1962): Laterality effects in audition. In: *Interhemispheric Relations and Cerebral Dominance*, edited by V. B. Mountcastle, pp. 177–195. Johns Hopkins Press, Baltimore.

Milner, B. (1963): Effects of different brain lesions on card sorting: The role of the frontal lobes. *Arch. Neurol.*, 9:90–100.

Milner, B. (1964): Some effects of frontal lobectomy in man. In: *The Frontal Granular Cortex and Behavior*, edited by J. M. Warren and K. Akert, pp. 313–334. McGraw-Hill, New York.

Milner, B. (1965): Visually-guided maze learning in man: Effects of bilateral hippocampal, bilateral frontal and unilateral cerebral lesions. *Neuropsychologia*, 3:317–338.

Milner, B. (1971): Interhemispheric differences in the localization of psychological processes in man. *Br. Med. Bull.*, 27:272–277.

Milner, B. (1974): Hemispheric specialization: Scope and limits. In: *The Neurosciences: Third Study Program*, edited by F. O. Schmitt and F. G. Worden, pp. 75–89. MIT Press, Cambridge, Massachusetts.

Milner, B. (1982): Some cognitive effects of frontal lobe lesions in man. In: *The Neuropsychology of Cognitive Function*, edited by D. E. Broadbent and L. Weiskrantz, pp. 211–226. The Royal Society, London.

Milner, B., and Petrides, M. (1984): Behavioural effects of frontal-lobe lesions in man. *Trends Neurosci.*, 7:403–407.

Milner, B., and Teuber, H-L. (1968): Alteration of perception and memory in man: Reflections on methods. In: *Analysis of Behavioral Changes*, edited by L. Weiskrantz, pp. 268–375. Harper & Row, New York.

Mirsky, A. F., and Orzack, M. H. (1977): Final report on psychosurgery pilot study. In: *Appendix—Psychosurgery: The National Commission for the Protection of Human Subjects Biomedical and Behavioral Research*, pp. II-1–168. DHEW Publication No. (OS)77-0002, Washington, D.C.

Mirsky, A. F., Primac, D. W., Marsan, C. A., Rosvold, H. E., and Stevens, J. R. (1960): A comparison of the psychological test performance of patients with focal and non-focal epilepsy. *Exp. Neurol.*, 2:75–89.

Mishkin, M. (1964): Perseveration of central sets after frontal lesions in monkeys. In: *The Frontal Granular Cortex and Behavior*, edited by J. M. Warren and K. Akert, pp. 219–241. McGraw-Hill, New York.

Mishkin, M. (1982): A memory system in the monkey. In: *The Neuropsychology of Cognitive Function*, edited by D. E. Broadbent and L. Weiskantz, pp. 85–95. The Royal Society, London.

Mishkin, M., and Bachevalier, J. (1983): Object recognition impaired by ventromedial but not dorsolateral prefrontal cortical lesions in monkeys. *Soc. Neurosci. Abstr.*, 9:29.

Mishkin, M., and Pribram, K. H. (1956): Analysis of the effects of frontal lesions in the monkey. II. Variations of delayed response. *J. Comp. Physiol. Psychol.*, 49:36–40.

Mishkin, M., Vest, B., Waxler, M., and Rosvold, E. (1969): A re-examination of the effects of frontal lesions on object alternation. *Neuropsychologia*, 7:357–363.

Mitchell-Heggs, N., Kelly, D., and Richardson, A. (1976): Stereotactic limbic leucotomy—a follow-up at 16 months. *Br. J. Psychiatry*, 128:226–240.

Mitchell-Heggs, N., Kelly, D., and Richardson, A. E. (1977): Stereotactic limbic leucotomy: Clinical, psychological and physiological assessment at 16 months. In: *Neurosurgical Treatment in Psychiatry, Pain, and Epilepsy*, edited by W. H. Sweet, S. Obrador, and J. G. Martin-Rodriquez, pp. 367–379. University Park Press, Baltimore.

Mohr, J. P. (1973): Rapid amelioration of motor aphasia. *Arch. Neurol.*, 28:77–82.

Mohr, J. P. (1976): Broca's area and Broca's aphasia. In: *Studies in Neurolinguistics*, Vol. 1, edited by H. Whitaker and H. Whitaker, pp. 201–236. Academic Press, New York.

Mohr, J. P., Pessin, M. S., Finkelstein, S., Funkenstein, H. H., Duncan, G. W., and Davis, K. R. (1978): Broca aphasia: Pathologic and clinical aspects. *Neurology (NY)*, 28:311–324.

Molliver, M. E., Grzanna, R., Lidov, H. G. W., Morrison, J. H., and Olschowka, J. A. (1982): Monoamine systems in the cerebral cortex. In: *Cytochemical Methods in Neuroanatomy*, edited by V. Chan-Palay and B. Palay, pp. 255–277. Alan R. Liss, New York.

Monakow, C. V. (1905): *Gehirnpathologie*. 2nd Ed. Holder, Vienna.

Money, J., Alexander, D., and Walter, H. T., Jr. (1965): *Manual for a Standardized Road-Map Test of Direction Sense*. Johns Hopkins University Press, Baltimore.

Moniz, E. (1937): Prefrontal leucotomy in treatment of mental disorders. *Am. J. Psychiatry*, 93:1379–1385.

Monrad-Krohn, G. H. (1947): Dysprosody or altered "melody of language." *Brain*, 70:405–415.

Monroe, R. R. (1970): *Episodic Behavioral Disorders*. Harvard, Cambridge, Massachusetts.

Moore, R. Y. (1982): Catecholamine neuron systems in brain. *Ann. Neurol.*, 12:321–327.

Mora, F., Avrith, D. B., Phillips, A. G., and Rolls, E. T. (1979): Effects of satiety on self-stimulation of the orbitofrontal cortex in the rhesus monkey. *Neurosci. Lett.*, 13:141–145.

Mora, F., Avrith, D. B., and Rolls, E. T. (1980): An electrophysiological and behavioural study of self-stimulation in the orbitofrontal cortex of the rhesus monkey. *Brain Res. Bull.*, 5:111–115.

Mori, E., and Yamadori, A. (1982): Compulsive manipulation of tools and pathological grasp phenomenon. *Clin. Neurol.*, 22:329–335.

Morlaas, J. (1928): *Contribution à l'Etude de l'Apraxie*, edited by A. Legrand. These, Paris.

Morrison, J. H., and Molliver, M. E. (1980): Cortical monoamine levels following frontal cortex ablation: A biochemical analysis using HPLC. *Soc. Neurosci. Abstr.*, 6:351.

Moruzzi, G., and Magoun, H. W. (1949): Brainstem reticular formation and activation of the EEG. *Electroencephalogr. Clin. Neurophysiol.*, 1:455–473.

Moscovitch, M. (1979): Information processing and the cerebral hemispheres. In: *Handbook of Behavioral Neurobiology, Vol. 2: Neuropsychology*, edited by M. S. Gazzaniga, pp. 379–446. Plenum, New York.

Moscovitch, M. (1982): Multiple dissociations of function in amnesia. In: *Human Memory and Amnesia*, edited by L. S. Cermak, pp. 337–370. Lawrence Erlbaum, Hillsdale, New Jersey.

Moscovitch, M., and Winocur, G. (1983): Contextual cues and release from proactive inhibition in young and old people. *Can. J. Psychol.*, 37:331–344.

Mountcastle, V. B. (1978): Brain mechanisms for directed attention. *J. R. Soc. Med.*, 71:14–28.

Mountcastle, V. B., Andersen, R. A., and Motter, B. C. (1981): The influence of attentive fixation upon the excitability of the light-sensitive neurons of the posterior parietal cortex. *J. Neurosci.*, 1:1218–1235.

Mountcastle, V. B., Lynch, J. C., Georgopoulos, A., Sakata, H., and Acuna, C. (1975): Posterior parietal association cortex of the monkey: Command functions for operations within extrapersonal space. *J. Neurophysiol.*, 38:871–908.

Muakassa, K. F., and Strick, P. L. (1979): Frontal lobe inputs to primary motor cortex: Evidence for four somatotopically organized "premotor" areas. *Brain Res.*, 177:183–188.

Munk, H. (1881): *Uber die Funktion der Grosshirnrinde: Gerammelte Mitteilunger den Jahren.* Hirschwald, Berlin.

Munk, H. (1890): *Ueber die Functionen der Grosshirnrinde.* Hirschwald, Berlin.

Murray, H. A. (1943): *Thematic Apperception Test.* Harvard University Press, Cambridge, Massachusetts.

Näätänen, R. (1982): Processing negativity: An evoked potential reflection of selective attention. *Psychol. Bull.*, 92:605–640.

Naeser, M. A. (1983): CT scan lesion size and lesion locus in cortical and subcortical aphasias. In: *Localization in Neuropsychology*, edited by A. Kertesz, pp. 63–119. Academic Press, New York.

Naeser, M. A., Alexander, M. P., Helm-Estabrooks, N., Levine, H. L., Laughlin, S. A., and Geschwind, N. (1982): Aphasia with predominantly subcortical lesion sites: Description of three capsular/putaminal aphasia syndromes. *Arch. Neurol.*, 39:2–14.

Naeser, M. A., and Hayward, R. W. (1978): Correlation between CT scan findings and the Boston Diagnostic Aphasia Exam. *Neurology (NY)*, 28:545–551.

Naeser, M. A., Hayward, R. W., Laughlin, S. A., and Zatz, L. M. (1981): Quantitative CT scan studies in aphasia. I. Infarct size and CT numbers. *Brain Lang.*, 12:140–164.

Naeser, M. A., Levine, H. L., Benson, D. F., Stuss, D. T., and Weir, W. S. (1981): Frontal leukotomy size and hemispheric asymmetries on computerized tomographic scans of schizophrenics with variable recovery. *Arch. Neurol.*, 38:30–37.

Nauta, W. J. H. (1964): Some efferent connections of the prefrontal cortex in the monkey. In: *The Frontal Granular Cortex and Behavior*, edited by J. M. Warren and K. Akert, pp. 397–409. McGraw-Hill, New York.

Nauta, W. J. H. (1971): The problem of the frontal lobe: A reinterpretation. *J. Psychiatr. Res.*, 8:167–187.

Nauta, W. J. H. (1972): Neural associations of the frontal cortex. *Acta Neurobiol. Exp. (Warsz.)*, 32:125–140.

Nauta, W. J. H. (1973): Connections of the frontal lobe with the limbic system. In: *Surgical Approaches in Psychiatry*, edited by L. V. Laitinen and K. E. Livingston, pp. 303–314. University Park Press, Baltimore.

Nelson, H. E. (1976): A modified card sorting test sensitive to frontal lobe defects. *Cortex*, 12:313–324.

New Webster's Dictionary (1975): Consolidated Book Publishers, New York.

Newcombe, F. (1969): *Missile Wounds of the Brain: A Study of Psychological Deficits*. Oxford University Press, London.

Newell, A. (1977): You can't play 20 questions with nature and win: Projective comments on the papers of this symposium. In: *Visual Information Processing*, edited by W. G. Chase, pp. 283–308. Academic Press, New York.

Nichols, I. C., and Hunt, J. M. (1940): A case of partial bilateral frontal lobectomy: Psychopathological study. *Am. J. Psychiatry*, 96:1063–1087.

Nielsen, J. M. (1936/1962): *Agnosia, Apraxia and Aphasia: Their Value in Cerebral Localization*. Hafner, New York.

Noguchi, H., and Moore, J. W. (1913): The demonstration of treponema pallidum in the brain in cases of general paralysis. *J. Exp. Med.*, 17:232–238.

Norman, D. A. (1981): Categorization of action slips. *Psychol. Rev.*, 88:1–15.

Ojemann, G., Fedio, P., and Van Buren, J. (1968): Amenia from pulvinar and subcortical parietal stimulation. *Brain*, 91:99–116.

Ojemann, G., and Ward, A. (1971): Speech representation in ventrolateral thalamus. *Brain*, 94:669–680.

Ojemann, G. A., and Whitaker, H. A. (1978): Language localization and variability. *Brain Lang.*, 6:239–260.

Oldendorf, W. H. (1980): *The Quest for an Image of the Brain*. Raven Press, New York.

Orbach, J., and Fischer, G. J. (1959): Bilateral resections of frontal granular cortex: Factors influencing delayed response and discrimination performance in monkeys. *Arch. Neurol.*, 1:78–86.

Orgogozo, J. M., and Larsen, B. (1979): Activation of the supplementary motor area during voluntary movement in man suggests it works as a supra-motor area. *Science*, 206:847–850.

Orzhekhovskaya, N. S. (1981): Fronto-striatal relationships in primate ontogeny. *Neurosci. Behav. Physiol.*, 11:379–385.

Oscar-Berman, M. (1973): Hypothesis testing and focusing behavior during concept formation by amnesic Korsakoff patients. *Neuropsychologia*, 11:191–198.

Oscar-Berman, M. (1975): The effects of dorsolateral-frontal and ventrolateral-orbitofrontal lesions on spatial discrimination learning and delayed response in two modalities. *Neuropsychologia*, 13:237–246.

Oscar-Berman, M. (1978): The effects of dorsolateral-frontal and ventrolateral-orbitofrontal lesions on nonspatial test performance. *Neuropsychologia*, 16:259–267.

Osmond, H. F. (1971): Personal recollections of lobotomy: In: *The Surgical Control of Behavior: A Symposium*, edited by A. Winter, pp. 38–41. Charles C Thomas, Springfield, Illinois.

Oxford English Dictionary: Compacted Edition (1979): Oxford University Press, London.

Paillard, J. (1982): Apraxia and the neurophysiology of motor control. In: *The Neuropsychology of Cognitive Function*, edited by D. E. Broadbent and L. Weiskrantz, pp. 111–134. The Royal Society, London.

Pandya, D. N., Dye, P., and Butters, N. (1971): Efferent cortico-cortical projections of the prefrontal cortex in the rhesus monkey. *Brain Res.*, 31:35–46.

Pandya, D. N., Karol, E. A., and Heilbronn, D. (1971): The topographic distribution of interhemispheric projections in the corpus callosum of the rhesus monkey. *Brain Res.*, 32:31–43.

Pandya, D. N., and Kuypers, H. G. J. M. (1969): Cortico-cortical connections in the rhesus monkey. *Brain Res.*, 13:13–36.

Pandya, D. N., Van Hoesen, G. W., and Mesulam, M-M. (1981): Efferent connections of the cingulate gyrus in the rhesus monkey. *Exp. Brain Res.*, 42:319–330.

Papez, J. W. (1937): A proposed mechanism of emotion. *Arch. Neurol. Psychiatry*, 38:725–743.

Partridge, M. (1950): *Pre-frontal Leucotomy*. Blackwell, Oxford.

Passingham, R. E. (1970): The neurological basis of introversion-extraversion: Gray's theory. *Behav. Res. Ther.*, 8:353–366.

Passingham, R. E. (1972): Non-reversal shifts after selective prefrontal ablations in monkeys (Macaca mulatta). *Neuropsychologia*, 10:41–46.

Paterson, A., and Zangwill, O. L. (1944): Disorders of visual space perception associated with lesions of the right cerebral hemisphere. *Brain*, 67:331–358.

Pease, D. M., and Goodglass, H. (1978): The effects of cuing on picture naming in aphasia. *Cortex*, 14:178–189.

Peled, R., Harnes, B., Borovich, B., and Sharf, B. (1984): Speech arrest and supplementary motor area seizures. *Neurology (NY)*, 34:110–111.

Penfield, W., and Evans, J. (1935): The frontal lobe in man: A clinical study of maximum removals. *Brain*, 58:115–133.

Penfield, W., and Jasper, H. (1954): *Epilepsy and the Functional Anatomy of the Human Brain*. Little, Brown, Boston.

Penfield, W., and Kristiansen, K. (1951): *Epileptic Seizure Patterns*. Charles C Thomas, Springfield, Illinois

Penfield, W., and Roberts, L. (1959): *Speech and Brain Mechanisms*. Princeton University Press, Princeton, New Jersey.

Penfield, W., and Welch, K. (1951): The supplementary motor area of the cerebral cortex: A clinical and experimental study. *AMA Arch. Neurol. Psychiatry*, 66:289–317.

Perlmutter, D., and Rhoton, Jr., A. L. (1978): Microsurgical anatomy of the distal anterior cerebral artery. *J. Neurosurg.*, 49:204–228.

Perret, E. (1974): The left frontal lobe of man and the suppression of habitual responses in verbal categorical behaviour. *Neuropsychologia*, 12:323–330.

Peterson, G. C. (1975): Organic brain syndromes associated with brain trauma. In: *Comprehensive Textbook of Psychiatry/II*, Vol. 1, 2nd Ed., edited by A. M. Freedman, H. I. Kaplan, and B. J. Sadock, pp. 1093–1094. Williams & Wilkins, Baltimore.

Peterson, H. O., and Kieffer, S. A. (1970): Neuroradiology. In: *Clinical Neurology*, Vol. 1, Chap. 2, edited by A. B. Baker and L. H. Baker. Harper & Row, Philadelphia.

Peterson, L., and Peterson, M. J. (1959): Short-term retention of individual verbal items. *J. Exp. Psychol.*, 58:193–198.

Petrides, M. (1982): Motor conditional associative-learning after selective prefrontal lesions in the monkey. *Behav. Brain Res.*, 5:407–413.

Petrides, M. (1985): Deficits on conditional associative-learning tasks after frontal- and temporal-lobe lesions in man. *Neuropsychologia*, 23:601–614.

Petrides, M., and Milner, B. (1982): Deficits on subject-ordered tasks after frontal- and temporal-lobe lesions in man. *Neuropsychologia*, 20:249–262.

Petrides, M., and Pandya, D. N. (1984): Projections to the frontal cortex from the posterior parietal region in the rhesus monkey. *J. Comp. Neurol.*, 228:105–116.

Petrie, A. (1952a): A comparison of the psychological effects of different types of operations on the frontal lobes. *J. Ment. Sci.*, 98:326–329.

Petrie, A. (1952b): *Personality and the Frontal Lobes*. Blakiston, New York.

Phelps, M. E., Huang, S. C., Hoffman, E. J., Selin, C., Sokoloff, L., and Kuhl, D. E. (1979): Tomographic measurement of local cerebral glucose metabolic rate in humans with (F-18) 2-fluoro-2-deoxy-D-glucose: Validation of method. *Ann. Neurol.*, 6:371–388.

Phelps, M. E., Mazziotta, J., Baxter, L., and Gerner, R. (1984): Positron emission tomographic study of affective disorders: Problems and strategies. *Ann. Neurol.* (Suppl.), 15:S149–S156.

Phillips, C. G., Zeki, S., and Barlow, H. B. (1984): Localization of function in the cerebral cortex: Past, present and future. *Brain*, 107:328–361.

Pick, A. (1903): On reduplicative paramnesia. *Brain*, 26:260–267.

Picton, T. W., and Hink, R. F. (1974): Evoked potentials: How? What? and Why? *Am. J. EEG Technol.*, 14:9–44.

Picton, T. W., Stuss, D. T., and Marshall, K. C. (1986): Attention and the brain. In: *The Brain, Cognition and Education*, edited by S. L. Friedman, K. A. Klivington, and R. W. Peterson. Academic Press, New York, pp. 19–79.

Pinéas, H. (1924): Hirnbefunde bei apraxie. *Zentralbl. Ges. Neurol. Psychiatr.*, 35:446. Referenced in Fisher, M. (1956): Left hemiplegia and motor impersistence. *J. Nerv. Ment. Dis.*, 123:201–218.

Pippard, J. (1955): Personality changes after rostral leucotomy: A comparison with standard prefrontal leucotomy. *J. Ment. Sci.*, 101:774–787.

Pisa, M., and Fibiger, H. C. (1983): Evidence against a role of the rat's dorsal noradrenergic bundle in selective attention and place memory. *Brain Res.*, 272:319–329.

Plum, F., and Posner, J. B. (1980): *The Diagnosis of Stupor and Coma*, 3rd Ed. Davis, Philadelphia.

Poeck, K., and Kerchensteiner, M. (1975): Analysis of the sequential motor events in oral apraxia. In: *Cerebral Localization*, edited by K. J. Zulch, O. Creutzfeldt, and B. C. Galbraith, pp. 98–109. Springer-Verlag, Berlin.

Pohl, W. (1973): Dissociation of spatial discrimination deficits following frontal and parietal lesions in monkeys. *J. Comp. Physiol. Psychol.*, 82:227–239.

Polimanti (1906): *Contributo alla fisiologia ed all'anatomia dei lobi frontali*. Referenced in Bianchi, L. (1922): *The Mechanism of the Brain and the Functions of the Frontal Lobes*. William Wood, New York.

Pollitt, J. D. (1960): Natural history studies in mental illness: A discussion based on a pilot study of obsessional states. *J. Ment. Sci.*, 106:93–112.

Polya, G. (1945): *How to Solve It*. Princeton University Press, Princeton, New Jersey.

Pontius, A. A. (1972): Neurological aspects in some type of delinquency especially among juveniles: Toward a neurological model of ethical action. *Adolescence*, 7:289–308.

Pontius, A. A., and Yudowitz, B. S. (1980): Frontal lobe system dysfunction in some criminal actions as shown in the narratives test. *J. Nerv. Ment. Dis.*, 168:111–117.

Pool, J. L., and Correll, J. W. (1958): Psychiatric symptoms masking brain tumor. *J. Med. Soc. N.J.*, 55:4–9.

Pool, J. L., Heath, R. G., and Weber, J. J. (1949): Topectomy: Surgical technique, psychiatric indications and postoperative management. *J. Nerv. Ment. Dis.*, 110:464–477.

Poppen, J. L. (1948): Technic of prefrontal lobotomy. *J. Neurosurg.*, 5:514–520.

Poppen, R. L., Pribram, K. H., and Robinson, R. S. (1965): Effects of frontal lobotomy in man on the performance of a multiple choice task. *Exp. Neurol.*, 11:217–229.

Popper, K. R., and Eccles, J. C. (1977): *The Self and Its Brain*. Springer-Verlag, Berlin.

Porrino, L. J., and Goldman-Rakic, P. S. (1982): Brainstem innervation of prefrontal and anterior cingulate cortex in the rhesus monkey revealed by retrograde transport of HRP. *J. Comp. Neurol.*, 205:63–76.

Porteus, S. D. (1950): *The Porteus Maze Test and Intelligence*. Pacific Books, Palo Alto, California.

Porteus, S. D., and Diamond, A. L. (1962): Porteus Maze changes after psychosurgery. *J. Ment. Sci.*, 108:53–58.

Porteus, S. D., and Kepner, R. DeM. (1944): Mental changes after bilateral prefrontal lobotomy. *Genet. Psychol. Monogr.*, 29:4–115.

Porteus, S. D., and Peters, H. N. (1947a): Maze Test validation and psychosurgery. *Genet. Psychol. Monogr.*, 36:3–86.

Porteus, S. D., and Peters, H. N. (1947b): Psychosurgery and test validity. *J. Abnorm. Soc. Psychol.*, 42:473–475.

Potter, H., and Butters, N. (1980): An assessment of olfactory deficits in patients with damage to prefrontal cortex. *Neuropsychologia*, 18:621–628.

Potter, H., and Nauta, W. J. H. (1979): A note on the problem of olfactory associations of the orbitofrontal cortex in the monkey. *Neuroscience*, 4:361–367.

Powell, T. P. S., Cowan, W. M., and Raisman, G. (1965): The central olfactory connexions. *J. Anat.*, 99:791–813.

Powers, W. T. (1973a): *Behavior: The Control of Perception*. Aldine, Chicago.

Powers, W. T. (1973b): Feedback: Beyond behaviorism. *Science*, 179:351–356.

Pratt, R. T. C. (1951): An investigation of the psychiatric aspects of disseminated sclerosis. *J. Neurol. Neurosurg. Psychiatry*, 14:326–336.

Pribram, K. H. (1950): Some physical and pharmacological factors affecting delayed response performance of baboons following frontal lobotomy. *J. Neurophysiol.*, 13:373–382.

Pribram, K. H. (1960): The intrinsic systems of the forebrain. In: *Handbook of Physiology, Vol. II: Neurophysiology*, edited by J. Field, H. W. Magoun, and V. E. Hall, pp. 1323–1344. American Physiological Society, Washington, D.C.

Pribram, K. H. (1961): A further experimental analysis of the behavioral deficit that follows injury to the primate frontal cortex. *Exp. Neurol.*, 3:432–466.

Pribram, K. H. (1967): The new neurology and the biology of emotion: A structural approach. *Am. Psychol.*, 23:830–838.

Pribram, K. H. (1973): The primate frontal cortex—executive of the brain. In: *Psychophysiology of the Frontal Lobes*, edited by K. H. Pribram and A. R. Luria, pp. 293–314. Academic Press, New York.

Pribram, K. H., Ahumada, A., Hartog, J., and Ross, L. (1964): A progress report on the neurological processes disturbed by frontal lesions in primates. In: *The Frontal Granular Cortex and Behavior*, edited by J. M. Warren and K. Akert, pp. 28–55. McGraw-Hill, New York.

Pribram, K. H., and Luria, A. R., editors (1973): *Psychophysiology of the Frontal Lobes*. Academic Press, New York.

Pribram, K. H., and Melges, F. T. (1969): The search for control. In: *Handbook of Clinical Neurology*, edited by P. J. Vinken and G. W. Bruyn, pp. 316–342. North Holland, Amsterdam.

Pribram, K. H., and Tubbs, W. E. (1967): Short-term memory, parsing, and the primate frontal cortex. *Science*, 156:1765–1767.

Prisko, L. (1963): Short-Term Memory in Focal Cerebral Damage. Ph.D. thesis, McGill University.

Quesney, L. F., Krieger, C., Leitner, C., Gloor, P., and Olivier, A. (1984): Frontal lobe epilepsy: Clinical and electrographic presentation. In: *Advances in Epileptology: XVth Epilepsy International Symposium*, edited by R. J. Porter, R. H. Mattson, A. A. Ward Jr., and M. Dam, pp. 503–508. Raven Press, New York.

Ramier, A-M., and Hécaen, H. (1970): Rôle respectif des atteintes frontales et de la latéralisation lésionnelle dans les déficits de la "fluence verbale." *Rev. Neurol. (Paris)*, 123:17–22.

Rasmussen, T. (1963): Surgical therapy of frontal lobe epilepsy. *Epilepsia*, 4:181–198.

Rasmussen, T., and Penfield, W. (1948): Movement of head and eyes from stimulation of human frontal cortex. *Assoc. Res. Nerv. Ment. Dis.*, 27:346–361.

Redlick, F. C., and Dorsey, J. F. (1945): Denial of blindness by patients with cerebral diseases. *Arch. Neurol. Psychiatry*, 53:407–417.

Rees, W. L. (1973): The value and limitations of psychosurgery in the treatment of psychiatric illness. *Psychiatr. Neurol. Neurochir.*, 76:323–334.

Reitan, R. M. (1955): Investigation of the validity of Halstead's measures of biological intelligence. *Arch. Neurol. Psychiatry*, 73:28–35.

Reitan, R. M. (1958): Validity of the trail-making test as an indication of organic brain damage. *Percept. Mot. Skills*, 8:271–276.

Reitan, R. M. (1964): Psychological deficits resulting from cerebral lesions in man. In: *The Frontal Granular Cortex and Behavior*, edited by J. M. Warren and K. Akert, pp. 295–312. McGraw-Hill, New York.

Reitan, R. M., and Davison, L. A., editors (1974): *Clinical Neuropsychology: Current Status and Applications*. Wiley, New York.

Reitman, F. (1946): Orbital cortex syndrome following leucotomy. *Am. J. Psychiatry*, 103:238–241.

Reivich, M., Kuhl, D., Wolf, A., Greenberg, J., Phelps, M., Ido, T., Casella, V., Fowler, J., Hoffman, E., Alavi, A., Som, P., and Sokoloff, L. (1979): The 18F fluorodeoxyglucose method for the measurement of local cerebral glucose utilization in man. *Circ. Res.*, 44:127–137.

Remington, F. B., and Rubert, S. L. (1962): Why patients with brain tumors come to a psychiatric hospital: A thirty year survey. *Am. J. Psychiatry*, 119:256–257.

Richter, C. P., and Hawkes, C. D. (1939): Augmentation spontanée d'activité et de nourriture chez les rats après l'ablation des pôles frontaux du cerveau. *J. Neurol. Psychiatry*, 2:231–242.

Richter, C. P., and Hines, M. (1938): Increased spontaneous activity produced in monkeys by brain lesions. *Brain*, 61:1–16.

Rickler, K. C. (1982): Episodic dyscontrol. In: *Psychiatric Aspects of Neurologic Disease*, Vol. II, edited by D. F. Benson and D. Blumer, pp. 49–73. Grune & Stratton, New York.

Riddle, M., and Roberts, A. H. (1978): Psychosurgery and the Porteus Maze tests: Review and reanalysis of data. *Arch. Gen. Psychiatry*, 35:493–497.

Riegele, L. (1931): De Cytoarchitektonic der Felder der Brocaschen region. *J. Psychol. Neurol.*, 42:496–514.

Riklan, M., and Levita, E. (1970): Psychological studies of thalamic lesions in humans. *J. Nerv. Ment. Dis.*, 150:251–265.

Rizzolatti, G., Matelli, M., and Pavesi, G. (1983): Deficits in attention and movement following the removal of postarcuate (area 6) and prearcuate (area 8) cortex in macaque monkeys. *Brain*, 106:655–673.

Roberts, A. H. (1976): Sequelae of closed head injuries. *Proc. R. Soc. Med.*, 69:137–140.

Roberts, D. C. S., Price, M. T. C., and Fibiger, H. C. (1975): The dorsal tegmental noradrenergic projection: An analysis of its role in maze learning. *J. Comp. Physiol. Psychol.*, 90:363–372.

Robin, A., and Macdonald, D. (1975): *Lessons of Leucotomy*. Henry Kimpton, London.

Robins, L. R. (1966): *Deviant Children Grown Up: A Sociological and Psychiatric Study of Sociopathic Personality.* Williams & Wilkins, Baltimore.

Robinson, A. L., Heaton, R. K., Lehman, R. A. W., and Stilson, D. W. (1980): The utility of the Wisconsin Card Sorting Test in detecting and localizing frontal lobe lesions. *J. Consult. Clin. Psychol.*, 48:605–614.

Robinson, D. A., and Fuchs, A. F. (1969): Eye movements evoked by stimulation of frontal eye fields. *J. Neurophysiol.*, 32:637–648.

Robinson, M. F. (1946): What price lobotomy? *J. Abnorm. Soc. Psychol.*, 41:421–436.

Robinson, M. F., and Freeman, W. (1954): *Psychosurgery and the Self.* Grune & Stratton, New York.

Robinson, R. G., and Benson, D. F. (1981): Depression in aphasic patients: Frequency, severity, and clinical-pathological correlations. *Brain Lang.*, 14:282–291.

Robinson, R. G., and Bloom, F. E. (1978): Changes in posterior hypothalamic self-stimulation following experimental cerebral infarction in the rat. *J. Comp. Physiol. Psychol.*, 92:969–976.

Robinson, R. G., Bloom, F. E., and Battenberg, E. L. F. (1977): A fluorescent histochemical study of changes in noradrenergic neurons following experimental cerebral infarction in the rat. *Brain Res.*, 132:259–272.

Robinson, R. G., Kubos, K. L., Starr, L. B., Rao, K., and Price, T. R. (1984): Mood disorders in stroke patients: Importance of location of lesion. *Brain*, 107:81–93.

Robinson, R. G., and Price, T. R. (1982): Post-stroke depressive disorders: A follow-up study of 103 patients. *Stroke*, 13:635–641.

Robinson, R. G., Shoemaker, W. J., Schlumpf, M., Volk, T., and Bloom, F. E. (1975): Effect of experimental cerebral infarction in rat brain on catecholamines and behavior. *Nature*, 255:332–334.

Robinson, R. G., Starr, L. B., Kubos, K. L., and Price, T. R. (1983): A two year longitudinal study of post-stroke mood disorders: Findings during the initial evaluation. *Stroke*, 14:736–741.

Robinson, R. G., and Szetela, B. (1981): Mood change following left hemispheric brain injury. *Ann. Neurol.*, 9:447–453.

Rogozea, R., and Ungher, J. (1968): Changes in orienting activity of cat induced by chronic hippocampal lesions. *Exp. Neurol.*, 21:176–186.

Roland, P. E. (1984): Metabolic measurements of the working frontal cortex in man. *Trends Neurosci.*, 7:430–435.

Roland, P. E., Larsen, B., and Lassen, N. A. (1980a): Supplementary motor area and other cortical areas in organization of voluntary movements in man. *J. Neurophysiol.*, 43:118–136.

Roland, P. E., Skinhoj, E., and Lassen, N. A. (1980b): Different cortical areas in man in organization of voluntary movements in extrapersonal space. *J. Neurophysiol.*, 43:137–150.

Ropper, A. H. (1982): Self-grasping: A focal neurological sign. *Ann. Neurol.*, 12:575–577.

Rosati, G., and DeBastiani, P. (1979): Pure agraphia: A discrete form of aphasia. *J. Neurol. Neurosurg. Psychiatry*, 42:266–269.

Rose, F. (1908): De l'apraxie des muscles céphaliques. *Sem. Med.*, 18:193–198. Referenced in Hécaen, H. (1981): Apraxias. In: *Handbook of Clinical Neuropsychology*, edited by S. B. Filskov and T. J. Boll, pp. 257–286. Wiley-Interscience, New York.

Rosenkilde, C. E. (1979): Functional heterogeneity of the prefrontal cortex in the monkey: A review. *Behav. Neural Biol.*, 25:301–345.

Ross, E. D. (1981): The aprosodias: Functional-anatomic organization of the affective components of language in the right hemisphere. *Arch. Neurol.*, 38:561–569.

Ross, E. D., Harney, J. H., de Lacoste-Utamsing, C., and Purdy, P. D. (1981): How the brain integrates affective and propositional language in a unified behavioral function: Hypothesis based on clinicoanatomic evidences. *Arch. Neurol.*, 38:745–748.

Ross, E. D., and Mesulam, M-M. (1979): Dominant language functions of the right hemisphere? Prosody and emotional gesturing. *Arch. Neurol.*, 36:144–148.

Ross, E. D., and Rush, A. J. (1981): Diagnosis and neuroanatomical correlates of depression in brain-damaged patients: Implications for a neurology of depression. *Arch. Gen. Psychiatry*, 38:1344–1354.

Ross, E. D., and Stewart, R. M. (1981): Akinetic mutism from hypothalamic damage: Successful treatment with dopamine agonists. *Neurology (NY)*, 31:1435–1439.

Rosvold, H. E. (1972): The frontal lobe system: Cortical-subcortical interrelationships. *Acta Neurobiol. Exp. (Warsz.)*, 32:439–460.

Rosvold, H. E., Mirsky, A. F., Sarason, I., Bransome, E. D., and Beck, L. H. (1956): A continuous performance test of brain damage. *J. Consult. Psychol.*, 20:343–350.

Rosvold, H. E., and Mishkin, M. (1950): Evaluation of the effects of prefrontal lobotomy on intelligence. *Can. J. Psychol.*, 4:122–126.

Rothman, M. (1906): Lichtheimsche motorische Aphasie. *Z. Klin. Med.*, 60:87–121.

Routtenberg, A. (1978): The reward system of the brain. *Sci. Am.*, 239:154–164.

Roux, J. (1899): *Arch. Neurol. (Paris)*, 8:177. Referenced in Denny-Brown, D. (1951): The frontal lobes and their functions. In: *Modern Trends in Neurology*, edited by A. Feiling, pp. 13–89. Butterworth, London.

Rubens, A. B. (1975): Aphasia with infarction in the territory of the anterior cerebral artery. *Cortex*, 11:239–250.

Ruch, T. C., and Fetz, E. E. (1979): The cerebral cortex: Its structure and motor functions. In: *Physiology and Biophysics, Vol. 1: The Brain and Neural Function*, edited by T. C. Ruch and H. D. Patton, pp. 53–122. Saunders, Philadelphia.

Ruch, T. C., and Shenkin, H. A. (1943): The relation of area 13 on the orbital surface of frontal lobes to hyperactivity and hyperphagia in monkeys. *J. Neurophysiol.*, 6:349–360.

Rudel, R. G., and Denckla, M. B. (1974): Relation of forward and backward digit repetition to neurological impairment in children with learning disabilities. *Neuropsychologia*, 12:109–118.

Rudnick, F. D. (1982): The paranoid-erotic syndromes. In: *Extraordinary Disorders of Human Behavior*, edited by C. T. H. Friedman and R. A. Fauget, pp. 91–120. Plenum, New York.

Ruesch, J. R. (1943): Intellectual impairment in head injuries. *Am. J. Psychiatry*, 100:480–496.

Ruesch, J. R., and Moore, B. E. (1943): Measurement of intellectual functions in acute stage of head injury. *Arch. Neurol. Psychiatry*, 50:165–170.

Ruff, R. L., and Arbit, E. (1981): Aphemia resulting from a left frontal hematoma. *Neurology (NY)*, 31:353–356.

Ruff, R. L., and Volpe, B. T. (1981): Environmental reduplication associated with right frontal and parietal lobe injury. *J. Neurol. Neurosurg. Psychiatry*, 44:382–386.

Russell, E. W. (1972): WAIS factor analysis with brain-damaged subjects using criterion measures. *J. Consult. Clin. Psychol.*, 39:133–139.

Russell, E. W., Neuringer, C., and Goldstein, G. (1970): *Assessment of Brain Damage. A Neuropsychological Key Approach*. Wiley-Interscience, New York.

Russell, W. R. (1951): Disability caused by brain wounds: A review of 1,166 cases. *J. Neurol. Neurosurg. Psychiatry*, 14:35–39.

Russell, W. R., and Espir, M. L. E. (1961): *Traumatic Aphasia: A Study of Aphasia in War Wounds of the Brain*. Oxford University Press, London.

Rutter, M. (1972): *Maternal Deprivation Reassessed*. Penguin, Harmondsworth.

Rylander, G. (1939): Personality changes after operations on the frontal lobes: A clinical study of 32 cases. *Acta Psychiatr. Neurol. [Suppl.]*, 20:3–327.

Rylander, G. (1948): Personality analysis before and after frontal lobotomy. *Res. Publ. Assoc. Nerv. Ment. Dis.*, 27:691–705.

Rylander, G. (1973): The renaissance of psychosurgery. In: *Surgical Approaches in Psychiatry*, edited by L. V. Laitinen and K. E. Livingston, pp. 3–12. University Park Press, Baltimore.

Samuels, J. A., and Benson, D. F. (1979): Some aspects of language comprehension in anterior aphasia. *Brain Lang.*, 8:275–286.

Sandifer, P. H. (1946): Anosognosia and disorders of body scheme. *Brain*, 69:122–137.

Sanides, F. (1970): Functional architecture of motor and sensory cortices in primates in the light of a new concept of a cortex evolution. In: *The Primate Brain*, edited by C. R. Noback and W. Montagna, pp. 137–208. Appleton, New York.

Sapolsky, R. M., and Eichenbaum, H. (1980): Thalamocortical mechanisms in odor-guided behavior. II. Effects of lesions of the mediodorsal thalamic nucleus and frontal cortex on odor preferences and sexual behavior in the hamster. *Brain Behav. Evol.*, 17:276–290.

Sato, M. (1971): Prefrontal cortex and emotional behaviors. *Folia Psychiatr. Neurol. Jpn.*, 25:69–78.

Scheibel, A. B. (1980): Anatomical and physiological substrates of arousal: A view from the bridge. In: *The Reticular Formation Revisited*, edited by J. A. Hobson and M. A. B. Brazier, pp. 55–66. Raven Press, New York.

Scheibel, M. E., and Scheibel, A. B. (1967): Structural organization of nonspecific thalamic nuclei and their projection toward cortex. *Brain Res.*, 6:60–94.

Scherer, I. W., Klett, C. J., and Winne, J. F. (1957): Psychological changes over a five year period following bilateral frontal lobotomy. *J. Consult. Psychol.*, 21:291–295.

Schiff, H. B., Alexander, M. P., Naeser, M. A., and Galaburda, A. M. (1983): Aphemia: Clinical-anatomic correlations. *Arch. Neurol.*, 40:720–727.

Schilder, P. (1924): Die encephalitis periaxialis diffusi (Nebst Bemerkungen uber die Apraxie des Lidschlusses). *Arch. Pyschiatr. Nervenkr.*, 71:327. Referenced in Fisher, M. (1956): Left hemiplegia and motor impersistence. *J. Nerv. Ment. Dis.*, 123:201–218.

Schilder, P. (1935): *The Image and Appearance of the Human Body.* International University Press, New York.

Schilder, P. (1939): The concept of hysteria. *Am. J. Psychiatry*, 95:1389–1413.

Schiller, F. (1947): Aphasia studied in patients with missile wounds. *J. Neurol. Neurosurg. Psychiatry*, 10:183–187.

Schrader, P. J., and Robinson, M. F. (1945): An evaluation of prefrontal lobotomy through ward behavior. *J. Abnorm. Soc. Psychol.*, 40:61–69.

Schulsinger, F. (1972): Psychopathy: Heredity and environment. *Int. J. Ment. Health*, 1:190–206.

Schwab, O. (1926): Uber Vorubergehende aphasische storungen nach Rindenexzision aus dem linken Stirnhirn bei Epileptikern. *Dtsch. Z. Nervenheilk.*, 94:177–184.

Schwartz, M. L., and Goldman-Rakic, P. S. (1984): Callosal and intrahemispheric connectivity of the prefrontal association cortex in rhesus monkey: Relation between intraparietal and principal sulcal cortex. *J. Comp. Neurol.*, 226:403–420.

Schwent, V. L., Hillyard, S. A., and Galambos, R. (1976): Selective attention and the auditory vertex potential. I. Effects of stimulus delivery rate. *Electroencephalogr. Clin. Neurophysiol.*, 40:604–614.

Scoville, W. B. (1949): Selective cortical undercutting as a means of modifying and studying frontal lobe function in man; preliminary report of 43 operative cases. *J. Neurosurg.*, 6:65–73.

Scoville, W. B., and Bettis, D. B. (1977): Results of orbital undercutting today: a personal series. In: *Neurosurgical Treatment in Psychiatry, Pain and Epilepsy*, edited by W. H. Sweet, S. Obrador, and J. G. Martin-Rodriguez, pp. 189–202. University Park Press, Baltimore.

Segarra, J. M. (1970): Cerebral vascular disease and behavior. 1. The syndrome of the mesencephalic artery (basilar artery bifurcation). *Arch. Neurol.*, 22:404–418.

Seidman, L. J. (1983): Schizophrenia and brain dysfunction: An integration of recent neurodiagnostic findings. *Psychol. Bull.*, 94:195–238.

Semmes, J., Weinstein, S., Ghent, L., and Teuber, H-L. (1963): Correlates of impaired orientation in personal and extrapersonal space. *Brain*, 86:747–772.

Senba, K., and Iwahara, S. (1974): Effects of medial septal lesions on the hippocampal electrical activity and the orienting response to auditory stimulation in drinking rats. *Brain Res.*, 66:309–320.

Shakow, D. (1963): Psychological deficit in schizophrenia. *Behav. Sci.*, 8:275–305.

Shallice, T. (1978): The dominant action system: An information-processing approach to consciousness. In: *The Stream of Consciousness*, edited by K. S. Pope and J. L. Singer, pp. 117–157. Plenum Press, New York.

Shallice, T. (1982): Specific impairments of planning. In: *The Neuropsychology of Cognitive Function*, edited by D. E. Broadbent and L. Weiskrantz, pp. 199–209. The Royal Society, London.

Shallice, T., and Evans, M. E. (1978): The involvement of the frontal lobes in cognitive estimation. *Cortex*, 4:294–303.

Shapiro, B. E., Alexander, M. P., Gardner, H., and Mercer, B. (1981): Mechanisms of confabulation. *Neurology (NY)*, 31:1070–1076.

Shapiro, B. E., Grossman, M., and Gardner, H. (1981): Selective processing deficits in brain damaged populations. *Neuropsychologia*, 19:161–169.

Sheer, D. E. (1956): Psychometric studies. In: *Studies in Topectomy*, edited by N. D. C. Lewis, C. Landis, and H. E. King, pp. 56–74. Grune & Stratton, New York.

Shiffrin, R. M., and Schneider, W. (1977): Controlled and automatic human information processing. II. Perceptual learning, automatic attending and a general theory. *Psychol. Rev.*, 84:127–190.

Shneider, R. C., Crosby, E. C., Bagchi, B. K., and Calhoun, H. D. (1961): Temporal or occipital lobe hallucinations triggered from frontal lobe lesions. *Neurology (NY)*, 11:172–189.

Shure, G. H., and Halstead, W. C. (1958): Cerebral localization of intellectual processes. *Psychol. Monogr.*, 72:1–40.

Silberpfennig, J. (1941): Contributions to the problem of eye movements: Disturbances of ocular movements with pseudohemianopsia in frontal lobe tumors. *Confin. Neurol.*, 4:1–13.

Silverberg, G. D., Castellino, R. A., and Goodwin, D. A. (1969): Porencephalic cysts demonstrated by encephalography with radioiodinated serum albumin. *N. Engl. J. Med.*, 280:315–316.

Sim, M., Turner, E., and Smith, W. T. (1966): Cerebral biopsy in the investigation of presenile dementia. *Br. J. Psychiatry*, 112:119–125.

Simon, H. (1981): Neurones dopaminergiques A10 et système frontal. *J. Physiol. (Paris)*, 77:81–95.

Skinhoj, E. (1965): Bilateral depression of CBF in unilateral cerebral diseases. *Acta Neurol. Scand. [Suppl. 14]*, 41:161–163.

Skinner, J. E., and Lindsley, D. B. (1967): Electrophysiological and behavioral effects of blockade of the nonspecific thalamo-cortical system. *Brain Res.*, 6:95–118.

Slomka, G., Tarter, R., and Hegedus, A. (1984): Agenesis of the frontal lobes: Neuropsychological sequelae. *Int. J. Clin. Neuropsychol.*, 6:12–16.

Smith, A. (1960): Changes in Porteus Maze scores of brain-operated schizophrenics after an eight-year interval. *J. Ment. Sci.*, 106:967–978.

Smith, A. (1962): Psychodiagnosis of patients with brain tumors. The validity of Hewson's ratios in neurological and mental hospital populations. *J. Nerv. Ment. Dis.*, 135:513–533.

Smith, A. (1964): Changing effects of frontal lesions in man. *J. Neurol. Neurosurg. Psychiatry*, 27:511–515.

Smith, A. (1966): Intellectual functions in patients with lateralized frontal tumours. *J. Neurol. Neurosurg. Psychiatry*, 29:52–59.

Smith, A. (1967): The serial sevens subtraction test. *Arch. Neurol.*, 17:78–80.

Smith, A., and Kinder, E. F. (1959): Changes in psychological test performances of brain-operated schizophrenics after eight years. *Science*, 129:149–150.

Smith, J. S., Kiloh, L. G., and Boots, J. A. (1977): Prospective evaluation of prefrontal leucotomy: Results at 30 months follow-up. In: *Neurosurgical Treatment in Psychiatry, Pain, and Epilepsy*, edited by W. H. Sweet, S. Obrador, and J. G. Martin-Roderiquez, pp. 217–224. University Park Press, Baltimore.

Smith, J. S., Kiloh, L. G., Cochrane, N., and Kljajic, I. (1976): A prospective evaluation of open prefrontal leucotomy. *Med. J. Aust.*, 1:731–735.

Smith, W. K. (1944): The frontal eye fields. In: *The Precentral Motor Cortex*, edited by P. C. Bucy, pp. 307–342. University of Illinois Press, Urbana.

Smythe, G. E., and Stern, K. (1938): Tumors of the thalamus. *Brain*, 61:339–360.

Snyder, S. H., Banerjee, S. P., Yamamura, H. I., and Greenberg, D. (1974): Drugs, neurotransmitters and schizophrenia. *Science*, 184:1243–1253.

Soniat, T. L. L. (1951): Psychiatric symptoms associated with intracranial neoplasms. *Am. J. Psychiatry*, 108:19–22.

Souques, A. (1928): Quelques cas d'anarthrie de Pierre Marie: Aperçu historique sur la localisation du langage. *Rev. Neurol (Paris)*, 2:319–368.

Soury, J. (1899): *Le système nerveux central*. Carré & Naud, Paris. Referenced in Bianchi, L. (1922): *The Mechanism of the Brain and the Functions of the Frontal Lobes*. William Wood, New York.

Sperry, R. (1985): Consciousness: Personal identity and the divided brain. In: *The Dual Brain: Hemispheric Specialization in the Human*, edited by D. F. Benson, E. Zaidel, and M. A. B. Brazier. Guilford Press, New York *(in press)*.

Sperry, R. W., and Gazzaniga, M. S. (1967): Language following surgical disconnection of the hemispheres. In: *Brain Mechanisms Underlying Speech and Language*, edited by F. L. Darley, pp. 108–121. Grune & Stratton, New York.

Spiegel, E. A., Wycis, H. T., Freed, H., and Lee, A. J. (1948): Stereoencephalotomy. *Trans. Am. Neurol. Assoc.*, 73:160–163.

Spiers, P. A. (1981): Have they come to praise Luria or to bury him? The Luria-Nebraska battery controversy. *J. Consult. Clin. Psychol.*, 49:331.

Spillane, J. D. (1942): Disturbances of body scheme: Anosognosia and finger agnosia. *Lancet*, 1:42–44.

Spreen, O. von (1956): Stirnhirnverletzte im Rorschach-Versuch. II. Statistische ergebnisse. *Z. Diagnost. Psychol. Personlichkeitsforsch.*, 4:146–173.

Spreen, O., and Benton, A. L. (1965): Comparative studies of some psychological tests for cerebral damage. *J. Nerv. Ment. Dis.*, 140:323–333.

Spreen, O., and Benton, A. L. (1969): *Neurosensory Center Comprehensive Examination for Aphasia*. University of Victoria Neuropsychology Laboratory, Victoria, B.C.

Squire, L. R. (1982): Comparisons between forms of amnesia: Some deficits are unique to Korsakoff's syndrome. *J. Exp. Psychol. [Hum. Learn. Mem.]*, 8:560–571.

Stamm, J. S. (1979): The monkey's prefrontal cortex functions in motor programming. *Acta Neurobiol. Exp.*, 39:683–704.

Stamm, J. S., and Kreder, S. V. (1979): Minimal brain dysfunction: Psychological and neurophysiological disorders in hyperkinetic children. In: *Handbook of Behavioral Neurobiology, Vol. 2: Neuropsychology*, edited by M. S. Gazzaniga, pp. 119–150. Plenum, New York.

Stedman's Medical Dictionary Illustrated (1979): Williams & Wilkins, Baltimore.

Stein, D. G., and Firl, A. C. (1976): Brain damage and reorganization of function in old age. *Exp. Neurol.*, 52:157–167.

Stein, S., and Volpe, B. T. (1983): Classical "parietal" neglect syndrome after subcortical right frontal lobe infarction. *Neurology (NY)*, 33:797–799.

Stengel, E. (1947): A clinical and psychological study of echo-reactions. *J. Ment. Sci.*, 93:598–612.

Stephens, R. B., and Stilwell, D. L. (1969): *Arteries and Veins of the Human Brain*. Charles C Thomas, Springfield, Illinois.

Stern, D. B. (1977): Handedness and the lateral distribution of conversion reactions. *J. Nerv. Ment. Dis.*, 164:122–128.

Sterne, D. M. (1969): The Benton, Porteus and WAIS digit span tests with normals and brain injured patients. *J. Clin. Psychol.*, 25:173–177.

Stevens, J. R. (1973): An anatomy of schizophrenia? *Arch. Gen. Psychiatry*, 29:117–189.

Stookey, B., Scarff, J., and Teitelbaum, M. (1941): Frontal lobectomy in the treatment of brain tumors. *Ann. Surg.*, 113:161–169.

Strecker, E. A., Palmer, H. D., and Grant, F. C. (1942): A study of frontal lobotomy. *Am. J. Psychiatry*, 98:524–532.

Stritch, S. J. (1969): The pathology of brain damage due to blunt head injuries. In: *The Late Effects of Head Injury*, edited by E. A. Walker, W. F. Caveness, and M. Critchley, pp. 501–526. Charles C Thomas, Springfield, Illinois.

Strom-Olsen, R., and Carlisle, S. (1970): Bi-frontal stereotactic tractotomy: A follow-up study of its effects on 210 patients. *Br. J. Psychiatry*, 118:141–154.

Strom-Olsen, R., Last, S. L., Brody, M. B., and Knight, G. C. (1943): Results of prefrontal leucotomy in 30 cases of mental disorder, with observations on surgical technique. *J. Ment. Sci.*, 89:165–181.

Strom-Olsen, R., and Northfield, D. W. C. (1955): Undercutting of orbital cortex in chronic neurotic and psychotic tension states. *Lancet*, 1:986–991.

Stroop, J. R. (1935): Studies of interference in serial verbal reactions. *J. Exp. Psychol.*, 18:643–662.

Struckett, P. B. A. (1953): Effect of prefrontal lobotomy on intellectual functioning in chronic schizophrenia. *Arch. Neurol. Psychiatry*, 69:293–304.

Stuss, D. T., Alexander, M. P., Lieberman, A., and Levine, H. (1978): An extraordinary form of confabulation. *Neurology (NY)*, 28:1166–1172.

Stuss, D. T., and Benson, D. F. (1983a): Emotional concomitants of psychosurgery. In: *Neuropsychology of Human Emotion*, edited by K. M. Heilman and P. Satz, pp. 111–140. Guilford Press, New York.

Stuss, D. T., and Benson, D. F. (1983b): Frontal lobe lesions and behavior. In: *Localization in Neuropsychology*, edited by A. Kertesz, pp. 429–454. Academic Press, New York.

Stuss, D. T., and Benson, D. F. (1984): Neuropsychological studies of the frontal lobes. *Psychol. Bull.*, 95:3–28.

Stuss, D. T., Benson, D. F., Kaplan, E. F., Della Malva, C. L., and Weir, W. S. (1984a): The effects of prefrontal leucotomy on visuoperceptive and visuoconstructive tests. *Bull. Clin. Neurosci.*, 49:43–51.

Stuss, D. T., Benson, D. F., Kaplan, E. F., Weir, W. S., and Della Malva, C. (1981a): Leucotomized and nonleucotomized schizophrenics: Comparison on tests of attention. *Biol. Psychiatry*, 16:1085–1100.

Stuss, D. T., Benson, D. F., Kaplan, E. F., Weir, W. S., Naeser, M. A., Lieberman, I., and Ferrill, D. (1983): The involvement of orbitofrontal cerebrum in cognitive tasks. *Neuropsychologia*, 21:235–248.

Stuss, D. T., Ely, P., Hugenholtz, H., Richard, M. T., LaRochelle, S., Poirier, C. A., and Bell, I. (1985): Subtle neuropsychological deficits in patients with good recovery after closed head injury. *Neurosurgery*, 17:41–47.

Stuss, D. T., Guberman, A., Nelson, R. F., and LaRochelle, S. (1984b): Longitudinal neuropsychological evaluation of three patients with paramedian thalamic infarcts. Presented at the International Neuropsychology Society Conference, Mexico City.

Stuss, D. T., Kaplan, E. F., and Benson, D. F. (1982a): Long-term effects of prefrontal leucotomy: Cognitive functions. In: *Neuropsychology and Cognition*, Vol. II, edited by R. N. Malatesha and L. C. Hartlage, pp. 252–271. Martinus Nijhoff, The Hague.

Stuss, D. T., Kaplan, E. F., Benson, D. F., Weir, W. S., Chiulli, S., and Sarazin, F. F. (1982b): Evidence for the involvement of orbitofrontal cortex in memory functions: An interference effect. *J. Comp. Physiol. Psychol.*, 96:913–925.

Stuss, D. T., Kaplan, E. F., Benson, D. F., Weir, W. S., Naeser, M. A., and Levine, H. L. (1981b): Long-term effects of prefrontal leucotomy: An overview of neuropsychologic residuals. *J. Clin. Neuropsychol.*, 3:13–32.

Stuss, D., and Richard, M. T. (1982): Neuropsychological sequelae of coma after head injury. In: *Coma: Physiopathology, Diagnosis and Management*, edited by L. P. Ivan and D. A. Bruce, pp. 193–210. Charles C Thomas, Springfield, Illinois.

Stuss, D. T., Sarazin, F. F., Leech, E. E., and Picton, T. W. (1983): Event-related potentials during naming and mental rotation. *Electroencephalogr. Clin. Neurophysiol.*, 56:133–146.

Stuss, D. T., and Trites, R. L. (1977): Classification of neurological status using multiple discriminant function analysis of neuropsychological test scores. *J. Consult. Clin. Psychol.*, 45:145.

Suzuki, H., and Azuma, M. (1977): Prefrontal neuronal activity during gazing at a light spot in the monkey. *Brain Res.*, 126:497–508.

Swiercinsky, D. (1978): *Manual for the Adult Neuropsychological Evaluation*. Charles C Thomas, Springfield, Illinois.

Talland, G. A., Sweet, W. H., and Ballantine, Jr., H. T. (1967): Amnesic syndrome with anterior communicating artery aneurysm. *J. Nerv. Ment. Dis.*, 145:179–192.

Tan, E., Marks, I. M., and Marset, P. (1971): Bimedial leucotomy in obsessive-compulsive neurosis: A controlled serial enquiry. *Br. J. Psychiatry*, 118:155–164.

Taveras, J. M., and Wood, E. H. (1976): *Diagnostic Neuroradiology*. Williams & Wilkins, Baltimore.

Taylor, L. B. (1979): Psychological assessment of neurosurgical patients. In: *Functional Neurosurgery*, edited by T. Rasmussen and R. Marino, pp. 165–180. Raven Press, New York.

Teasdale, G., and Mendelow, D. (1984): Pathophysiology of head injuries. In: *Closed Head Injury. Psychological, Social and Family Consequences*, edited by N. Brooks, pp. 4–36. Oxford University Press, Oxford.

Teuber, H. L. (1955): Physiological psychology. *Annu. Rev. Psychol.*, 6:267–296.

Teuber, H. L. (1959): Some alterations in behavior after cerebral lesions in man. In: *Evolution of Nervous Control from Primitive Organisms to Man*, edited by A. D. Bass, pp. 157–194. American Association for the Advancement of Science, Washington, D.C.

Teuber, H-L. (1964): The riddle of frontal lobe function in man. In: *The Frontal Granular Cortex and Behavior*, edited by J. M. Warren and K. Akert, pp. 410–444. McGraw-Hill, New York.

Teuber, H-L. (1966): The frontal lobes and their function: Further observations on rodents, carnivores, subhuman primates and man. *Int. J. Neurol.*, 5:282–300.

Teuber, H-L. (1972): Unity and diversity of frontal lobe functions. *Acta Neurobiol. Exp. (Warsz.)*, 32:615–656.

Teuber, H-L., Battersby, W. S., and Bender, M. B. (1949): Changes in visual searching performance following cerebral lesions. *Am. J. Physiol.*, 159:592.

Teuber, H-L., Battersby, W. S., and Bender, M. B. (1951): Performance of complex visual tasks after cerebral lesions. *J. Nerv. Ment. Dis.*, 114:413–429.

Teuber, H-L., Corkin, S., and Twitchell, T. E. (1977): A study of cingulotomy in man. In: *Appendix— Psychosurgery: The National Commission for the Protection of Human Subjects of Biomedical and Behavioral Research*, pp. III-i–87. DHEW Publ. No. (OS)77–0002, Washington, D.C.

Teuber, H-L., and Proctor, F. (1964): Some effects of basal ganglia lesions in subhuman primates and man. *Neuropsychologia*, 2:85–93.

Teuber, H-L., and Weinstein, S. (1956): Ability to discover hidden figures after cerebral lesions. *Arch. Neurol. Psychiatry*, 76:369–379.

Thiebaut, M. M. F., and Guillaumat, L. (1945): Hémianopsie relative. *Rev. Neurol. (Paris)*, 77:129.

Thorndike, E. L. (1911): *Animal Intelligence: Experimental Studies*. Macmillan, New York.

Thurstone, L. L., and Thurstone, T. (1943): *The Chicago Tests of Primary Mental Abilities*. Science Research Associates, Chicago.

Tijssen, C. C., Tavy, D. L. J., Hekster, R. E. M., Bots, G. T. A. M., and Evdtz, L. J. (1984): Aphasia with a left frontal interhemispheric hematoma. *Neurology (NY)*, 34:1261–1264.

Tilney, F. (1928): *The Brain, From Ape to Man*. Hoeber, New York.

Tognola, G., and Vignolo, L. A. (1980): Brain lesions associated with oral apraxia in stroke patients: A clinico-neuroradiological investigation with the CT scan. *Neuropsychologia*, 18:257–272.

Tonkonogy, J., and Goodglass, H. (1981): Language function, foot of the third frontal gyrus, and rolandic operculum. *Arch. Neurol.*, 38:486–490.

Tow, B. M. (1955): *Personality Changes Following Frontal Leucotomy.* Medical Publishers, Oxford.

Trends in Neurosciences (1984): 7(11):403–454.

Trimble, M. R., and Grant, I. (1982): Psychiatric aspects of multiple sclerosis. In: *Psychiatric Aspects of Neurologic Disease*, Vol. II, edited by D. F. Benson and D. Blumer, pp. 279–299. Grune & Stratton, New York.

Trites, R. L. (1977): *Neuropsychological Test Manual.* Ronalds Federated, Montreal.

Trost, J., and Canter, G. J. (1974): Apraxia of speech in patients with Broca's aphasia. *Brain Lang.*, 1:63–79.

Tubbs, W. E. (1969): Primate frontal lesions and the temporal structure of behavior. *Behav. Sci.*, 14:347–356.

Tucker, D. M. (1981): Lateral brain function, emotion, and conceptualization. *Psychol. Bull.*, 89:19–46.

Tucker, D. M., Watson, R. T., and Heilman, K. M. (1977): Discrimination and evocation of affectively intoned speech in patients with right parietal disease. *Neurology (NY)*, 27:947–950.

Tulving, E. (1985): Memory and consciousness. *Can. Psychol.*, 26:1–12.

Tyler, H. R. (1969): Disorders of visual scanning with frontal lobe lesions. In: *Modern Neurology: Papers in Tribute to Derek Denny-Brown*, edited by S. Locke, pp. 381–393. Little, Brown, Boston.

Tzavaras, A., Albert, M. L., and Hécaen, H. (1972): Essai de dissociation des déficits de la perception spatiale élémentaire au cours de lésions corticales. *Rev. Neurol. (Paris)*, 129:60–62.

Uemura, E., and Hartmann, H. A. (1978): RNA content and volume of nerve cell bodies in human brain. I. Prefrontal cortex in aging normal and demented patients. *J. Neuropathol. Exp. Neurol.*, 37:487–496.

Ungerleider, L. G., and Brody, B. A. (1977): Extrapersonal spatial orientation: The role of posterior parietal, anterior frontal, and inferotemporal cortex. *Exp. Neurol.*, 56:265–280.

Valenstein, E. S. (1973): *Brain Control: A Critical Examination of Brain Stimulation and Psychosurgery.* Wiley, New York.

Valenstein, E. S. (1977): The practice of psychosurgery: A survey of the literature (1971–1976): In: *Appendix; Psychosurgery: The National Commission for the Protection of Human Subjects of Biomedical and Behavioral Research*, pp. I-i to I-183. DHEW Publication (OS)77–002, Washington, D.C.

Van Bogaert, L., and Martin, P. (1929): Sur deux signes du syndrôme de déséquilibration frontale: L'apraxie de la marche et l'atonie statique. *Encephale*, 24:11–18.

Van Hoesen, G. W., Pandya, D. N., and Butters, N. (1975): Some connections of the entorhinal (area 28) and perirhinal (area 35) cortices of the rhesus monkey. II. Frontal lobe afferents. *Brain Res.*, 95:25–38.

Van Zomeren, A. H., Brouwer, W. H., and Deelman, B. G. (1984): Attentional deficits: The riddles of selectivity, speed, and alertness. In: *Closed Head Injury: Psychological, Social and Family Consequences*, edited by N. Brooks, pp. 74–107. Oxford University Press, Oxford.

Venables, P. H. (1963): The relationship between level of skin potential and fusion of paired light flashes in schizophrenic and normal subjects. *J. Psychiatr. Res.*, 1:279–287.

Victor, M., Adams, R. D., and Collins, G. H. (1971): *The Wernicke-Korsakoff Syndrome.* Davis, Philadelphia.

Vidor, M. (1951): Personality changes following prefrontal leucotomy as reflected by the Minnesota Multiphasic Personality Inventory and the results of psychometric testing. *J. Ment. Sci.*, 97:159–173.

Von Bonin, G., and Bailey, P. (1947): *The Neocortex of Macaca mulatta.* University of Illinois Press, Urbana.

Von Crammon, D., and Jurgens, V. (1983): The anterior cingulate cortex and the phonatory control in monkey and man. *Neurosci. Biobehav. Rev.*, 7:423–425.

Von Economo, C. (1929): *The Cytoarchitectonics of the Human Cerebral Cortex.* Oxford University Press, New York.

Von Stockert, T. R., and Bader, L. (1976): Some relations of grammar and lexicon in aphasia. *Cortex*, 12:49–60.

Vowels, L. M., and Gates, G. R. (1984): Neuropsychological findings. In: *Multiple Sclerosis: Psychological and Social Aspects*, edited by A. F. Simons, pp. 82–90. Heinemann, London.

Vygotsky, L. S. (1962): *Thought and Language*, edited and translated by E. Hanfmann and G. Vakar. MIT Press, Cambridge, Massachusetts.

Wade, M. (1947): Effect of sedatives upon delayed response in monkeys following removal of prefrontal lobes. *J. Neurophysiol.*, 10:57–61.

Waggoner, R. W., and Bagchi, B. K. (1954): Initial masking of organic brain changes by psychic symptoms. *Am. J. Psychiatry*, 110:904–910.

Walch, R. (1956): Uber die Aufgaben der Hirnverletzenheime nach den Bundesversorgungsgesetz. In: *Das Hirntrauma*, edited by E. Rehwald, pp. 461–468. Thieme, Stuttgart.

Walker, A. E., and Jablon, S. (1959): A follow-up of head-injured men of World War II. *J. Neurosurg.*, 16:600–610.

Walsh, K. W. (1977): Neuropsychological aspects of modified leucotomy. In: *Neurosurgical Treatment in Psychiatry, Pain, and Epilepsy*, edited by W. H. Sweet, S. Obrador, and J. G. Martin-Rodriquez, pp. 163–174. University Park Press, Baltimore.

Walsh, K. W. (1978): *Neuropsychology. A Clinical Approach.* Churchill Livingstone, Edinburgh.

Walter, W. G. (1973): Human frontal lobe function in sensory-motor association. In: *Psychophysiology of the Frontal Lobes*, edited by K. H. Pribram and A. R. Luria, pp. 109–122. Academic Press, New York.

Walter, W., Cooper, R., Aldridge, V. J., McCallum, W. C., and Winter, A. L. (1964): Contingent negative variation: An electric sign of sensorimotor association and expectancy in the human brain. *Nature*, 203:380–384.

Warren, J. M. (1964): The behavior of carnivores and primates with lesions in the prefrontal cortex. In: *The Frontal Granular Cortex and Behavior*, edited by J. M. Warren and K. Akert, pp. 168–191. McGraw-Hill, New York.

Warrington, E. K., Logue, V., and Pratt, R. T. C. (1971): The anatomical localisation of selective impairment of auditory verbal short-term memory. *Neuropsychologia*, 9:377–387.

Watson, R. T., Andriola, M., and Heilman, K. M. (1977): The EEG and neglect. *J. Neurol. Sci.*, 34:343–348.

Watson, R. T., and Heilman, K. M. (1979): Thalamic neglect. *Neurology (NY)*, 29:690–694.

Watson, R. T., and Heilman, K. H. (1983): Callosal apraxia. *Brain*, 106:391–403.

Watson, R. T., Heilman, K. M., Cauthen, J. C., and King, F. A. (1973): Neglect after cingulectomy. *Neurology (NY)*, 23:1003–1007.

Watson, R. T., Heilman, K. M., Miller, B. D., and King, F. A. (1974): Neglect after mesencephalic reticular formation lesions. *Neurology (NY)*, 24:294–298.

Watson, R. T., Valenstein, E., and Heilman, K. M. (1981): Thalamic neglect: Possible role of the medial thalamus and nucleus reticularis in behavior. *Arch. Neurol.*, 38:501–506.

Waziri, R. (1978): The Capgras phenomenon: Cerebral dysfunction with psychosis. *Neuropsychobiology*, 4:353–359.

Webster's New Collegiate Dictionary (1979): Merriam-Webster, Springfield, Massachusetts.

Wechsler, D. (1945): A standardized memory scale for clinical use. *J. Psychol.*, 19:87–95.

Wechsler, D. (1955): *Manual for the Wechsler Adult Intelligence Scale.* Psychological Corporation, New York.

Wechsler, I. S. (1952): *A Textbook of Clinical Neurology.* Saunders, Philadelphia.

Wehler, R., and Hoffman, H. (1978): Intellectual functioning in lobotomized and non-lobotomized long term chronic schizophrenic patients. *J. Clin. Psychol.*, 34:449–451.

Weigl, E. (1941): On the psychology of so-called processes of abstraction. *J. Abnorm. Soc. Psychol.*, 36:3–33.

Weinberg, J., Diller, L., Gerstman, L., and Schulman, P. (1972): Digit span in right and left hemiplegics. *J. Clin. Psychol.*, 28:361.

Weinstein, E. A. (1969): Patterns of reduplication in organic brain disease. In: *Handbook of Clinical Neurology*, Vol. 3, edited by P. J. Vinken and G. W. Bruyn, pp. 251–257. North Holland, Amsterdam.

Weinstein, E. A., and Cole, M. (1963): Concepts of anosognosia. In: *Problems of Dynamic Neurology*, edited by L. Halpern, pp. 254–273. Hebrew University Medical School, Jerusalem.

Weinstein, E. A., and Kahn, R. L. (1950): Syndrome of anosognosia. *Arch. Neurol. Psychiatry*, 64:772–791.

Weinstein, E. A., and Kahn, R. L. (1955): *Denial of Illness: Symbolic and Physiological Aspects.* Charles C Thomas, Springfield, Illinois.

Weinstein, E. A., Kahn, R. L., and Sugarman, L. A. (1952): Phenomenon of reduplication. *Arch. Neurol. Psychiatry*, 67:808–814.

Weinstein, S., and Teuber, H-L. (1957): Effects of penetrating brain injury on intelligence test scores. *Science*, 125:1036–1037.

Weintraub, M. I. (1983): *Hysterical Conversion Reactions*. Spectrum, New York.

Weiskrantz, L. (1978): A comparison of hippocampal pathology in man and other animals. In: *Functions of the Septohippocampal System*. Ciba Symposium No. 58. Elsevier, Amsterdam.

Welch, K., and Stuteville, P. (1958): Experimental production of unilateral neglect in monkeys. *Brain*, 81:341–347.

Welt, L. (1888): Ueber Charakterveranderungen des Menschen infolge von Lasionen des Stirnhirns. *Dtsch. Arch. Klin. Med.*, 42:339–390.

Wheeler, L., Burke, C. J., and Reitan, R. M. (1963): An application of discriminant functions to the problem of predicting brain damage using behavioral variables. *Percept. Mot. Skills*, 16:417–440.

Wiesendanger, M. (1983): Cortico-cerebellar loops. In: *Neural Coding of Motor Performance*, edited by J. Massion, J. Paillard, W. Schultz, and M. Wiesendanger, pp. 41–53. Springer-Verlag, Berlin.

Will, B. E., and Rosenzweig, M. (1976): Effets de l'environnement sur la récupération fonctionnelle après lésions cérébrales chez les rats adultes. *Biol. Behav.*, 1:5–16.

Willett, R. A. (1960): The effects of psychosurgical procedures on behavior. In: *Handbook of Abnormal Psychology: An Experimental Approach*, edited by H. J. Eysenck, pp. 566–610. Basic Books, New York.

Williams, P. L., and Warwick, R. (1975): *Functional Neuroanatomy of Man*. W.B. Saunders, Philadelphia.

Winner, E., and Gardner, H. (1977): The comprehension of metaphor in brain-damaged patients. *Brain*, 100:717–729.

Winocur, G., Oxbury, S., Roberts, R., Agnetti, V., and Davis, C. (1984): Amnesia in a patient with bilateral lesions to the thalamus. *Neuropsychologia*, 22:123–143.

Winokur, G., and Crowe, R. R. (1975): Personality disorders. In: *Comprehensive Textbook of Psychiatry*, Vol. 2, 2nd Ed., edited by A. M. Freedman, H. I. Kaplan, and B. J. Sadock, pp. 1279–1297. Williams & Wilkins, Baltimore.

Wise, S. P., and Strick, P. L. (1984): Anatomical and physiological organization of the non-primary motor cortex. *Trends Neurosci.*, 7:442–446.

Wolff, B. B. (1960): The application of the Hewson ratios to the WAIS as an aid in the differential diagnosis of cerebral pathology. *J. Nerv. Ment. Dis.*, 131:98–109.

Wundt, W. (1873–1874): *Grundzuge der Physiologischen Psychologie*. Englemann, Leipzig.

Wurtman, R. J., and Growdon, J. H. (1980): Dietary enhancement of CNS neurotransmitters. In: *Neuroendocrinology*, edited by D. T. Krieger and J. C. Hughes, pp. 59–65. Sinauer Associates, Sunderland, Massachusetts.

Wurtz, R. H., and Mohler, C. W. (1976): Enhancement of visual responses in monkey striate cortex and frontal eye fields. *J. Neurophysiol.*, 39:766–772.

Yacorzynski, G. K., Boshes, B., and Davis, L. (1947): Psychological changes produced by frontal lobotomy. *Res. Publ. Assoc. Nerv. Ment. Dis.*, 27:642–657.

Yacorzynski, G. K., and Davis, L. (1945): An experimental study of functions of the frontal lobes in man. *Psychosom. Med.*, 7:97–107.

Yakovlev, P. I. (1962): Morphological criteria of growth and maturation of the nervous system in man. *Res. Publ. Assoc. Nerv. Ment. Dis.*, 39:3–46.

Yakovlev, P. I., and Lecours, A-R. (1967): The myelogenetic cycles of regional maturation of the brain. In: *Regional Development of the Brain in Early Life*, edited by A. Minkowski, pp. 3–70. Blackwell, Oxford.

Yamamoto, P., and Ueki, S. (1977): Characteristics in aggressive behavior induced by midbrain raphe lesions in rats. *Physiol. Behav.*, 19:105–110.

Yeterian, E. H., and Van Hoesen, G. W. (1978): Cortico-striate projections in the rhesus monkey: The organization of certain cortico-caudate connections. *Brain Res.*, 139:43–63.

Yin, T. C., and Mountcastle, V. B. (1977): Visual input to the visuomotor mechanisms of the monkey's parietal lobe. *Science*, 197:1381–1383.

Zaidel, E. (1976): Auditory vocabulary of the right hemisphere following brain bisection or hemidecortication. *Cortex*, 12:191–211.

Zaidel, E. (1982): Reading in the disconnected right hemisphere: An aphasiological perspective. In: *Dyslexia: Neuronal, Cognitive and Linguistic Aspects, Wenner-Grem Symposium on Dyslexia*, edited by Y. Zotterman, pp. 67–91. Pergamon Press, Oxford.

Zangwill, O. L. (1949): Review: Brain and intelligence; a quantitative study of the frontal lobes, by W. C. Halstead. *Q. J. Exp. Psychol.*, 1:147.

Zangwill, O. L. (1966): Psychological deficits associated with frontal lobe lesions. *Int. J. Neurol.*, 5:395–402.

Zatorre, R. J. (1985): Discrimination and recognition of tonal melodies after unilateral cerebral excisions. *Neuropsychologia*, 23:31–41.

Zubin, J. (1975): Problems of attention in schizophrenia. In: *Experimental Approaches to Psychopathology*, edited by M. L. Kietzman, S. Sutton, and J. Zubin, pp. 139–166. Wiley, New York.

Zurif, E. B., and Caramazza, A. (1976): Psycholinguistic structures in aphasia: Studies in syntax and semantics. In: *Studies in Neurolinguistics*, edited by H. Whitaker and H. A. Whitaker, Vol. I, pp. 261–292. Academic Press, New York.

Zurif, E. B., Caramazza, A., and Myerson, R. (1972): Grammatical judgements of agrammatic aphasics. *Neuropsychologia*, 10:405–417.

Subject Index